PRESENTED TO S.C.B.U.

BY.

DRS. A. CONNORS & R. MEHTA

Clinics in Developmental Medicine Nos. 84/85

Neurological Evaluation of Infants and Children

HENRY W. BAIRD, M.D.

Professor of Pediatrics
Temple University School of Medicine
Attending Pediatrician (Neurology)
St. Christopher's Hospital for Children
Philadelphia

ELEANORA C. GORDON, M.D.

Honorary Staff
St. Christopher's Hospital for Children
Philadelphia

Medical illustrations by
LARRY STEIN

1983

Spastics International Medical Publications

LONDON: William Heinemann Medical Books Ltd.

PHILADELPHIA: J. B. Lippincott Co.

ISBN 0433 01130 0

Printed in England at THE LAVENHAM PRESS LTD., Lavenham, Suffolk

Contents

Foreword

One of the most successful of the early Clinics in Developmental Medicine was *Neurological Examination of Children*, written by the late Richmond S. Paine with the help of Professor Thomas E. Oppé. This book has guided many paediatricians and paediatric neurologists through the hazards of the neurological examination of children. The approach of that volume was a broad one; Richmond Paine provided the neurological detail, which Professor Oppé put into the broader paediatric ambience. We are very grateful to Professor Oppé for allowing us to use material from that earlier volume in the present one. At the time of his death, Richmond Paine had already begun to revise the book, realising even then that changes had occurred in the expectations of parents of children coming for a neurological examination.

S.I.M.P. are very grateful to Henry Baird and Eleanora Gordon for taking on the difficult task of preparing this completely new text for our series. I am sure it will be as useful to present and future paediatricians as the previous volume was to older generations. Indeed, the needs of parents and children have changed over the years, and the change in title from 'examination' to 'evaluation' stresses the need now for the examiner not only to record signs of neurological dysfunction but also to be able to say what it means in terms of the child's actual functioning within the community. During the last 15 years, while the 'traditional' paediatric neurological patient has continued to come forward for evaluation (*i.e.* the child who has to be assessed because of some clear-cut neurological disorder, such as epilepsy or the possibility of a tumour), there has been an enormous increase in the number of children presenting with a learning and/or behaviour disorder, which the client's family and friends feel has a neurological basis. The authors present clear-cut ways for assessing children who present with these problems.

This book is *not* a textbook of paediatric neurology; the decision about how to handle the problem once the child has been evaluated—in terms of management and care—is not discussed. However, the clinician will make an appropriate start with the evaluation outlined in this book, and a solid basis for future management and care will have been established.

MARTIN BAX

Preface

This book is written to help pediatricians carry out a neurological evaluation of an infant or child. Its intent is to assist both the general physician who has an interest in pediatric neurological problems and the young physician who wishes to develop skills in developmental pediatrics, neurology and rehabilitation.

The evaluation may be a standard medical consultation or it may be needed to help the family and professionals in other disciplines provide the best possible comprehensive program for the child in his community. The physician must be able to perform a skilled neurological evaluation, and to make sure that the recommendations based on that assessment are carried out. In order to accomplish the latter, the physician must be familiar with community resources, and be able to communicate any findings effectively to the family and other professionals.

The examination and procedures described are those which a general practitioner or pediatrician can be expected to do in the office or clinic within the limits of available time, space and equipment. Acute and major neurological problems requiring hospital admission are beyond the scope of this book. It is not intended to be a textbook of pediatric neurology and does not describe the management of neurological conditions. Rather, the emphasis is on a logical approach to the identification of the child's problem and the assessment of the child's needs.

The experienced physician will order only those diagnostic procedures which have a specific bearing on the child's problem, and will strike a reasonable balance between searching too far for answers and not looking at all. Until specific etiologies are known, treatment is unlikely to be entirely successful. Developmentally disabled children are more vulnerable and are more easily affected adversely by inappropriate therapy. Through observation and carefully selected studies, the physician hopes to find acceptable solutions to very complex problems.

The assessment may be complicated by the fact that no two people agree on the child's main needs. For example, a child with trisomy 21 (Down syndrome) will present many facets. The physician will see the medical problems, but may wish to have a geneticist count the chromosomes, an ophthalmologist treat the myopia, an otolaryngologist improve the chronic rhinitis and the conductive hearing loss, and a cardiologist check the heart murmur. A parent may feel that all problems would be solved 'if only he could talk', and so wish for speech therapy. The school might want an exact definition of learning skills to facilitate proper classroom placement. The social worker wants to evaluate the effect on the family of having a retarded child, and the community asks 'Can he be independent? Who will support him? Who will protect him?'. Meanwhile, what are the child's own desires? He wishes to be accepted—by all.

CHAPTER 1

The Basic Neurological Evaluation: General Considerations

The referral

A satisfactory evaluation includes not only a synthesis of previous information with the findings of the current examination, but also a definition of priorities in a way that is useful to the child and family. The physician will want to know relevant information concerning the past from the family and from other resources—medical, educational and social. The reason for the evaluation must be defined and expectations must be discussed with the family. The basic neurological examination might need to be supplemented with additional studies, laboratory tests and consultations. A working diagnosis is reached, and recommendations are made for immediate and long-term needs. The scope of the assessment should depend on the purpose for which it is requested. If the referring source, the examining physician and the family are clear about the purpose of the visit from the beginning, the evaluation will be efficient and productive.

Referrals for neurological evaluation may be primarily for diagnosis. Conditions such as developmental delay, spasticity, motor weakness or seizures may have been noted or suspected by the referring physician or the family. Sometimes a change in well-defined existing conditions requires thorough evaluation. For example, a change in frequency, severity or type of convulsive disorder must be studied, or loss of a previously acquired skill must be explained.

There may also be a need for a reassessment of a well-defined problem, the emphasis being on current management and long-term planning rather than on diagnosis. The needs of a severely physically handicapped child, for example, may be quite different at eight years of age from what they were at four years of age. Sometimes assessments are sought because the child without definite neurological symptoms has difficulty in adapting to the home and community environment. Evaluations may be needed for school difficulties (both behavioral and academic), or for hyperactivity or a personality change.

The setting

A family bringing a child for neurological evaluation is likely to be anxious and apprehensive. The parents may have travelled a long way, their expectations may be unclear, and the child may be irritable, tired or scared.

A good neurological evaluation can be done almost anywhere, but the results are likely to be much more satisfactory if the setting and routine are designed to mitigate the stress of the visit. This requires efficient organization to ensure a short waiting-time.

There should be space available for testing motor skills (walking a straight line, climbing steps, hopping, running) and for testing visual acuity. There should be privacy from the rest of the office or clinic, and space should be available for interviewing both the parents without the child and the child without the parents. Nearby washrooms should have facilities appropriate for children and be fully accessible for a disabled person in a wheelchair; indeed, the entire office or clinic should be accessible and barrier-free.

The physician should establish an examination routine which is efficient, personal and without interruptions. Sometimes an assessment is part of a teaching program in a medical center: then the examining physician must develop a teaching method which will be instructive but will not unduly slow down the examination or impose on the family's privacy.

Sometimes there is an obvious need for alternative evaluations, by psychologists and physical therapists for example. If too much is scheduled for one day the child and family may become exhausted and confused, yet if the consultations are scheduled for another day the child might appear quite differently to other consultants, or the family might fail to attend. If preliminary material, sent before the child is seen, indicates the need for multiple consultations, then some way must be found to avoid duplication of effort. The preliminary information can be circulated, the consultants can sit in for the initial history-taking, and they can work with the child while the physician gets supplementary information from the parents. This approach requires some flexibility by all concerned, but it is far preferable to the rigidly scheduled 'processing' approach in which each consultant in succession sees the child for 30 minutes.

Time required for evaluation

The time required to evaluate a child depends on how long the problems have existed, their severity, and the amount of interpretation and planning necessary. Often one visit is enough, but occasionally a second one is necessary if diagnostic laboratory tests and special studies are needed, or if for some reason a satisfactory examination cannot be performed. *The time taken for the assessment must be appropriate for its purpose.*

The first third of the visit should be regarded as an 'overview', in which the problems or complaints are discussed and an effort made to establish rapport with the child and family. Easy questions about the past are asked first and a history is developed. At this point the scope of the task should become apparent. The next third of the visit is taken up by a structured examination. The last third is devoted to clarifying details, presenting an opinion to the family, arranging for additional studies, filling out forms and making recommendations. 45 minutes would be a minimum time to allow for the examination; however, for a complicated problem an initial assessment could take as long as 90 minutes.

Subsequent visits are likely to be much shorter, since there is less emphasis on examination and history-taking and more on the interpretation of results gleaned from additional information.

Recording the information

No single recording form will suit everyone. Preference depends on training and habit. Some examiners prefer structured, direct questions which can serve as reminders and ensure that nothing is omitted from the history. This check-list type of examination form is easier for the less experienced to use, but some families dislike answering questions asked from a form and feel that the questioner is not really interested in their problems.

Other physicians feel constricted by a rigid set of questions and prefer a loosely-organized form which permits a free flow of ideas. They will work out a technique which is suitable for their needs. Once a preference is established the approach should be consistent, or essential material will be omitted.

If the child is active during the visit, only brief notes are practicable during the examination and much of the written work must be done after the examination is over.

The form of the final report of the assessment will vary according to the purpose of the assessment. When parents have access to their child's records, the physician must bear in mind that the written report must be consistent with the discussions held with the family.

Equipment

The choice of equipment considered necessary for a satisfactory neurological evaluation is based on the examiner's preferences, experience and training. Obviously, it must also be appropriate for the age of the child and for the purpose of the examination. Basic medical diagnostic equipment is supplemented by testing objects found useful in eliciting certain responses. Specific presenting symptoms, such as school difficulties or unusual problems, may require additional, specialized test materials.

A list of useful equipment is presented below as a guide.

Some standard medical equipment
Reflex hammer (pediatric)
Blood-pressure cuffs—small and large
Tuning fork (frequency 256)
Narrow enamelled-steel retractable tape-measure (make sure edges are not sharp)
Two- to four-cell flashlight with cuff for transillumination[1]

Additional testing equipment
Safety pin
Sterile cotton
Coins—small and large
Stove-bolts and nuts—small and large for testing fine motor co-ordination (Fig. 1)

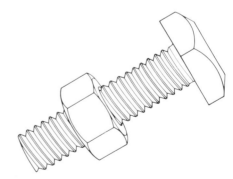

Fig. 1. A stove bolt is one test for assessing manual dexterity and co-ordination. This is not a standardized test; it is used primarily for observation.

Rubber ball about 8cm (3in) in diameter
White thread
Pencil and paper
Material for testing smell: toothpaste, orange, cinnamon
Material for testing taste: sugar, salt, vinegar, quinine
Large indestructible toy, such as red plastic dump-truck
Paper cups, to be used as occluders for visual screening
Wooden 3cm (1in) cubes
Material for gross testing of hearing: cellophane (candy wrapper), bell, high-pitched rattle, cup and spoon, STYCAR picture cards/Reed test[2]
Finger puppets
Red lens
Moving spring toy (inexpensive, so that it can be replaced frequently)

Variety of small toys (*e.g.* doll, car, chair) for 18-month to four-year developmental screening

Special testing material
Denver Developmental Screening Test forms and equipment[3]
Vineland Social Maturity Scale[4]
Peabody Picture Vocabulary Test[4]
Slosson Drawing Co-ordination Test for children and adults[5]
Slosson Standardized Word Lists[5]
Bender Visual Motor Gestalt Test[6]
Standard Snellen Test Chart[7]
Miniature Snellen Chart (hand-held)[8]
Titmus Stereo Tests[9]
Ishihara's Tests for color blindness[10]
Manuals for the STYCAR vision, hearing and language tests[11]

[1]'Transdapter' may be obtained by writing to Medical Dept., Ross Laboratories, Columbus, Ohio 43216.
[2]Reed Test obtainable from Royal National Institute for the Deaf, 105 Gower Street, London WC1. England.
[3]Forms and manual obtainable from Lodoca Project and Publishing Foundation, Inc., East 51st and Lincoln Street, Denver, Colorado 80216.
[4]American Guidance Service, Inc., Publishers Building, Circle Pines, Minnesota 55014*
[5]Slosson Educational Publications, 140 Pine Street, East Aurora, N.Y. 14052.
[6]Grune & Stratton, Inc., 111 Fifth Avenue, New York, N.Y. 10003.*
[7]National Society for the Prevention of Blindness, Inc., 79 Madison Avenue, New York, N.Y. 10016.
[8]Matalene Surgical Instrument Co., Inc., 141 East 44th Street, New York, N.Y. 10017.
[9]Titmus Optical Co., Inc., Petersburg, Virginia 23803.†
[10]Kanehare Shuppan Co. Ltd., Tokyo, Japan.* ‡
[11]NFER-Nelson Publishing Co. Ltd., Darville House, 2 Oxford Road East, Windsor, Berkshire SL4 1DF, England.

*Also obtainable from NFER-Nelson Publishing Co. Ltd., Darville House, 2 Oxford Road East, Windsor, Berkshire SL4 1DF, England.
†Also obtainable from Graham Field, Inc., 415 2nd Avenue, New Hyde Park, N.Y. 11040.
‡Also obtainable from Stereo Optical Co., 3539 N. Kenton Ave., Chicago, Ill. 60641.

CHAPTER 2

The History

A medical history is a factual account of what has already occurred. Although it can never be complete, a good history will tell the physician all he or she needs to know. Its length, detail and the time required to obtain it are secondary in importance to its accuracy and clarity. The parents and the child must feel that the examiner has the time, interest and ability to help them. The physician who makes proper introductions and who greets the child by name, no matter what the age, will convey an attitude of concern and interest.

Parents usually are clear about what they want, what they feel is wrong and what they have been told is wrong. Occasionally, however, a family will have been shunted from one clinic to another without having been given a clear notion of the purpose of their visits. In this case the examiner must take the time to explain the reasons for the referral.

Many parents welcome the opportunity to write down their ideas, especially if this can be done before the visit. Home movies, family photographs and baby books are often useful, and parents should be encouraged to provide them. A form for recording the parents' impressions can be mailed to them at the time the appointment is made.

The examiner must exercise tact and discretion, especially when taking a history in the presence of the child. Questioning on sensitive subjects is best reserved for a time when the parents can be interviewed alone.

Sometimes a child is accompanied by a social worker, who may or may not have a close relationship with the child. Information given by a social worker is more likely to emphasize family and environmental factors. A foster parent may provide a very objective view of the child's current level of performance but is less likely to know much about earlier development or the medical history.

Written records can be extremely valuable in providing hard data, but considerable care is needed in evaluating them. Typewritten material often has been condensed or edited almost beyond recognition, and there is tremendous variation in how information is obtained and recorded. The examiner must learn to scan the material quickly for relevant dates and facts, and where possible written records should be gone over before the child's visit. Even written material obtained after the child's examination can provide a useful check on the history as given by the family. However, history recorded from written material rather than from direct questioning should be identified as such.

The presenting problem

The physician needs to ascertain the family's perception of the problem. How old was the child when the symptoms began? Was the onset insidious? How urgent are the symptoms? Have the symptoms changed during the past days, weeks or months?

Are the symptoms influenced by the time of day, the setting, activity, or change in environment? Are the symptoms growing worse? Have there been any changes in the child's appetite, energy or activities? Has anything like it been seen before in the family? Has anyone who cares for the child been ill? Have there been any stresses or upheavals within the family? What other evaluations have been carried out, and what therapy tried? What do the family and referring source expect from this evaluation?

Sometimes open-ended questions to the parent yield better results than routine factual inquiries. For example, it is better to ask 'When did *you* feel something was wrong?' than 'How long has your child had this problem?', and 'What do *you* think caused the problem?' is preferable to 'What is the reason given for the problem?'.

If verbal, a child can describe feelings and symptoms, and a child's memory for the time and sequence of events may be more accurate than the parents'.

The time of onset of symptoms can be determined by association with specific events in the child's life—when the child entered school, moved to a new house, went on vacation, acquired a new sibling, and so on.

One group of symptoms might concern a deviation from an expected accomplishment, *i.e.* the family is concerned because they feel that there has been a delay in sitting up, walking or talking. The physician must decide whether the lack of accomplishment actually exists. If it does exist, is it caused by general developmental delay, by the loss of a previous skill or by the presence of a motor, sensory or emotional handicap? Are the child's accomplishments delayed in all areas or is there a lag in one area alone?

The loss of a previous skill should be established beyond doubt. This is best done by asking for specific accomplishments which may have been lost rather than simply by asking vague questions concerning the 'weakness': the baby who could hold a bottle and sit up can no longer do so; a child can no longer hold a fork, draw, tie shoes, dress or climb the stairs.

A second category of presenting problems includes various symptoms which can cause concern, among them headaches and possible seizures (Chapter 7), tics and other involuntary movements (Chapter 5), and difficulties with co-ordination (Chapter 5).

The physician must evaluate the symptoms and assess whether concern is justified, as well as ascertaining whether the symptom has a functional cause, is a manifestation of an organic neurological problem or is caused by systemic disease.

Some parental concerns are not based on specific neurological symptoms, but rather deal with the child's adjustment at home, in the community and at school. In this case the physician must evaluate not only the child but also his relationship to his family and his environment.

Associated neurological problems

Often neurological problems are not clear-cut, and more than one disability may exist. For example, a child with apparent cerebral palsy also may have seizures and experience difficulties in school. Although the motor handicap is the presenting problem, the physician must also evaluate the status of the convulsive disorder and its therapy and seek the reasons behind the learning difficulty.

Previous evaluations

All previous evaluations and therapies should be documented in the child's chart for future reference. If the present referral is the most recent of a long series of evaluations, the physician may wonder why the others were unsuccessful.

General medical history

The general medical history should emphasize those aspects of the child's health history which might have neurological significance. The order of the questions and the detail necessary are flexible, and depend on the personal preference and technique of the examiner, the age of the child and the significance of certain aspects of the history to the over-all problem.

Although the parents' account of the presenting problem may be accurate, it is well known that recall of other parts of the history may be less certain. Parents are notoriously vague about remembering the time of developmental achievements, unless very recently acquired. Inaccuracies may be caused by parental bias, misinterpretation of the question, anxiety, or simple lapse of memory.

Good co-operation and accurate recall may be expected if easy questions requiring affirmative answers are asked first. Even a routine question may elicit an answer or comment which opens up a whole new and important line of inquiry.

The material covered in the following sections of the general medical history must be adapted to suit the evaluation. Both the age of the child and the nature of the problem should influence the amount of time spent on various portions of the history. For example, a careful chronicle of events occurring during the neonatal period obviously is vital in the evaluation of an infant or very young child with developmental delay, but this can be skimmed over when taking the history of a 10-year-old youngster who was entirely healthy and well-adjusted before beginning to complain of dizzy spells.

The history form should list specific items to be covered in a conventional history, such as obstetrical and neonatal details, immunizations, childhood diseases, and a review of systems. The following discussion includes comments on the significance of the material covered, together with suggestions for detailed questioning where appropriate.

Mother's pregnancy and labor; delivery; neonatal period

There will be much variation both in the detail available and the reliability of the account of events preceding and surrounding the birth of the child. Some mothers will be very vague about details of the pregnancy and ignorant about specifics of delivery. In contrast, young couples trained in childbirth education are extremely familiar with all details of the pregnancy, labor and delivery. Most mothers will remember whether, and in what way, the pregnancy was *different* from any of her other pregnancies, and most are quite clear about the length and quality of labor, the gestation period and the birthweight. As a rule, mothers are asked about 'any abnormality of fetal movements', but their response may be worthless unless the mother *spontaneously* comments that the fetal movements were different from previous pregnancies or that they changed or stopped.

Events of possible neurological significance include obstetrical complications during pregnancy, labor or delivery which could result in anoxia; prematurity; a history of maternal illness, infection or injury; radiation during pregnancy; and a history of infection or contagious disease in any member of the household during the mother's pregnancy. Social factors can be significant. The age of the mother at delivery is also important.

Drug or alcohol ingestion during pregnancy may have an effect on the fetus and lead to difficulties in delivery and in neonatal care (Smithells 1979). A history of irregular or delayed prenatal care or of precipitate labor somewhere outside a delivery room should alert the physician to be on the lookout for any signs of developmental delay.

Obvious medical problems in the hospital newborn unit also should be recorded. If seizures occurred, at what age were they observed? What studies were done? What was thought to be the cause, and how were they treated? Seizures which occur before 72 hours of age usually have a better prognosis than those occurring subsequently. Were there any difficulties with feeding or sucking? Such difficulties in the hospital newborn unit are a non-specific but valuable pointer to the baby who is at risk neurologically. The mother should be asked if there was anything *different* about the hospital routine. Was she allowed to see the baby at the usual time? Was there anything unusual about the care given? Did the people responsible for the child seem unusually concerned? How long did mother and baby stay in hospital? If there was a serious problem and the baby was in an intensive care unit, how often did she visit, and did she participate in the baby's care?

Infancy (up to 24 months)

Questioning about infancy should begin with general inquiries. Did the baby thrive? Were there many minor illnesses, such as colds? Did the baby have any problems with feeding or night waking?

A question about the baby's 'personality' can provide a clue to abnormal behavior. Excessive irritability, crying or lethargy are all significant, and comparison with the behavior of other members of the family at a similar age can be helpful. Responses to the question 'What makes the baby smile and laugh?' can indicate the amount of social stimulation and familial affection received by the baby. An infant who cannot be made to smile or laugh or who is generally unresponsive may have a serious problem, possibly severe developmental delay or a sensory deficit, or may be understimulated.

A toddler with a history of constant activity might be simply an exuberant personality; on the other hand, he could be showing early signs of a behavior problem (see Chapter 9).

Immunizations

Questions about immunizations are asked primarily to see if any severe or unusual reaction could have neurological significance. If a reaction *did* occur, was the child in good health when the immunization was given? The possible association of infantile myoclonic seizures with a reaction to pertussis vaccination is well known

(Baird and Borofsky 1957, Kulenkampff *et al.* 1974, Fenichel 1982). The physician who does a neurological evaluation has a responsibility for the 'whole child', and should have a general interest in the prevention of handicapping conditions. Therefore the physician should make sure that any immunizations which are inadequate or lacking are completed.

Childhood diseases, serious illnesses, injuries

The neurologically impaired child is medically, physically and psychologically vulnerable to illnesses, injuries and stresses that might not affect his or her normal peers (Rutter *et al.* 1970). Questions are asked about childhood diseases and serious illnesses to determine any possible neurological significance and to see what effect the illness had on the child. How severe was the illness? Was the child's reaction to it greater than that expected for an average child? Does the child always react to illness with unusual intensity or high fever? Did the illness have any perceptible influence on development, academic progress, personality or social activities?

A recital of injuries suffered may suggest that the child is accident-prone. The physician must then decide whether the unusual number of cuts, bruises, bumps, burns or fractures are caused by the activities of a high-spirited child who is much more daring than his peers, or are the result of problems with co-ordination or sensory impairment. It is important to determine whether the risks taken by the child are appropriate for age or whether they indicate lack of awareness of danger, poor impulse control, or 'acting out' behavior. The environment also must be considered as a factor in the succession of injuries. Have reasonable safety precautions been taken? Has supervision been adequate? Is the neighborhood safe?

The physician also should consider the possibility of child abuse as a cause of unusual or frequent injuries. A handicapped child is especially vulnerable, because parents with limited child-rearing skills cannot always meet the challenge of providing the necessary and time-consuming care. Of course, child abuse can cause a neurological disability and may explain a bizarre group of neurological symptoms which do not fit a recognizable condition or syndrome. Tactful, non-judgmental questions may expose the problem: 'Do you ever feel you can't stand him another minute?'; 'What do you do when you feel that way?'; 'How do you control him'?; 'Do other people at home feel the same way about him?'; 'How do they manage him?'.

Hospital admissions

For possible future reference, a careful history should contain details of admissions to hospital, with dates, names of hospitals and reasons for admission. If the child were very young, it would be useful to know whether the mother stayed in hospital with the child. Assessment of the child's reactions to the stay in hospital and of any problems encountered in care may yield useful information about the child's response to stress. A list of hospital admissions also can be an objective indication of the severity of health problems, the difficulty in over-all health care, and of the emotional drain on the family. In the United States, frequent stays in hospital can be a serious financial drain, as well.

General health and review of systems

An over-all view of the child's current well-being can be pieced together from answers to inquiries about general health, together with a review of the systems. The physician should ask the proper questions, and they may not be concerned directly with the nervous system, since certain neurological conditions are associated with health problems. For example, a child with trisomy 21 (Down syndrome) often is myopic, may have congenital heart-disease, and may have frequent upper-respiratory infections which can lead to middle-ear disease and conductive hearing-loss.

A review of systems also affords an insight into the general health of the family and the family's attitude toward illness and invalidism. Questions about the child's health can be extended to the health of family members: 'Who else has allergies?; Your mother?; Does she live with you?; Isn't it lucky she can be such a help to you?; How old is she?. Usually such questions are asked when dealing with the family history, but often useful information is elicited in this indirect way. If such questions indicate that there are areas of concern about the family's health, further questions can be asked later.

Eating habits are important in the child's health and care, and can also affect the rest of the family. Is the diet sensible and reasonable, considering the age of the child and the nature of his handicap? Does the child enjoy eating, and are his eating skills appropriate for his age? Does the child eat with the rest of the family? If not, why not? Does preparation of the diet or feeding the child cause undue trouble for the parent or caretaker? Are food and eating ever used in a power struggle between parent and child?

Good sleeping habits are also basic to the child's well-being and any disturbance or difficulty can create a serious problem in the household. Does the child's pattern of rest and sleep allow the parents adequate unbroken rest? Does the child sleep in a crib with the sides up or in a single-bed? Are the sides necessary? Does the child share a bedroom or bed with parents or siblings? Must bedroom windows or doors be locked to keep the child in? Is bedtime pleasurable or a battle?

Medication

A complete list of current medication, including vitamins, should be obtained.

Developmental history

Any evaluation of a neurological problem must include an opinion about whether or not a child is developmentally normal. Developmental normality is based on the evidence that physical growth, mental ability, motor skills, language, social behavior and emotional stability are those expected for the child's age. The developmental history is the first step in this assessment. The physician must determine whether the parental version of the history indicates that the infant or child is on schedule for normal development. If discrepancies emerge, the formal neurological evaluation should seek an explanation.

Of course the amount of time spent in obtaining a developmental history depends on the age of the child. Inquiries about developmental milestones in infancy and early childhood are necessary with the parents of a baby or toddler, and for any child who is suspected of developmental delay. On the other hand, a child who is doing satisfactory grade-level work in school, whose size and physical skills are appropriate for age and who participates in social activities is probably normal, and relatively little emphasis need be placed on the minutiae of development.

The physician's evaluation of the developmental history must be based on experience and a thorough knowledge of child development. Invaluable resources are Illingworth's *The Development of the Infant and Young Child* (1966) and *Basic Developmental Screening* (1977), and Knobloch and Pasamanick's edition of Gesell and Amatruda's *Developmental Diagnosis* (1974).

Most parents remember only the most obvious milestones, and recollection of the first-born's accomplishments usually are more detailed than those of later children, unless a special problem existed with another child. Very few parents can remember exactly when the baby rolled from front to back, or transferred an object from one hand to the other. Common answers to questions about development are that the baby 'seemed normal' or that a particular skill was acquired 'at the usual time'.

Hart and colleagues (1978) did a study on the extent of recall of developmental events among a group of mothers attending a child-health clinic. They reported that the number of mothers able to recall milestones decreased in proportion to the length of time since the developmental event. Walking was the best-remembered milestone, and the time of smiling the least well recalled. A 'baby book', recording accomplishments, usually is more reliable than a mother's recall. Indirect questions may help: 'How does this one compare with your other children?'; 'What was he doing on his first birthday?'; 'Did she talk before she walked?'.

Although the parents' account of the child's development may be incomplete, inaccurate, vague or biased, the examiner nevertheless should make an effort to elicit the information. The parents' responses will reveal something about their expectations of the child, and in any case the final opinion about the child's development will be based on much more than the history. The astute physician will place the parents' responses in the proper perspective.

It is wise to emphasize positive aspects of development; to record what the child *can* do. Can he feed himself a cracker? Can he walk with one hand held? Can an older child ride a bicycle, swim, skate, build models, go to the store, handle money? Is the child helpful and responsible around the house? No matter how handicapped, every child can be a source of pride and pleasure. The questioning about development can proceed much more smoothly if the parents feel that the physician is looking for strengths rather than limitations.

The examiner should be alert for any sign which indicates that a previous skill has been lost. Regression in development can be an ominous indication of a degenerative disease or of a neuromuscular problem.

A developmental history for a baby or young child, or for a child suspected of developmental delay, includes questions about traditional developmental accomplishments which the mother might be likely to remember. The examiner must be certain that the parent fully understands the question: a 'social smile' may mean one thing to the physician and quite another to the parent. It must be emphasized that the range of normal development is large, and physical and social maturation are influenced by many factors. An apparent discrepancy must be evaluated in relation to all other findings, and a particular presenting problem—for example, delay in talking (see Chapter 9)—will require detailed questioning in one area.

A socially responsive smile occurs when, without being tickled or touched, the baby smiles in response to a smile or greeting from another person. The baby is said to sit alone when he can sit in the crib or on the floor, without support, for five seconds or more. The baby who stands erect and unsupported for 10 seconds or more is standing alone. A baby walks alone when he takes five or more steps without holding on to anything or anyone.

The developmental history also should include information about the child's personality, behavior, social adjustment and family relationships. Chapter 8 gives profiles of behavior and accomplishments expected of babies and young children at the ages of four weeks, 12 weeks, 24 weeks, 12 months and 24 months.

Other questions about development include skills in self-care (feeding, dressing, toilet habits), locomotion (walking, running, climbing stairs) and the emergence of language. Table XX (p. 165) lists activities and skills expected of children between the ages of two and five years.

A child whose language skills develop normally but whose motor skills are significantly delayed should be checked carefully for a lag in motor development. Significant delay in both motor and language skills suggests retardation, a severe physical handicap or severe deprivation. Normal motor development with delayed language could indicate retardation, a communication disorder or a serious emotional problem.

Sometimes skills are not learned because of lack of opportunity, for example if there are no stairs to learn to climb, or the mother does not encourage a child to learn to dress because 'it would take too long'. Perhaps the observed delayed development is a result of poor care, lack of stimulation or deprivation.

There is wide variation in attitudes toward bladder and bowel training and in methods for their accomplishment. In the absence of serious delay, the exact time of mastery of bladder and bowel control is not as important as how it was managed. Methods and expectations of toilet-training might give clues about parental attitudes toward child-rearing. A mother who is rigid about toilet training might also be a strict disciplinarian. One who believes in *laissez faire* might be incapable of setting limits on behavior. The physician should seek an explanation if satisfactory bladder and bowel control were or are significantly delayed.

Tactful questioning should be done about any current behavior problems such as enuresis, encopresis, excessive temper tantrums or difficulty with discipline. It is important to know whether the child has such a problem, and how the family copes with it.

An effort should be made to learn how a school-age child spends time at home, at school and in the community. If possible, questions about activities, hobbies, friends and preferences should be asked of the child: 'What did you do yesterday, starting from the time you got up?'; 'What do you like to do most?'; 'What do you like to do least?'; 'What is your best friend like?'; 'What do you want to do when you grow up?'. Questions about friends are especially important, since a seriously emotionally disturbed child is not likely to have many friends.

By asking about activities and community interests, the physician will be perceived by the child and family as someone who is interested in them as people, not merely as a family with a child who has a 'presenting problem'.

Education

Educational success is based on the acquisition of skills or academic achievement which are appropriate for the child's ability, and on a satisfactory adjustment to the school and the people in it. Some examiners like to start with the earliest pre-school experience and work forward. Others prefer to describe the present school experience and work backward. Does the child participate in extracurricular activities? Does the child have friends at school? Is the child's behavior at school different from that at home? What is the school like? How far away is it? (Chapter 9 gives suggestions for detailed questions when the presenting problem involves educational difficulty.)

Family history and home environment

The section on 'family history' obviously should include basic information about neurological conditions among other family members which might have a bearing on the presenting problem. The family's familiarity with a neurological condition in a relative can increase the reliability of the history. A mother who has seizures herself, or who has seen seizures in another child or relative, is likely to give an accurate and detailed account of seizures in her own child. Evidence that a relative may have been similarly affected requires clarification. Also of potential significance are relatives who died early in life, required institutional care or attended a special clinic. The presence of inherited diseases in the family might necessitate a formal genetic history (see Appendix C).

The family 'constellation' shows the place of the child in that family. It has been often said that 'no two children in the family inherit the same set of parents'. The first-born may have inexperienced parents with high expectations, whereas the last-born invariably is compared with his or her siblings. All of the child's actions, reactions, adjustments and accomplishments depend on where and how the child fits in. The home environment includes not only parents and siblings, but also all others who live under the same roof. Often it is helpful to draw a diagram of the family group, represented by circles and squares, in order to identify the members living in the same household; their ages, occupations, relationships; and close relatives and friends. For example, a grandparent who is a chronic invalid could be the cause of additional stress on the mother of a handicapped child, whereas a sprightly, tolerant, wise grandparent could be a tower of strength.

The academic and occupational records of siblings are important, in that they provide clues about family expectations. Siblings' school placements might show a family pattern of educational difficulties. Serious health problems in a sibling might be an additional strain on the mother.

Special questions on the environment need to be asked when the child is in foster care: how long has the child been with the foster mother?; what are her qualifications and experience?; what are the problems of other children in the house; and how old are they?

Family stress

Medical, financial or social stresses within the family sometimes have a direct or indirect bearing on the child's presenting problem or on planning for comprehensive care. The physician should be alert for clues in the history or in observation which suggest the existence of such serious stresses.

Agencies involved in care and counseling

Medical, financial and social problems can cause a family to become involved with several different public and private agencies dealing with care, counseling and financial subsidy. It is extremely important to acquaint oneself with these agencies currently working with the family so that responsibility for follow-up may be delineated, and appropriate information properly routed.

Summary

The physician obtains a first impression of the nature of the problem on the basis of the information gained from discussion with the child and family, and from indirect observation of the child while the history is being taken. Sometimes parents do not mention obvious things, such as a small head, strabismus, post-operative scars, cuts, bumps, bruises and chronic skin lesions. By tactful questioning, the physician should determine the extent of the parents' knowledge about these: the condition might or might not be relevant, but it should be accounted for. The examiner must then make a judgment about the scope, direction, emphasis and content of the examination, bearing in mind that the time available is limited and that the attention-span of the child and of the family will decrease.

On the basis of the first impression, several decisions must be made. These should indicate whether the assessment needs to emphasize diagnosis or planning. If the need is for diagnosis, has the condition been recognized previously, and is it progressive or static? The history will provide helpful clues; for instance a sudden disability suggests a vascular phenomenon; loss of a previously acquired skill may suggest a degenerative disease or brain tumor.

The nature of the history will dictate the scope and extent of the subsequent examination, some parts of which may need to be only brief. A history suggestive of a vascular phenomenon necessitates careful examination of cranial-nerve function, whereas a child presenting with a reading problem in school requires careful developmental assessment, with less time spent on examining cranial nerves. The history should also reveal whether the family's perception of the problem is realistic and sympathetic.

CHAPTER 3

The Preliminaries

Very few physicians have ever done a complete neurological examination, for it is impossible to test every part of every nerve. The physician must do the best possible evaluation to define the problem and to determine what needs to be done about it. The particular technique and emphasis will be dictated by the nature of the problem, the health, co-operation and disability of the child, the time available, and the attention-span of all concerned.

Neurological and developmental literature abounds with methods of examination and assessment. The experienced examiner will have developed an individual technique which is comfortable, efficient and valid. Although the sequence and content may vary according to the situation, the examiner's general method should remain constant from patient to patient.

The method described on the following pages represents an approach which regards the child as having a problem, not a label, and the examination is based on the recognition of abnormalities which will explain the problem. The steps in the examination are considered in a definite order for use with a co-operative child who can follow directions. The order is designed to assure maximum comfort and efficiency for the child and physician (see Appendix A). It is not a ritual analysis of separate components of the nervous system.

The examination given in the following pages is one which, in general, is applicable to children over three years of age, although many of the steps can and should be included in the evaluation of younger children. (Details of a special approach and interpretation for the examination of infants and very young children up to two years of age are given in Chapter 8.) Adaptation will have to be made for special situations, such as lack of co-operation or limitations imposed by the child's disability. Confidence can be built and co-operation obtained if easy tasks are done first. For example, a child with a motor handicap could be tested first in verbal skills with a Peabody Picture Vocabulary Test, in which he is likely to do well, while a child with a verbal problem might feel more at ease starting with tests of motor function.

It is important to praise the child when he does something well, even the simplest task, and usually this will encourage him to co-operate with further tasks. This is just as important for a school-aged child as for a younger one.

In the following pages specific step-by-step directions for the examination are followed at appropriate intervals by discussion of the significance of the procedures and the findings. The astute clinician will vary the order of the examination to suit the particular child's needs, so the ordering of the following chapters is arbitrary to some extent. Commonly, for example, an examination may begin with looking at the child's head and making observations about cranial nerves (Chapter 4), followed by some of the less 'threatening' items to do with the development of young children (Chapter 8), then perhaps come back to sections of Chapter 5. However, the logic of

15

the order of the various chapters is to progress from the neurological evaluation to children with particular problems and the examination of infants and children at various ages.

A systematic general physical examination, with emphasis appropriate to the problem, is an integral part of the neurological examination.

The 'unco-operative' child

Sometimes a child will be violently 'unco-operative' and will struggle against any type of examination, or will be withdrawn and immobile and resist examination by refusing to interact in any way. If the success of the examination seems to be in jeopardy because of these reactions, the physician must put the problem into perspective. Is the behavior typical for the child or of recent onset? Does the child behave this way at home? Is the behavior unrelated to the presenting medical complaint or is the behavior part of the problem? If it is not part of the medical problem, is it the result of anxiety, fear, previous bad experience with physicians, or just plainly manipulative?

Usually the child can be won over if time and patience permit, and time spent talking informally with the child and playing with books and toys may be well invested. Sometimes a modified approach ('This is the best we can do') will have to be used: in that case the period of indirect observation is especially valuable, and careful questioning about daily living can establish whether or not the child can see, hear, eat, chew, swallow, talk and move around, and whether the child is thought to be functioning at the appropriate developmental level. Obviously, the decision about whether to reschedule the examination, win the child over, or settle for an incomplete examination depends on the reasons for the examination, the personalities involved and the time available.

The indirect examination

The indirect examination begins as soon as the child enters the room and it continues throughout the history-taking, the formal examination and the discussion with the family. Clinical impressions gathered through observation are substantiated by formal testing. Careful observation will provide a starting point for the examination by indicating which areas might be abnormal. Can eye-contact be established with the child?

Bear in mind that the child's stature or head circumference, for example, may reflect a familial trait ('look at the parents').

Does the child look like the rest of the family? Is his general appearance unusual enough to suggest a particular syndrome or a general neurodevelopmental disorder? Is physical development symmetrical? Is the child approximately the size expected for his chronological age? Is his apparent developmental level appropriate? Is he thriving, or chronically or acutely ill? Is he tired, toxic or hungry? Is there any obvious congenital defect, or unusual skin pigmentation? How does he communicate? Does he respond to questions? Does he swallow milk or juice without difficulty? Can he feed himself a cracker and chew it easily? Is his facial expression unusual? How does he move? Is his choice of locomotion that expected for his age? Is he agile or clumsy? Is he in constant motion or rooted to a chair? Does he explore the room with curiosity and pleasure, or is he intent on instant destruction? Does he look at and play with toys? Is there a strong hand-preference? Is he apathetic, depressed, anxious and fearful, or chatty and euphoric? Is the attention-span so short that examination will be difficult? How does he get along with his family? Do the parents echo each of the examiner's questions, answer for the child, interpret each question and give the child the answer? Are they obviously supportive and loving, or distant and hostile?

The child's appearance may be such that a specific condition or syndrome immediately comes to mind. For example, a girl who enters the examining room with her right leg swinging out, scraping the toe of her shoe on the floor, and whose arm is held tight to her body with the elbow flexed, the forearm pronated and the wrist flexed, has a right hemiplegia. The appearance of the child with typical trisomy 21 (Down syndrome) varies somewhat according to age and race, but the combination of brachycephalic head, upward slant of the eyes, epicanthal folds, low-set ears and extremities which are short in proportion to the trunk, is so characteristic that the diagnosis is suggested immediately.

Sometimes the general appearance may suggest a syndrome or condition but the examiner cannot be sure and must check the literature after the clinical appraisal. Classification of syndromes can be based on morphology, genetics, biochemistry or symptoms. The examiner should be familiar with the major common syndromes and should have one or more references available, for example *Birth Defects Atlas and Compendium* (Bergsma 1979) or *Developmental Defects and Syndromes* (Salmon 1978). Other visible physical abnormalities may indicate a non-specific neuro-developmental disorder.

A clinical impression can be reinforced by experience, and by a matching photograph and a description in the literature. The diagnosis should be supported by appropriate objective tests, such as radiological studies, chromosomal analyses and laboratory studies. If the cause of the child's unusual appearance has been established already, the examiner should look for other associated handicaps which might affect good comprehensive care.

Certain physical attributes can give clues to a particular condition: a strong 'barn-like' odor about the child indicates the need to check for phenylketonuria; sebaceous adenomata and butterfly erythema suggest tuberous sclerosis (Fig. 2); a port-wine hemangioma may be associated with the Sturge-Weber syndrome (Fig. 3); and scattered bruises and scars should alert the physician to the possibility of child abuse. (Skin signs are discussed further in Chapter 4).

Although a great deal of valuable information can be gained from observation alone, the examiner should beware of snap judgments and *café-au-lait* red-herrings. Clues and leads should be investigated, but often they provide only a guide to the direction and scope of the examination.

Beginning the examination: weighing and measuring
Directions

Begin by noting the child's name, and what version of it he prefers to be called. Most children have a decided preference. Establish good rapport with a younger child by exchanging 'gifts'. A tape-measure can be traded for a car or doll, then returned.

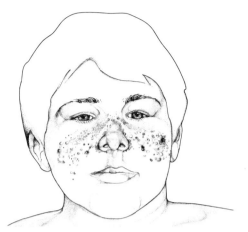

Fig. 2. Tuberous sclerosis: sebaceous adenomata are evident, flesh-colored or as pink nodules, typically in the nasolabial folds, cheeks and chin.

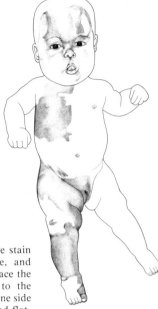

Fig. 3. Sturge-Weber syndrome. Port-wine stain (nevus flammeus) is present on the face, and sometimes on the body, at birth. On the face the stain usually follows a similar pattern to the trigeminal nerve. Usually it is confined to one side of the body, and is sharply demarcated and flat. In the area of the stain the lips appear to be thickened.

Draw an older child into conversation about something of obvious interest—a book he has with him or a school or team insignia on a jacket or shirt. Try to establish eye contact, without staring.

Observe the child's co-ordination when climbing onto the scale. Note his ability to follow directions. Check gross vision of older children by asking them to read off the values on the scale.

Have the child sit on the mother's lap, or, if older, on the examiner's table, with his legs hanging over the edge (to observe movement disorders or asymmetry). Take his blood pressure.

Discussion

Weighing and measuring. Participation in weighing and measuring gives the physician an opportunity to interact with and handle the child. It is usually a good place to start, but can be deferred if the child appears to be frightened. Dressing and undressing are also parts of the examination: they test co-ordination and independence, and even may reveal family attitudes. (The common procedure of having an aide strip, weigh and measure the child, and perhaps leave him shivering in

18

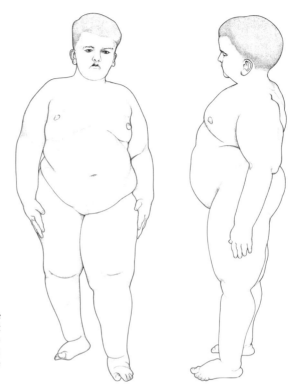

Fig. 4. Prader-Willi syndrome. The face has excessive fat, the mouth turns down at corners; genitalia are small and under-developed, testicles are undescended; hands and feet are small and patients are obese.

a hospital gown to await the physician, is deplorable, and is mentioned here only to be condemned.)

The exact procedure of weighing and measuring depends on the clinic or office facilities (for example, where the scale is located), but it should be consistent. If the scale is down the hall from the examination room the child can be weighed clothed, but without shoes or leg-braces. Any physical problem which precludes standard measurements being taken should be noted on the record. Measurements of head circumference and chest (taken until two years of age) should be recorded in both centimeters and inches, and weight in both kilograms and pounds. The results should be reproducible to 0.5lb or 0.2kg. Measurements should be plotted on a graph or chart giving percentiles or standard deviations. If the child's height or weight is below the 3rd percentile or above the 97th percentile for sex and age, further study is indicated.

Short stature could be the result of chronic disease, neurological disorder (*e.g.* cerebral palsy) or severe physical and emotional deprivation. It could be caused by a spinal abnormality; it could be endocrine in origin, as in hypothyroidism; or it could be an inherited or a chromosomal disorder such as gonadal dysgenesis. The physician should look for other abnormalities which suggest a syndrome.

Obesity can result from severe limitation of physical activity imposed by the child's disability; it could be dietary; or it may be an integral part of a particular condition, such as the syndromes of Laurence-Moon-Biedl or Prader-Willi (Fig. 4).

CHAPTER 4

Examination of the Skin, Head and Cranial Nerves

Most infants and children are more comfortable if examined in the presence of their parents. Many older children prefer to be examined without their parents being present, and to have some time alone with the physician. Toddlers usually feel more secure on the mother's lap and the examination can begin there.

THE SKIN

Directions

Inspect the skin for any unusual pigmentation, nevi, bruises or other evidence of injury.

Discussion

There are several skin signs which may be associated with neurological disorders. The Sturge-Weber syndrome is a combination of an upper facial vascular nevus (port-wine stain), and a thin-walled vascular nevus on the surface of the cerebral cortex, often accompanied by ocular glaucoma on the affected side, and epilepsy occurs in 90 per cent of cases.

The presence of *café-au-lait* spots, which are oval, irregular pale-brown lesions distributed asymmetrically over trunk and extremities, may indicate neurofibromatosis. The lesions may be insignificant in the newborn period but grow in size and number with age. More than six of these larger than 1cm in size, accompanied by soft cutaneous.or subcutaneous nodules, constitutes strong evidence of neurofibromatosis (an autosomal dominant with variable penetrance). Because a bony defect of the orbit allows the tumor to recede, the proptosis commonly seen in neurofibromatosis in childhood often disappears when the child lies flat.

Tuberous sclerosis is characterized by one or more hypopigmented leaf-like patches on the skin, by adenoma sebaceum in a butterfly distribution over nose and face, and shagreen patches (often lumbo-sacral) which may appear in late childhood. The skin signs alone should alert one to this disorder; there may be accompanying myoclonic seizures and a modified hypsarrhythmia in the EEG.

Other neurocutaneous syndromes are linear nevus (a sebaceous waxy yellow midline linear vertical lesion, which is elevated and usually on the forehead or chin, lip and nose), von Hippel-Lindau (retinal angiomata and cerebellar hemangio-blastoma), giant-cell nevus (a pigmented hairy nevus on the trunk) and ataxia-telangiectasia (progressive choreoathetosis associated with decreased immuno-globulins (IgA amd IgE)). In the last condition cutaneous telangiectasia are prominent in the antecubital and popliteal areas. These conditions have been associated with mental retardation but the precise relationship of the skin manifestations with those of the central nervous system is poorly understood (Menkes 1980).

THE HEAD: SIZE, SHAPE AND HAIR

Directions

Inspect the head for size, shape and symmetry. Measure the head circumference with a steel tape, encircling the head just above the eyebrows and around the maximum point of the occiput posteriorly. Take the measurement several times and use the greatest value. Palpate the sutures, and judge the size and tension of the anterior fontanelle, if present. Palpate and inspect the scalp for dimples, tufts of hair, bony prominences, depressions and tenderness. Note the quantity, texture and distribution of hair.

Discussion

Head size

The definition of an abnormally large or small head is based on statistics and is arbitrary. A normal child can have a head circumference which is borderline in either direction. The size of the infant's or child's head is determined by the growth of the cranial contents and the structure of the cranial bones. The rate of growth is influenced by heredity, general health, function of other systems (cardiac and endocrine) and the child's age and weight. For a baby whose height is above the 97th percentile, the head circumference will usually also follow to above the 97th percentile, although with a lag of a few weeks. A growth curve can document the progress of the child and reveal any deviations from expected growth.

A measurement that is statistically abnormal should be supplemented by observation and measurement of parents and siblings. After two years of age, the head circumference should be smaller than the chest circumference.

Microcephaly (see Table I) conventionally is defined as a head circumference more than 2SD below the mean, or below the third percentile for age, sex and gestation. Except for small head-size associated with craniosynostosis, microcephaly is always synonymous with microencephaly, an under-growth of the brain. Microcephaly may be a primary defect in brain development or it may be secondary to noxious influences which occur during pregnancy, in the perinatal period or in early infancy. Adverse influences include congenital infections, radiation, anoxia, difficult delivery and severe malnutrition.

Macrocephaly (see Table II) is defined as a head circumference of more than 2SD above the mean, or above the 97th percentile for age, sex and gestation. The term simply denotes 'large head', which may derive from a variety of causes. The terms megalencephaly and macroencephaly can be used to describe large and heavy brains, sometimes associated with morphological abnormalities and mental retardation (Lawrence 1964), but also found in people of normal intellect (Lorber and Priestley 1981).

Evaluation of the rate of enlargement and other evidence of neurological impairment will determine whether the condition is progressive, as in hydrocephalus, subdural hematoma or effusion, or a brain tumor. It is a pathological sign if the circumference is increasing rapidly, and may also be if it is above the 97th percentile and continues parallel to this. However, if the rate of increase in head circumference

21

TABLE I
Disorders associated with microcephaly

Primary (prenatal)	*Secondary (perinatal or postnatal)*
Genetic	Infection
Chromosomal	Trauma
Maternal irradiation	Metabolic
Intra-uterine infection or anoxia	Anoxia
Exposure to chemicals *in utero* (aminopterin)	
Maternal metabolic illness (diabetes mellitus, phenylketonuria)	

TABLE II
Disorders associated with macrocephaly

Achondroplasia	'Primary' (familial or unknown etiology)
Cerebral gigantism	Pseudotumor cerebri
Hydranencephaly	Subdural effusions
Hydrocephalus:	Miscellaneous (associated with increased
Dandy-Walker syndrome, cysts,	intracranial pressure or increase in
tumors, aqueductal stenosis,	ratio of CSF production to resorption):
A-V malformations, post-infectious,	lead, vitamin A disorders,
post-traumatic	hypo-parathyroidism, steroid ingestion,
Increased size of cerebral hemispheres:	genetic congenital heart-disease,
leukodystrophies, neural	environmental deprivation
ectodermoses (Sturge-Weber,	
neurofibromatosis, tuberous sclerosis)	

is decelerating it should be sufficient to observe a child without resorting to drastic measures.

Rarely, increasing head circumference without increased intracranial pressure or ventricular size may be the first evidence of a leukodystrophy (Canavan disease, Alexander disease or Van Bogaert-Bertrand disease). Computed tomography findings of symmetrical, low-density white matter in Canavan disease (spongy degeneration of the brain) seem to be characteristic.

An abnormally large head may be static, and can be an associated finding in many conditions, including cerebral malformations, lipidoses, achondroplasia osteopetrosis, mucopolysaccharidoses, tuberous sclerosis and cerebral gigantism (Sotos syndrome).

Head shape

The shape of the head may provide useful clues about underlying pathology. Hydrocephalus is characterized by frontal bossing. An infant with bilateral subdural hematoma may have biparietal enlargement. Unilateral parietal enlargement may be seen after trauma. Occipital prominence is characteristic of the Dandy-Walker syndrome (Fig. 5).

The term *brachycephalic* ('brachys': short) is used to describe a head that is short and wide with a broad flattened forehead. It is a characteristic finding in Down

22

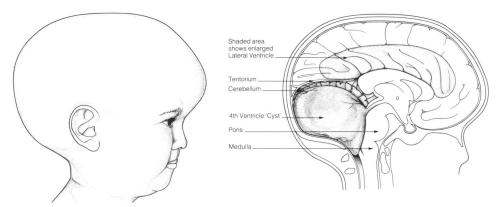

Shaded area
shows enlarged
Lateral Ventricle

Tentorium
Cerebellum

4th Ventricle 'Cyst'

Pons

Medulla

Fig. 5. Dandy-Walker syndrome. *(Left)* The head is large, with prominent occiput. *(Right)* This figure [redrawn from Ingraham and Watson 1954] shows a large 'cyst' of the 4th ventricle, probably associated with obstruction of the foramina of Luschka and Magendie (not identified). The cerebellum and tentorium are displaced upward; and pons, medulla and upper cervical cord are flattened and displaced anteriorly because of 'cystic' enlargement of 4th ventricle.

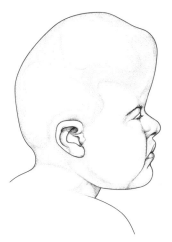

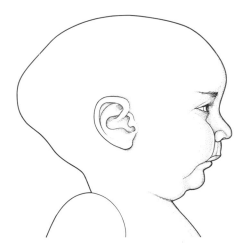

Fig. 6. Brachycephaly due to premature closure of the coronal sutures, which prevents antero-posterior growth but allows lateral growth, resulting in a foreshortened head.

Fig. 7. Scaphocephalic head: premature closure of the sagittal suture prevents lateral growth but allows anteroposterior growth, resulting in a long, narrow head.

syndrome. Brachycephaly also results from premature closure of the coronal suture (Fig. 6). *Scaphocephaly* ('skaphe': skiff) and *dolichocephaly* ('dolichos': long) both denote a long narrow head (Fig. 7). Positional flattening of a premature infant's soft skull may occur because weak neck-muscles preclude changes in position. This scaphocephaly in a premature baby may persist into adult life (Baum and Searls 1971). Premature closing of the sagittal suture is also a cause of scaphocephaly, since the skull grows in an anteroposterior direction along the path of least resistance.

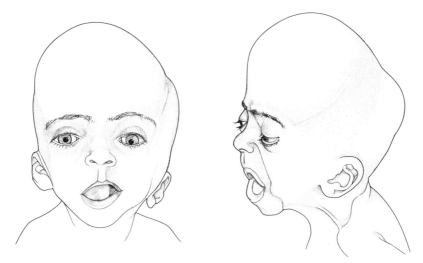

Fig. 8. Crouzon syndrome. The head has a wide, flat, high forehead, with early simultaneous synostosis of the coronal, sagittal and metopic sutures (oxycephaly), resulting in progressive cranial stenosis and hypoplasia of facial bones. The eyes have an 'anti-mongolian' slant and are exophthalmic, with hypertelorism.

Premature fusion of all cranial sutures directs the upward expansion of the skull against the region of the anterior fontanelle, where there is least resistance: oxycephaly ('oxys': sharp), a pointed head, is the result. Premature closure of a cranial suture may be unilateral, resulting in asymmetry. Craniosynostosis of varying degrees may be a finding in some syndromes, such as those of Crouzon (Fig. 8) and Apert (Fig. 9).

During the first year of life, some babies may have some degree of positional asymmetry (plagiocephaly) because of lying most of the time with the head turned to one side, perhaps initially to look toward the centre of the room or toward the light, rather than toward the wall. The infant's soft skull soon becomes flattened on one side of the occiput and it is then uncomfortable to lie in any other posture. Positional asymmetry is exaggerated in infants who have failed to achieve sitting balance by the normal age, in the presence of infantile torticollis, or in deprived children who are kept in their cots for long periods. It is important to distinguish positional asymmetry (in which one occiput is flatter and the ipsilateral frontal region more prominent but the two hemicrania are of equal volume) from the quite different situation in which one hemicranium is larger than the other, making one suspect intracranial hematoma or another expanding lesion on that side.

The anterior fontanelle

Usually the anterior fontanelle is closed by the age of 18 months, but the upper limit of normal closure is 29 months (Acheson and Jefferson 1954). A small or absent fontanelle might be a result of craniosynostosis and should be investigated. A persistently open fontanelle could be caused by hypothyroidism, increased intra-

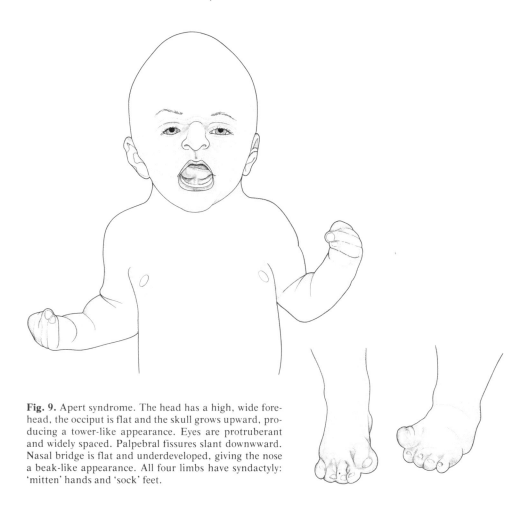

Fig. 9. Apert syndrome. The head has a high, wide forehead, the occiput is flat and the skull grows upward, producing a tower-like appearance. Eyes are protruberant and widely spaced. Palpebral fissures slant downwward. Nasal bridge is flat and underdeveloped, giving the nose a beak-like appearance. All four limbs have syndactyly: 'mitten' hands and 'sock' feet.

cranial pressure because of hydrocephalus, a tumor, a subdural hematoma, or pseudotumor cerebri. Severe growth retardation, which mimics hypopituitarism, can result from emotional and social deprivation, and an affected child may develop bulging of the anterior fontanelle and separation of the sutures during the catch-up phase of growth.

Findings on palpation

The usual findings from palpation are one or more bony prominences, which eventually may prove to be without significance. Bony depression or actual openings in the skull may be felt, which may be old depressed fractures, congenital anomalies such as biparietal foramina (usually harmless unless very large), or a variety of other lesions. Local tenderness of the skull to pressure most often reflects a recent injury of some kind, but it is well to bear in mind that occipital tenderness, particularly if greater on one side than on the other, is a sign of posterior fossa tumor which has been overlooked.

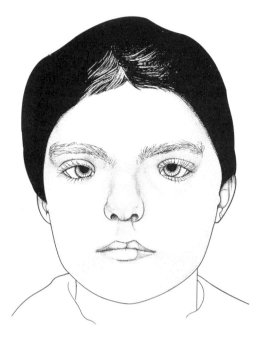

Fig. 10. Waardenburg syndrome. The medial canthi and lacrimal point are displaced laterally, but the distance between the pupils and outer canthi is normal (pseudohypertelorism). The nasal root is broad and the lips are prominent, with a cupid's bow. The eyes are an iridescent pale blue and there is a white forelock.

Hair

Hair that is coarser than expected for the age of the child may indicate congenital hypothyroidism. 'Kinky hair' is a characteristic of Menkes syndrome (together with slow growth, progressive cerebral degeneration, abnormalities of copper metabolism and X-linked recessive inheritance): the electron-microscopic hair findings are pili torti, trichorrhexis nodosa and monilethrix (Taylor and Green 1981). Hair abnormalities are also found in association with argininosuccinic aciduria and some cases of sensorineural hearing loss.

Alopecia can be caused by a drug such as sodium valproate, by acute stress, or it may be the result of constant hair-pulling by an emotionally disturbed child. A white forelock is sometimes seen in children with the Waardenburg syndrome (Fig. 10). The hair of a child with untreated phenylketonuria is always a lighter color than that of the parents and siblings. A low hair-line occurs in platybasia and in the Klippel-Feil syndrome. Alopecia areata is probably an autoimmune disorder: it is also found in association with other autoimmune disturbances (hypoparathyroidism, Addison's disease, thyroiditis, pernicious anemia, ovarian agenesis and steatorrhea).

INTRACRANIAL BRUITS

Although intracranial bruits are a frequent incidental finding among normal children (Moore and Baumann 1969), the examiner should become experienced in the technique of auscultation in order to be able to recognize the rare but significant abnormal sound. Although the diagnostic information is rarely specific, transmission of vascular sounds to the skull may be striking. The murmurs may seem very unusual to those who are not familiar with the normal variety of sounds.

Directions

Place a bell-type stethoscope over the temporal, mastoid, parietal and frontal areas, and over each eyelid. Compare the quality and timing of the sounds from each side of the skull. Listen for bruits in both carotid arteries. Compress each carotid artery to see if the bruit is obliterated. Ask the child to move his head into various positions.

Discussion

Almost all bruits are systolic. Obliteration of the bruit by compression of the carotid artery will help distinguish the true intracerebral bruit from transmitted cardiac murmurs, as well as from a venous hum, which is more continuous and influenced by a change in the position of the head. Systolic bruits which are heard over the distribution of the superficial temporal artery should be checked to determine whether they continue after digital compression of the artery.

The quality of the bruit itself is one of the best criteria for the experienced examiner, since pathological bruits have a characteristic quality which is difficult to describe but has been compared to 'footsteps in an empty church'. However, it is difficult—and usually impossible—to distinguish by auscultation alone the entirely innocuous bruit from that resulting from an intracranial vascular malformation or vascular tumor, or from bruits associated with hyperthyroidism, transmitted cardiac murmurs, or pyrexia alone. If an arteriovenous malformation within the skull has been detected by other means (CT scan or angiogram), often it is possible to associate this finding with auscultatory changes. These sounds tend to be more constant and less affected by changes in position. Auscultation can be misleading for an inexperienced examiner: for example, a child with an uncomplicated febrile seizure could be erroneously considered to have an arteriovenous malformation because of a 'murmur in the skull'.

TRANSILLUMINATION

Transillumination of the head is a routine part of the neurological examination *of all children under a year of age*, and even up to two or three years of age if hydrocephalus, porencephaly or other congenital malformation is suspected. The procedure requires proper equipment and some time and trouble, but it should be done if developmental delay is suspected and the cause is uncertain. A two- to four-cell flashlight with a special cuff to constrict the light is sufficient if the room is dark. More sophisticated transilluminators, such as the Chun gun* (Fig. 11), provide a dependable source of light of consistent intensity. These instruments are convenient and safe if used as directed (McArtor and Saunders 1979). A red light in the examining room or on the light source will speed the examiner's adaptation to the dark. The extent of transillumination varies with the intensity of the light source used and the examiner should 'calibrate' the instrument by examining normal infants. If the margins of transillumination are questionable the area should be measured.

*See p.4 for supplier's address.

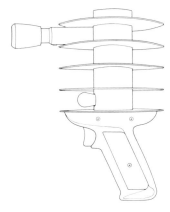

Fig. 11. The Chun gun. (A two- to four-cell flashlight with special adaptor-cuff for transillumination is an alternative method, but is difficult to standardize.)

Directions

Shine the test light on your own hand to check intensity and temperature, and transilluminate your own hand between the distal ends of the metacarpal bones to make sure your adaptation to the dark is complete. Apply the flashlight to the frontal, parietal and occipital regions on either side of the child's head. Transilluminate any abnormal protruding area. A small halo of light around the flashlight is normal and the size of this depends to some extent on the power of the light. Up to 3.5cm may be normal in very young infants and the halo is usually wider at the front of the head than at the back. It should not be mistaken for an abnormal collection of fluid.

Discussion

Total transillumination of the cranial vault may occur with hydranencephaly (Fig. 12). Light from a source in the occipital midline may be seen in the child's pupils and often in the nares. Extreme hydrocephalus also yields total transillumination. Porencephaly may be deduced from a large local area of illumination, though the appearance of an old subdural effusion is similar. In contrast, a fresh subdural hematoma often reduces the normal halo on the affected side. Non-localized excessive transillumination over the frontal regions may reflect cortical atrophy, with an excess of subarachnoid fluid, but this should be interpreted with caution. For example, an area up to 3.5cm (1¼in) may be normal in the frontal area of a premature infant. Encephaloceles usually transilluminate, unlike cephalhematomata and the moderate protrusion of the normal brain which may take place through large fused biparietal foramina. A subdural puncture followed by leakage of subarachnoid fluid under the scalp, or infiltration of fluid from an intravenous infusion of a scalp vein, can produce dramatic 'transillumination', which may be largely confined to one side if the patient has been lying with that side dependent. In view of the serious implications of marked cerebral malformations, suspicious transillumination usually indicates the need for confirmatory tests which provide objective documentation, such as EEG, angiography, air encephalography, radioactive isotopes or CT scan.

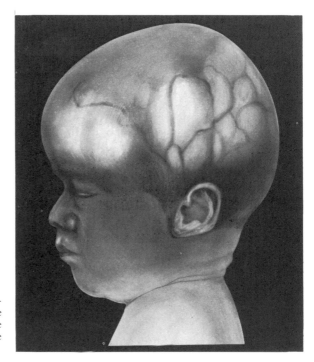

Fig. 12. Transillumination of hydran-cephalic infant. In a dark room, the examiner places the Chun gun on the side of the child's head to see the malformation.

THE FACE

Directions

Look closely at the child's face to see if there are any features which suggest congenital malformations or well-defined syndromes. Pay attention to the spacing of the eyes. If the interorbital distance appears unusually wide or narrow, measure the distance between the center of both pupils with the eyes looking straight ahead (Table III). Note excessively sparse, thick or confluent eyebrows. Note whether the palpebral fissure slants upward or downward in relation to its lateral aspect. Note the bridge and contour of the nose, and the size and shape of the mouth. Determine whether the mandible is large or small in proportion to the skull. Inspect the ears for abnor-

TABLE III

Interpupillary distances (mm)

Months	Mean	Range	Years	Mean	Range
Birth	38	33-45	3	49	42-54
3	42	36-48	5	50	44-56
6	43	38-50	7	52	46-58
9	45	39-52	10	54	48-60
12	46	39-52	13	56	48-62
18	47	40-53			
24	48	41-54			

From Goodman and Gorlin (1977).

29

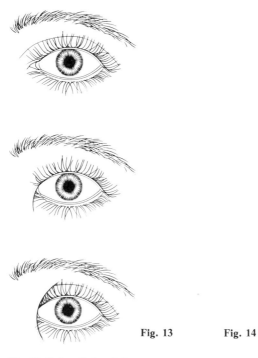

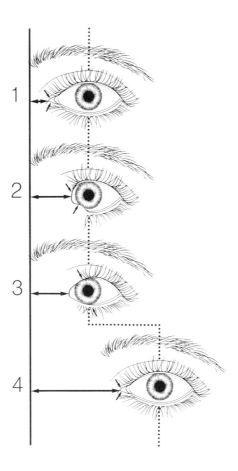

Fig. 13   **Fig. 14**

Fig. 13. Epicanthal variations.

Fig. 14. Distance of pupil to midline: **1** 'normal'; **2** primary telecanthus; **3** telecanthus plus temporal displacement of puncta (note arrows); **4** pure telecanthus with hypertelorism. [Redrawn after Pashayan *et al.* 1973.]

Fig. 15. Proportional measurements of the face. SHP = sagittal high point of the skull; G = glabella, the most prominent point of the frontal bone in the midsagittal plane; N = nasion, the point marking the intersection of the midsagittal plane and a tangential line connecting the superior palpebral sulci; NT = nasion terminalis, tip of the nose; SN = subnasale, the point at which the nasal septum merges with the upper lip in the midsagittal plane—this corresponds to the highest point of the philtrum (the vertical groove in the median portion of the upper lip); C = cornulabialis, corner of the lips; M = mentum, midline long prominence of the mandible. **1** = distance superior head point (SHP) to nasal bridge (N); **2** = distance N to subnasion (SN); **3** = distance to corner of mouth (C); **4** = distance C to mandibular prominence (M).

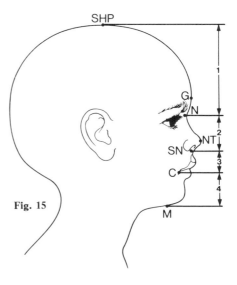

Fig. 15

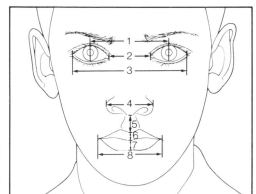

Fig. 16. Common facial differences: **1** inter-pupillary distance; **2** inter-medial canthi distance; **3** inter-lateral canthi distance; **4** distance between external border of nostrils; **5** midline nasal furrow; **6** midline upper lip; **7** midline lower lip; **8** distance between lateral margins of lips.

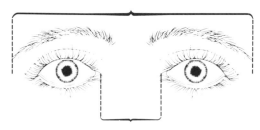

Fig. 17. Hypertelorism, characterized by excessive distance between the eyes and broadened nasal bridge.

malities of the pinna and external auditory meatus, and for the presence of pre-auricular tags or dimples. Determine the position of the ears on the skull by checking the level of the external auditory meatus relative to the alae nasi when the head is level. It can be difficult to write a description of an unusual facies. 'Characteristic' facies are those that can be described in such a way that others can recognize them. Photographs can be helpful but their usefulness is limited unless measurements are included. Figures 13-16 show landmarks that may be helpful.

Discussion

Holoprosencephaly, hypertelorism, hypotelorism

Holoprosencephaly describes a broad spectrum of facial anomalies which reflect defective formation of the forebrain, and can include hypotelorism (interorbital ridge distance less than 1 cm), bilateral cleft lip with absent philtrum and palatal abnormalities. The extent of the anomalies suggests the extent of the forebrain defects. (Trisomy 13-15 is one cause.)

Hypertelorism (Fig. 17) refers to an increased interpupillary or interorbital distance compared with normal values for age, sex and race. It may occur sporadically or it may be secondary to many conditions, including gigantism, Crouzon disease and Hurler syndrome.

Pseudohypertelorism can be due to telecanthus, which is defined as an increased distance between the medial canthi of the palpebral fissures. It can also result from increased ocular or nasal soft tissues (primary telecanthus) or from an increase in the bony interorbital distance (secondary telecanthus). Often it erroneously gives the impression of squint. Placement of the puncta (the openings of the tear ducts) should also be noted: they are usually located medially in both the upper and lower lids. Displaced puncta, in addition to telecanthus, have been reported in the Waardenburg and other syndromes.

Hypotelorism has been described as a feature of heredofamilial brachial plexus neuropathy (Dunn *et al.* 1978).

The first arch syndrome

This syndrome describes a group of conditions with a common embryonic defect—a malformation of the first branchial arch—giving rise to abnormal development of the eye, ear, zygoma and mandible. These conditions include Treacher-Collins syndrome (Fig. 18), Pierre-Robin syndrome (Fig. 19), mandibulo-facial dysostosis, deformities of the external and middle ear, congenital deafness, hypertelorism, cleft lip and cleft palate. Clinical manifestations vary, but deafness is such a common finding in the first arch syndrome that it must be carefully established whether the child has adequate hearing. The size and shape of the mouth give clues to a particular syndrome: for example, a 'carp' mouth is seen in the Cornelia De Lange syndrome and a small mouth is characteristic of trisomy 18.

A mandible which is large in proportion to the skull occurs in the basal-cell nevus syndrome. A small jaw is associated with both Treacher-Collins and Pierre-Robin syndromes. In the latter, the combination of micrognathia and glossoptosis produces a small airway, which in infancy can cause considerable mechanical difficulty with feeding and respiration. Micrognathia (Fig. 20) combined with microcephaly and microphthalmos has occurred among the offspring of women who received radiation therapy during pregnancy.

Anomalies of the external ear may indicate middle-ear malformation and deafness. Renal anomalies are also associated with external-ear malformation, and cerebral anomalies occur in association with low-set ears and missing aural cartilage with far greater than random frequency (Aase 1980).

The National Collaborative Perinatal Project (NCPP) has provided data on over 50,000 infants followed from the prenatal period to seven years of age. These data indicate that microtia (small size) and other malformations of the pinna are uncommon. The distribution of all external-ear and branchial-cleft malformations are: pre-auricular sinus 8.3/1000, pre-auricular tags 1.7/1000, microtia 0.3/1000, other malformed pinna 1.14/1000, and branchial-cleft sinus 0.2/1000.

The definition of low-set ears is based on features of the face, which may cause difficulty if the features have been altered by associated malformations. A line from the lateral corner of the orbit, which is perpendicular to the plane of the face, should intersect the helical root. Traditionally, artists use a horizontal line from the eyebrow to the upper edge of the helix and a parallel line from the base of the subnasale to the lower ear insertion. The normal length of the ear at birth for fullterm infants is 34-43mm, at three months it is 38 to 50mm, at six months 39-55mm, and at 12 months 39-55mm (Melnick and Myrianthopoulos 1979).

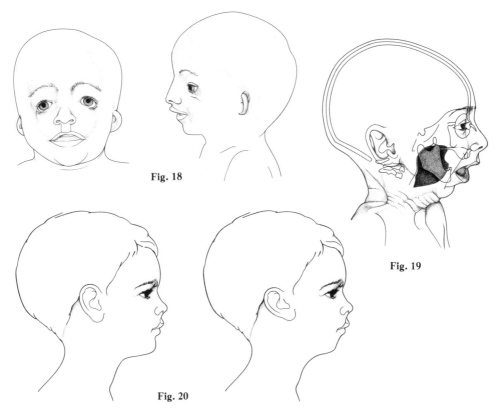

Fig. 18

Fig. 19

Fig. 20

Fig. 18. Treacher-Collins syndrome, in which the palpebral fissures slant downward, there is hypoplasia of the malar and zygoma areas and a small, retracted chin. There are eyelid colobomas, usually on the outer third of the lower lid. The nose appears to be large because of the retracted chin. The ears are poorly formed.

Fig. 19. Pierre-Robin syndrome. The face has a small, receding chin and the ears are low-set. The mandible is hypoplastic and receding, causing the tongue to fall backward into the pharynx, obstructing the epiglottis, preventing normal respiration and causing respiratory distress.

Fig. 20. Micrognathia *(right)* compared with normal. The chin recedes and the lower jaw is small. This condition may occur alone or in association with other defects, and may lead to mechanical difficulties with feeding during early life.

Malformations of the ear are associated with hearing loss and middle-ear anomalies, but the loss may occur only on the opposite side. A malformed ear in one family member makes hearing loss significantly more likely in other members of the family. Although it is generally accepted that ear anomalies are associated with renal abnormalities, this was not a striking finding in the NCPP series. Microtia (small ear) may be associated with trisomy 21 (small, square, thickened ear), Treacher-Collins syndrome (malar and mandibular hypoplasia, down-slanting palpebral fissures, defect of lower eyelid, malformation of external ear), oculoauriculovertebral dysplasia, Apert syndrome (craniosynostosis, irregular midfacial hypoplasia, hypertelorism, syndactyly, broad distal thumb and toe), Bixler syndrome (hypertelorism, cleft lip/palate, mild syndactyly) and the thalidomide syndrome. In this last syndrome the etiology of the ear anomalies in experimental animals is believed to be hemorrhage in selective embryological areas from which the ear is known to develop.

THE EYES

LIDS, CONJUNCTIVAE, SCLERAE, IRIDES, PUPILS

Directions

Have the child sit comfortably at eye level. Make eye contact in a friendly manner. Note whether the child shows any unusual mannerisms which might indicate diplopia, such as compensatory head tilting, covering one eye or squinting. Look to see if the eyes are straight in a neutral position. Look for ptosis. Note obvious abnormalities of the iris, cornea and pupils. Check the sclerae for telangiectasia and jaundice. Note the size of the globes and feel the tension by pressing gently on the eyeballs over closed lids: increased intraocular tension causes the globe to feel like a marble.

Shine a light on the pupils to check the position and symmetry of the light reflex and the pupillary response. The light should reflect symmetrically just to the medial side of the center of the pupils. Check the response to accommodation by bringing the light in toward the child's nose and looking for convergence and pupillary constriction.

Have the child reach for an object or toy. Observe whether he can fix his vision on the toy and note the skill in reaching for and grasping it. Look for tremors or abnormal associated movements. Test for an intact corneal reflex by touching the cornea with a twist of sterile cotton-wool and looking for movement of the lid on the opposite side.

Discussion

Eye contact

Eye contact is a basic form of communication which often is taken for granted. Children with strabismus from early life may not be looked at because the parents or other adults may find it difficult and uncomfortable, so these children have a poor start in developing normal communication. Children and adults seek attention and communicate by establishing eye contact. It is well known that instructions from parent to child, teacher to child and employer to employee are most effective if eye contact is made. Reluctance to make eye contact is associated with deference or deviant behavior.

Ptosis

Ptosis may be congenital or hereditary. It is often bilateral. The Marcus-Gunn phenomenon describes a form of congenital ptosis in which there is a reflex elevation of the lid in response to movement of the jaw. Voluntary elevation is preserved and upward gaze is normal. Whether congenital or of early onset, ptosis is a prominent symptom of myasthenia gravis (see Fig. 32, p. 85). It increases with fatigue and may be asymmetrical.

Slight ptosis associated with paralysis of the superior tarsal muscle is associated with paralytic lesions of the cervical sympathetic chain (Horner syndrome, see Fig. 31, p. 80). However, the upper lip droops only to or slightly below the upper margin of the pupil and usually the child can raise the lid completely by voluntary effort. The pupil is small and reactive, and the lower eyelid is elevated slightly ('upside-down ptosis'). Complete ptosis, with paralysis of the third nerve and of the levator palpebrae superioris, is more extreme and the palpebral fissure may be completely closed. Partial cases occur and are more easily recognized if one watches the contraction of the frontalis muscle as the child attempts to open his eyes. This is said not to occur in cases of hysterical ptosis. True ptosis must be differentiated from an abnormally wide palpebral fissure on the opposite side caused by paresis of the seventh nerve and the orbicularis oculi, and from lid-lag associated with hyperthyroidism.

Exophthalmos

Bilateral exophthalmos usually is the result of hyperthyroidism and, if marked, presents no difficulty in recognition. Unilateral exophthalmos frequently has neurological significance. In doubtful cases, diagnosis is helped by the presence of lid-lag, reduced ability to converge, increased width of the palpebral fissure and infrequent spontaneous blinking. Unilateral exophthalmos can occur in hyperthyroidism, but usually it indicates localized intraorbital or intracranial disease. Examples are retrobulbar masses within the orbit (*e.g* neuroblastoma, rhabdomyosarcoma, sarcoid, nasopharyngioma, neurofibroma, optic glioma), orbital cellulitis, deformities of the skull, thromobisis of the cavernous sinus (with paralysis of the third, fourth and sixth cranial nerves and of the first two divisions of the fifth) and intracranial tumors of the anterior fossa.

It is often stated that pulsating exophthalmos is characteristic of arteriovenous fistula in the cavernous sinus, but in many instances there is no pulsation. Exophthalmos may also pulsate if caused by an intracranial aneurysm or a vascular malformation elsewhere. Auscultation of the eye and surrounding region for bruit is particularly important. Exophthalmos and enophthalmos may be stimulated, respectively, by macrophthalmos (congenital enlargement of the globe) and by microphthalmos. Enophthalmos can be part of the syndrome of paralysis of the cervical sympathetic chain, but it can also occur with atrophy of intraorbital tissue. Microphthalmos is related to a variety of conditions. It may be a feature of a chromosomal aberration (trisomy 13-15) or the result of infections such as toxoplasmosis or congential rubella: if accompanied by a white pupil, it may be a sign of retrolental fibrovascular mass.

The term 'buphthalmos' is used to describe the enlargement of the eye and corneal clouding seen in infantile glaucoma.

Conjunctivae and sclerae

Conjunctival telangiectasia may suggest ataxia telangiectasia as a basis of a child's ataxic gait. Telangiectasia also occur on the ears. Blue sclerae are found in osteogenesis imperfecta.

The irides

Bilateral abnormalities of the iris usually are inherited developmental defects associated with nystagmus, poor vision, photophobia and a predilection for the development of glaucoma. Sporadic aniridia sometimes is associated with the sporadic form of Wilms tumor.

Heterochromia of the iris may be congenital. If there is an old paralytic lesion of the cervical sympathetic chain, the eye on the affected side may be hypopigmented in comparison with the other. In glaucoma the iris of the affected eye may be lighter. The Waardenburg syndrome includes heterochromia as one of its manifestations. Kayser-Fleischer rings, pathognomonic of Wilson disease, may be visible as green-gold or muddy yellow-brown discoloration of the cornea. Definitive diagnosis of Kayser-Fleischer rings may require examination with a slit-lamp. The rings are caused by the deposition of copper in Descemet's membrane.

Brushfield spots (Fig. 21) are white or yellowish dots, less than 1mm in diameter, which are arranged in a ring around the irides, concentric with the pupil and located nearer the outer border of the irides than the pupils. They are seen in a fair percentage of normal children, but are particularly characteristic of trisomy 21 (Down syndrome), in which they appear in more than 90 per cent of cases, although they tend to disappear with age and often are not detectable above six years of age. Usually Brushfield spots are seen in blue irides rather than brown.

Coloboma is a defect in the iris which may arise from faulty closure of the fetal fissure. It is often found in the six o'clock position, giving a 'keyhole' effect. It is unusual for vision to be affected unless the defect extends back to the optic nerve.

The corneal reflex

The corneal reflex is elicited by the examiner's touching the child's cornea with a clean gauze or fiber wick. Watch for the prompt contraction of the pupil on the same side and on the opposite side. A wisp of cotton may be sufficient to elicit the reflex.

This reflex tests the integrity of the first branch of the fifth cranial-nerve. In a well child, absence of corneal sensation may be an isolated unilateral finding, without apparent significance. However, absence of the corneal reflex may be associated with a pontine tumor. In an unconscious child, the loss of corneal sensation is an ominous sign of midbrain dysfunction. The reflex may be lost for between five and 60 minutes following intravenous administration of diazepam. Decreased corneal sensation may also occur in familial dysautonomia.

The pupils

Once the newborn period is passed, the pupils usually are larger than in adult life and react vigorously to light and to accommodation. Excessively small pupils are seen during deep coma and in some cases of increased intracranial pressure, acute brain-stem lesions involving interruption of dilator fibres, and during sleep. Very slight

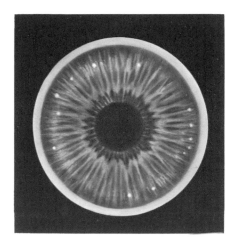

Fig. 21. Brushfield spots are aggregates of stromal fibers which form a ring around the iris near the limbus. They tend to disappear with age.

constriction normally occurs during the expiratory phase of respiration. Mydriasis in children is defined as a pupillary diameter greater than 5mm. Dilatation of the pupils occurs with anxiety, fear, sexual arousal, pain and in certain stages of coma, and with some lesions of the midbrain.

The pupils of near-sighted individuals may be somewhat dilated, just as those of far-sighted people may be constricted. The pupils are fixed and dilated during a seizure. Atropine or some other mydriatic used for ophthalmological examination may cause inequality and sluggish response, even after several days. Intravenous diazepam given for status epilepticus can result in a non-reactive pupil, which may be associated with an absent corneal reflex for several hours. Slightly oval or eccentric pupils may be a harmless normal variation; frequently they are seen during recovery from induced mydriasis.

Hippus, or rhythmic dilatation and constriction of the pupils, is usually of no diagnostic significance. Inequality of the pupils also may be a harmless congenital anomaly.

The most important implication of a dilated, fixed pupil is a possible paralytic lesion of the third cranial nerve. Paralysis of the parasympathetic fibers of the third nerve may result either from lesions in the orbit or from involvement of the nerve in the superior orbital fissure, in the cavernous sinus or in its intracranial course. Dilatation that is unresponsive to light, as well as marked in degree, is a particularly important sign of increased intracranial pressure.

With lesions of the third nerve, both direct and consensual responses are absent on the affected side but remain intact in the opposite eye. The pupil of an eye made blind by an ocular lesion or a lesion in the optic nerve does not constrict to light, nor does that of the opposite eye consensually, but the blind eye may show consensual pupillary constriction when the opposite eye is stimulated. The Argyll-Robertson pupil was of considerable diagnostic importance before congenital syphilis became so uncommon. The combination of absent pupillary constriction to light and pre-servation of the response to accommodation is not pathognomonic of syphilis of the

37

central nervous system; it can occur in postencephalitic states, syringobulbia, lesions in the region of the pineal body or superior colliculus, and in disseminated sclerosis. Absence of reflex miosis to light is also seen in the Adie syndrome, a ciliary ganglion lesion which may be associated with absence of tendon reflexes, leading to further confusion with syphilis of the central nervous system. However, in the Adie syndrome the pupil usually is slightly dilated in average room-light, whereas the Argyll-Robertson pupil is small and relatively invariable in size. The pupillary abnormality is also unilateral in the majority of Adie cases. The myotonic Adie-syndrome pupil is excessively sensitive to methacholine chloride ('Mecholyl')—another differential test.

The Marcus-Gunn pupillary response (not the Marcus-Gunn phenomenon of congenital ptosis) differentiates unilateral optic-nerve dysfunction from non-organic visual loss, simple strabismus or opacities in the media. The pupil on the affected side constricts less in response to light stimulation than does the normal eye.

Paralytic lesions of the cervical sympathetic system or of the C8 and T1 roots produce unilateral miosis, which is probably the most specific feature of the Claude Bernard-Horner syndrome. Other features uncommonly encountered without miosis include slight ptosis (much less than is seen with paralytic lesions of the parasympathetic fibers in the third nerve), suppression of perspiration on the affected side of the face, and enophthalmos.

EXTRA-OCULAR MOVEMENTS, VISUAL FIELDS, CRANIAL NERVES 3, 4, 6

Directions

Test the movements of both eyes together by moving a toy, a flashlight or a dangling tape-measure from side to side, up and down in the midline and diagonally across the bridge of the nose. Look for free, unrestricted, smooth visual pursuit. Note any muscle restriction or nystagmus. Test each eye alone in a similar fashion by holding a light in one hand and using the other to cover one eye. Most children over the age of three years will tolerate occlusion of one eye with an eye-patch. If the child is apprehensive, hold the light in one hand and cover the eye by pretending to brush back a lock of hair. Look for latent strabismus by noting slight movement of the non-covered eye as the cover is applied (the eye with strabismus is the one that moves), and also when the cover is removed.

If the child is co-operative, repeat the cover test with the child looking up, down and at both a near and a far target in order to bring out latent strabismus in these positions, which may not show up when the child is looking straight ahead.

Do a rough check on the integrity of the visual fields by asking the child to fix his eyes on the bridge of your nose. Note the point at which the child's eyes deviate toward and fix on an object, such as a dangling tape-measure, when it is brought from behind the child's head forward into the field of vision. This is the probable limit of the visual field. Test an older child by asking him to indicate when he sees your finger enter each quadrant of his visual field; also ask how many fingers he sees.

Check for diplopia by asking if the child sees one or more toy or pencil when one is held in front of him and moved up to the left, up to the right, down to the left and down to the right. Use a red lens to test for diplopia in an older child. Cover the eye with the lens and ask the child to look at a white light. A single red-white image

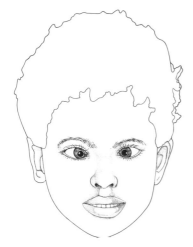

Fig. 22. The child with strabismus cannot fix both eyes simultaneously on the same point. Strabismus may be divergent, convergent, upward or downward, unilateral or alternating. (Note asymmetrical position of 'light reflex' on pupil.)

should be seen. If ocular palsy is present, both a red and a white image will be seen. If the child can do so, ask him to describe the position of the red and white image as the position of the light source is changed. Also note the pupillary response to light.

Discussion

Visual fields

Usually perimetry and tangent screen examinations are unnecessary to detect the common visual-field defects of children, which are chiefly homomynous hemianopia (mainly accompanying spastic hemiparesis) and bitemporal hemianopia in the presence of tumors in the region of the optic chasm. However, those tests can be done on surprisingly young children by an experienced ophthalmologist with time and patience.

Strabismus

The term 'conjugate' is used to describe eye movements which are functioning in parallel, whether the movements are normal or abnormal (coarse, fine, rapid, slow).

The term 'strabismus' (squint) means that the ocular axes are not parallel, so the axes of the two eyes cannot be fixed simultaneously on the same point (Fig. 22). However, in the common non-paralytic strabismus of childhood, either affected eye can be moved through the complete range of motion if tested separately. The deviation may be divergent (external) or convergent (internal), upward or downward, unilateral or alternating (in the last, the patient can fix with either eye but the opposite eye deviates).

The term 'heterotropia' is used for manifest strabismus, when non-parallelism is obvious with both eyes open. It must be differentiated from pseudostrabismus—a false appearance of strabismus because of a flat nasal bridge, narrow interpupillary distance or epicanthic folds. Esotropia is convergent strabismus and exotropia divergent: hypertropia refers to vertical deviation.

'Heterophoria' refers to latent strabismus, in which the eyes appear to be straight

TABLE IV
Actions of external ocular muscles

	Abduction (out)	Adduction (in)	Elevation (up)	Depression (down)	Intorsion (turn up)	Extorsion (turn down)
Lateral rectus; cranial nerve 6	+					
Medial rectus; cranial nerve 3		+				
Superior rectus; cranial nerve 3		+	+		+	
Inferior rectus; cranial nerve 3		+		+		+
Inferior oblique; cranial nerve 3	+		+			+
Superior oblique; cranial nerve 4		+		+	+	

when fixing on objects but deviate when either eye is covered. Again, hyperphoria indicates a tendency to vertical deviation, esophoria to inward and exophoria to outward deviation. Esophoria and exophoria are often found in patients with hyperopia and myopia, respectively.

Internal strabismus is common between three and six years of age. It may be caused by excessive convergence as a result of the accommodation necessary to overcome a refractive error. Owing to early suppression of the visual image of the squinting eye, diplopia is not a feature of common strabismus in childhood. The development of amblyopia makes early recognition of strabismus and prompt referral to an ophthalmologist highly desirable. While non-paralytic strabismus is not necessarily of any further neurological significance, it should be mentioned that strabismus is considerably more common among children with organic brain syndromes than among the general population.

Ocular palsies

Paralytic ocular motor disorders can be evidence of brain tumors, inflammatory disease, neurodegenerative disease and developmental defects. The causes are numerous, and include developmental anomalies, infection, tumors, vascular disorders, trauma, neuromuscular disorders and myogenic problems. The majority of ocular palsies occurring in children can be traced to cranial-nerve dysfunction (Table IV). Congenital cranial-nerve palsies may indicate the syndrome of congenital infection, birth trauma or developmental anomalies. Acquired cranial-nerve palsies are most often a sign of a serious pathological process.

The third cranial nerve innervates the medial rectus (a pure adductor of the eye), the superior and inferior recti and the inferior oblique, as well as the levator palpebrae superioris and the constrictor pupillae muscles.

With paralysis of the third nerve, the affected eye deviates laterally and slightly downward. In children, complete paralysis of the third nerve (if confirmed by further examination of eye movements) usually is the result of some affection of the nerve outside the midbrain. The ipsilateral eye is the one involved. If the paralysis is partial, interpretation is more difficult, for there is a surprising amount of dispute and confusion about the anatomical arrangements of the fibers. Paralysis of the third nerve also results in ptosis of the upper lid and dilatation of the pupil. Nuclear lesions of the third nerve often involve only one or more of its extra-ocular muscles, with or without ptosis or internal ophthalmoplegia (that is, the pupillary reactions and accommodation remain normal). Infranuclear lesions usually result in complete paralysis unless the lesion is within the orbit itself. Increasing intracranial pressure or trauma are the commonest causes of third nerve palsy in children.

The fourth nerve supplies only the superior oblique, and the sixth nerve the lateral rectus. The external rectus is a pure abductor but the superior and inferior recti and oblique muscles have functions of both vertical movement and rotation or torsion. Paralysis of the fourth nerve produces relatively little change in the position at rest during forward gaze in the midline, although there may be slight elevation of the eye, which becomes more obvious as the eye is adducted. There is no accurate basis for distinction between nuclear and infranuclear lesions of the fourth nerve, except that the former produce contralateral and the latter ipsilateral paralysis. Isolated fourth-nerve palsies are rare among children.

Paralysis of the sixth cranial nerve produces medial deviation of the affected eye during midline forward gaze. In abducens paralysis of recent onset, the child usually rotates the head slightly laterally toward the paretic side in order to avoid diplopia. Paralysis of the third or fourth nerve is associated with tilting rather than turning the head, the occiput being tilted toward one shoulder and the face directed toward the opposite side and slightly upward. After noting the asymmetrical posture of the head, if the examiner reverses it manually the primary deviation which results from the paralytic strabismus will become more obvious. A nuclear sixth-nerve palsy is almost always accompanied by involvement of the closely adjacent seventh nerve. *Paralysis of the sixth nerve is a common, non-specific sign of increased intracranial pressure.* The long course of the nerve from the pons to the eye renders it especially vulnerable to pressure or trauma.

The nuclei of the third, fourth, sixth and seventh cranial nerves are close to the median longitudinal bundle, and complicated syndromes are more commonly encountered than isolated nuclear palsies. Apparent paralysis of eye movement must also be distinguished from weakness associated with ocular or orbital disease, refractive errors and strabismus based on muscular imbalance or myasthenia gravis. The presenting signs of myasthenia gravis may be ocular muscle palsy and ptosis.

Skew deviation of the eyes, in which one eye (usually the ipsilateral one) is turned downward and inward while the other deviates outward and upward, is occasionally encountered in disease of the brain stem or cerebellum or of other structures in the posterior fossa, but its anatomical basis is the subject of debate.

Conjugate deviation, or gaze largely directed to one side, may be due to either a contralateral irritative lesion or to an ipsilateral paralytic lesion in one of the cortical centers for eye movements. Various areas of the diencephalon, brain stem and cerebellum are also involved in ocular deviation. Deviation of the eyes to the opposite side is conceivable with small irritative mass lesions in the opposite hemisphere, but clinically, irritative deviation is associated chiefly with Jacksonian, focal or simultaneous unilateral seizures. In these circumstances it is usually accompanied by turning of the head in the same direction as the eyes. At rest, recovery from the deviation usually takes place within a few weeks, although lateral gaze to command may be affected for a much longer period (not following movements or reflex movement). Destructive or paralytic cortical lesions cause deviation of the eyes toward the side of the lesion. Irritative lesions are uncommon in the pons and mid-brain, but if they occur they produce ipsilateral deviation of the eyes. Destructive lesions at this level are associated with contralateral deviation, but usually this is only slight. (Paresis of gaze toward the side of the lesion is more obvious in most cases.) Abnormal positioning of the head may occur with either brain-stem or cortical lesions.

Supranuclear disturbances of eye movements affect conjugate gaze rather than individual eye-movements. Paralysis of conjugate upward gaze is associated with lesions at the level of the medial lemniscus (Parinaud syndrome), and may be encountered with pineal tumors as well as with encephalitis, vascular lesions, disseminated sclerosis and other abnormalities in the same region.

The most common impairment of eye movements resulting from lesions of the median longitudinal bundle is anterior (or superior) internuclear ophthalmoplegia, appearing on lateral gaze as paralysis of adduction of the contralateral eye (usually adduction is preserved in convergence), together with monocular nystagmus of the abducting eye and sometimes a degree of paresis in abduction. Convergence may also be affected if the lesion is in the midbrain. Posterior inferior internuclear ophthalmoplegia is supposed to consist of paresis of abduction of the contralateral eye, which may converge normally, but there is doubt as to the existence of this entity. Diverse intrinsic lesions of the brain stem may produce internuclear ophthalmoplegia; disseminated sclerosis is by far the most common, although among young children one should entertain other diagnoses.

Oculomotor apraxia

Occasionally children are seen with a presumably congenital disability, characterized by loss of volitional control of eye movements, frequently with nystagmus, loss of smooth following from side to side, or other neurological abnormalities, but with preservation of random movements of the eyes. Cogan and Adams (1953) have termed this 'oculomotor apraxia', the features of which are: some defect of voluntary horizontal eye-movements and also of horizontal attraction movements of the eyes, together with normal and full random eye-movements; characteristic jerking movements of the head, which may aid in positioning the eyes when used voluntarily; a defect in the quick phase of opticokinetic nystagmus; controversion or lag of the eyes on rotation of the head to the opposite direction or on a vertical axis (the doll's eye phenomenon); and reading difficulties in most, if not all, children who are old enough to be able to read. All of the early cases reported were males (Altrocchi and Menkes 1960). Most of the children had normal vertical eye-movements but absent or defective following movements in the horizontal plane, and at least a history of awkwardness of gait. Usually the signs were symmetrical. The anatomical basis of the condition was unknown, and there was no known treatment.

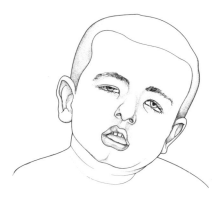

Fig. 23. Moebius syndrome. The face is expression-less, the eyes are open awake or sleeping because of weak orbicularis oculi muscles. A convergent squint is common and the mouth usually hangs open.

Eye-righting reflex and the doll's eye phenomenon

When the neck is flexed, extended and rotated, the eyes should move concomitantly, that is they should look in the direction of rotation and upward if the head is extended, down if flexed. This is the eye-righting reflex, which ensures adjustment of eye movements to compensate for turning the head. Absence of the eye-righting reflex signifies brain-stem injury, but the appearance of the reflex may be delayed for a few weeks in normal premature and fullterm infants.

The confusing term doll's eye phenomenon is used to describe the absence of eye movements in response to rotation of the head (*i.e.* the doll's eyes are fixed or painted), or the apparent turning of the eyes in the opposite direction to rotation. (The eyes stay still while the head is rotated laterally, giving the appearance of movement in a direction opposite to rotation.) If the child is comatose, the doll's eye phenomenon signifies brain-stem injury.

Syndromes involving cranial nerves

A number of syndromes have been described which involve the third, fourth and sixth cranial nerves. Some of these are the result of congenital anomalies which usually are non-progressive and more or less innocuous to the patient, but their recognition is important in the exclusion of more serious diseases. When examining a baby with apparent partial congenital ptosis, the alert physician will ask to see the family's baby photographs for comparison with the baby's present condition.

In the Moebius syndrome (Fig. 23) there is paralysis of the external recti (rarely only on one side), associated with paresis or paralysis of the facial musculature. It has been debated whether this is due primarily to aplasia of the nuclei in the brain stem or aplasia of the muscles themselves. Other ocular muscles may be involved, and many other congenital anomalies in various areas of the body may co-exist. Paralysis limited to both external recti sometimes is referred to as the Gerhardt syndrome. In the Duane syndrome the lateral rectus muscles are replaced largely by fibrous tissue, and the palpebral fissure widens as the child attempts lateral gaze (which is limited) and narrows as he adducts. There is retraction and elevation of the globe on adduction. There may also be fibrosis of the levator palpebrae superioris. The Gradenigo syndrome consists of paralysis of one lateral rectus, with tenderness or swelling behind the ipsilateral ear, and indicates inflammatory disease in the petrous pyramid.

There are several acquired syndromes of ocular-nerve paresis with involvement of the long tracts of the brain stem. The Benedikt syndrome includes ipsilateral oculo-motor paralysis with contralateral tremor, ataxia or some kind of hyperkinesis in the upper extremity, and reflects involvement of the third nerve as it passes through the red nucleus. In the Weber syndrome there is involvement of the third nerve as it passes through the cerebral peduncle, including paralysis of the third nerve on one side and a contralateral hemiparesis. The syndrome of Millard and Gubler is ipsi-lateral sixth-nerve paralysis (usually plus the seventh) and contralateral pyramidal hemiparesis. The syndrome of Foville is possibly a variation of this: it consists of hemiparesis on one side with opposite facial paralysis, ipsilateral to the lesion, and paresis of lateral gaze, attributed by some to involvement of the para-abducens nucleus. There are several variations of the syndrome of Raymond-Cestan, including paresis of ipsilateral conjugate gaze on deviation of the eyes to the opposite side, contralateral hemiparesis, and sometimes contralateral sensory deficit to touch, passive movement or position. The contralateral sensory deficit indicates involvement of the medial lemniscus, which is also affected occasionally in some of the other syn-dromes mentioned. All these combinations reflect an intrinsic lesion of the brain stem.

In children this lesion unfortunately is most frequently an intrinsic glioma infil-trating the brain stem, and is inoperable. (Such tumors usually produce papilloedema relatively late, in contrast to most other tumors in the posterior fossa.) Onset usually is gradual over several weeks or months, but may be as short as a week in a few cases. Careful contrast studies are needed to confirm the diagnosis by showing posterior displacement of the fourth ventricle and aqueduct. Infiltrating gliomata of the mid-brain, pons and medulla also may produce a large number of other cranial-nerve signs, chiefly crossed with respect to the long-tract signs in the extremities. However, there may be bilateral and very irregular patchy involvement.

Another syndrome with similar implications is that of Nothnagel, in which there is unilateral third-nerve paralysis with ipsilateral ataxia resulting from involvement of the brachium conjunctivum and its connections. The so-called syndrome of the inter-penduncular space consists of bilateral third-nerve paresis with spastic tetraparesis of the limbs. In the absence of other evidence of intrinsic involvement, this could be due to pressure from an extrinsic lesion on the cerebral peduncles and oculomotor nerves.

Monocular diplopia

Monocular diplopia is usually psychogenic but can occur with cataracts, sub-luxation of the lens, retinal detachment, and (rarely) cerebral lesions, with dissociation of visual projection. Double images of different size or shape but not different position (aniseikonia) result from some intra-ocular abnormality and not from dys-function of the ocular muscles.

Nystagmus

Classification

Nystagmus is an involuntary movement of the eyeball, which may be either

44

rhythmic or non-rhythmic (pendular), and may be associated with disease of the cere-bellum and its central connections, the eye or the inner ear. In certain circumstances it may also be produced as a normal phenomenon. Rhythmic nystagmus is characterized by alternate slow and quick components, resulting in a jerky, unequal repeated move-ment. Pendular nystagmus consists of more or less regular, equal to-and-fro move-ments to either side of a central point. Nystagmus is also classified in terms of direction: horizontal, vertical, oblique, rotatory or mixed. It is important to note the approximate speed, which may vary from 10 to as many as 100 oscillations per minute. The approximate amplitude should also be noted. Movements of smallest amplitude are often brought to the examiner's attention only during ophthalmoscopic examination or by covering the eye with a +20 diopter lens which magnifies the nystagmus and eliminates fixation. Generally, fine nystagmus is the term applied to excursions of less than 1mm and coarse nystagmus to excursions of more than 3mm.

The effect of the position of the eyes on the nystagmus should also be noted. The least intensity (first-degree) is present only when the child looks in the direction of the quick component; second-degree nystagmus is present in the neutral position and third-degree when looking in the direction of the slow component. Latent nystagmus appears only when one eye is covered, there being no abnormal movement when both eyes are used together. Because it may be impossible for a child's eyes to move in full range if there is paresis of an extra-ocular muscle, descriptions of nystagmus should include a remark on the extent of any limitation.

Congenital nystagmus

Congenital nystagmus is present at birth but usually it is not apparent for two or three months. It may be minimal in one position, and the baby may adapt by tilting the head very early in life. The nystagmus is pendular at rest, changing to jerky movements on lateral gaze. Occasionally the infant's head may oscillate as he attempts to fix on a specific object. Congenital nystagmus often is associated with poor visual acuity. It may be hereditary and associated with other signs and symptoms such as ocular albinism. The *Birth Defects Atlas and Compendium* (Bergsma 1979) lists over 40 birth defects associated with nystagmus.

Sensory deprivation nystagmus

Sensory deprivation nystagmus ('ocular nystagmus') is not present at birth. It is pendular and may be either coarse or rapid. The coarse, slow, searching movements are characteristic of amaurosis or poor vision, either ocular or cortical, acquired before the age of fixation. Ocular nystagmus can be seen in such conditions as congenital cataract and corneal opacities. Searching movements of smaller amplitude, or pendulous to-and-fro nystagmus, may occur with any serious impairment of visual acuity acquired in early childhood, or probably as late as the age of six years. Defective vision acquired in later childhood or adult life does not produce ocular nystagmus unless macular vision is specifically affected; the movements then are aimless and slower, and probably represent attempts at fixation rather than a true nystagmus. Ocular albinism is characterized by a sensory deprivation nystagmus caused by the lack of foveal function. Horizontal nystagmus caused by a posterior fossa lesion usually is associated with head tilt and other signs and symptoms.

Downbeat and see-saw nystagmus

Downbeat nystagmus describes increased downward movement on lateral gaze or in the midline primary position. It is associated with cervico-medullary pathology, such as the Arnold-Chiari malformation or platybasia.

See-saw nystagmus, in which one eye-movement is upward while the other is downward, may be congenital, but if it is acquired, then chiasmal lesions accompanied by bitemporal hemianopia should be suspected.

Vestibular nystagmus

Vestibular nystagmus is a pathological form of the normally inducible labyrinthine nystagmus. It varies with head position, tends to have a rotatory component and is most evident at rest. It is accompanied by vertigo and nausea. It can result from either exaggeration or depression of the function of the semicircular canals, vestibular nerves or vestibular nuclei. Unless associated with infections of the middle ear, labyrinthitis is an uncommon cause of nystagmus in children. The slow phase of the nystagmus is toward the affected side. However, labyrinthine nystagmus is soon compensated and lasts only a few weeks, even after total destruction of one labyrinth or one vestibular nerve. In the early acute stage there should always be a degree of vertigo as well. The Menière syndrome is associated with hydrops of the semicircular canals, including paroxysms of vertigo and progressive hearing loss, as well as nystagmus. It is found rarely, if at all, in children. Neoplasms, demyelinating processes and other lesions in the brain stem may produce nystagmus because of involvement of the vestibular nuclei, the median longitudinal bundle or other structures. Vertical or rotatory 'cog-wheel' nystagmus is particularly characteristic of these processes. Nystagmus also may accompany lesions of the spinal cord, at least down to the second cervical segment, and it occurs with tumors, syringomyelia and other lesions, probably as a result of involvement of the median longitudinal bundle.

Cerebellar nystagmus

In cerebellar nystagmus the eyes tend to be positioned slightly away from the affected side when at rest. Lateral gaze produces nystagmus with the quick component in the direction of gaze, and the slow component toward the position of rest. The nystagmus is more pronounced when the patient looks toward the side of the lesion.

Physiological nystagmus

While nystagmus normally is never present at rest, in certain circumstances it can be induced in normal individuals. Horizonal gaze nystagmus (also called end-point or physiological nystagmus) should be seen only on far gaze on either side. Fatigue nystagmus is sustained but fixation nystagmus ceases after five or six jerks. Another variety of end-point nystagmus results from attempting to fixate the eyes beyond the limits of the binocular visual field, although this does not occur in every normal individual. This nystagmus of eccentric fixation is accentuated by fatigue.

Toxic nystagmus

Sedation or the administration of anticonvulsant drugs, especially phenytoin, may induce horizontal nystagmus. This toxic nystagmus may also be found after overdoses of nicotine and quinine, and in lead poisoning.

Opticokinetic nystagmus

This type of nystagmus is experienced by persons watching the landscape from a moving vehicle, and for this reason is sometimes referred to as railway nystagmus. The slow phase is in the direction of the moving field of vision or of the movement of stripes on a rotating drum, with the quick phase in the opposite direction. Among infants and young children, the presence of opticokinetic nystagmus can be used as a criterion of cortical vision. However, children with general developmental retardation may take weeks or months to respond to a moving tape-measure or striped drum, so such failure should not be accepted in itself as sufficient proof of cortical blindness.

Labyrinthine nystagmus

This is a normal physiological response to stimulation of the semicircular canals by rotation or by changes in temperature produced by irrigating the auditory canal with warm or cold water. The slow phase corresponds to the direction of movement of the endolymph, with the rapid phase in the opposite direction.

Some people can induce voluntary nystagmus by deliberate effort, usually involving convergence and fixation. It is rapid and pendular and can be sustained only for brief periods of time.

Other involuntary eye-movements

Abnormal eye-movements other than nystagmus chiefly comprise paroxysmal, involuntary conjugate deviation of the eyes, most often upward. These oculogyric crises are characteristic of postencephalitic Parkinsonism in adults, but in children they sometimes occur in other postencephalitic states. It is important to distinguish these from petit mal fits. Quick, jerky, violent shooting movements of the eyes in various directions, but particularly upward, may be associated with acute idiopathic cerebellar ataxia of childhood (Dyken and Kolár 1968).

Ocular bobbing movements are irregular and not rhythmic. The initial movement is down and the return is relatively slow. Other ocular oscillations include opsoclonus, which are multidirectional but conjugate; the irregular ocular flutter of acute cerebellar disease; and the saccadic movements associated with instability of fixation. The last-mentioned are irregular 'square-wave' jerks away from the center and back again. They are involuntary, rapid, abrupt, and occur simultaneously in both eyes.

FUNDUSCOPIC EXAMINATION: CRANIAL NERVE 2

Directions

A funduscopic examination requires patience, a darkened room and a good ophthalmoscope. Direct the child's attention away from the light by asking him to look at a picture on the wall directly opposite. Use a dim light on the ophthalmoscope for the first minute or two while explaining the procedure. Start with a setting of $+20$ to examine the cornea and lens for ulcerations, opacities, clouding and cataracts. Gradually move to a setting of 0 to bring the retina and the optic-nerve head into focus. Locate the macula and note any abnormalities in it or the surrounding area. Note the caliber, pulsations and distributions of the retinal vessels. Look for abnormal deposits, abnormalities of pigmentation, and hemorrhage. Examine the optic-nerve head by checking its size, color and surrounding structures. If the disc appears to be elevated, try to measure the number of diopters of papilloedema by assessing the difference between the power of the lens of the ophthalmoscope used to bring the disc itself into optimal focus and the power of the lens used to focus on the surrounding area.

Discussion

The cornea

Corneal ulceration may be present in the Riley-Day syndrome (familial dysautonomia), as a result of lack of tears and hypoesthesia. It may also occur in herpes zoster, herpes simplex and varicella infections. Corneal opacities or clouding are associated with some birth defects, including trisomy 18, the mucopolysaccharidoses and the mucolipidoses. Congenital cataracts can be hereditary, or they may be a manifestation of intra-uterine infection (rubella, toxoplasmosis), an inborn error of metabolism (galactosemia), or a component of a diverse group of conditions of different origins (Lowe syndrome, pseudohypoparathyrodism).

The retina

Examination of the retinae may disclose retrolental fibroplasia, choreoretinitis or other abnormalities. Healed choreoretinitis is suggestive of old toxoplasmosis or cytomegalic inclusion disease, but can result from other infections and must be differentiated from congenital retinal colobomata. Retinal angiomatosis may suggest von Hippel-Lindau disease, and phakomatous lesions occur in some patients with tuberous sclerosis. Narrowing of the caliber of the retinal artery is an early sign of retinal degeneration.

Retinal deposits of pigment have differing explanations. Black deposits of pigment in the peripheral retina of stellate (bone corpuscle) shape are typical of retinitis pigmentosa (more properly, pigmentary degeneration of the retina), which is a feature of Laurence-Moon-Biedl syndrome and of other familial disorders of the nervous system. Retinitis pigmentosa must be distinguished from the flagstone-shaped blocks of melanosis retinae (a harmless congenital anomaly), from 'pepper and salt' retina (when it is present to a marked degree), and from the hyperpigmentation which often accompanies cerebromacular degenerations (Table V).

Progressive external ophthalmoplegia is said to occur if only those fibers supplying the extra-ocular muscles are involved. Its principal feature is an expressionless face (the facies of facial diplegia) and it occurs in various non-specific disorders. Because retinal degeneration is associated with some of these descriptions, observation of the optic fundi may enable identification of the specific clinical disorder. Retinitis pig-

TABLE V
Examples of disorders associated with retinitis pigmentosa

A-β-lipoproteinemia (Bassen-Kornzweig syndrome):
    autosomal recessive inheritance, acanthocytosis, hereditary degenerative neuromuscular disease with ataxia, intestinal malabsorption and cutaneous sensory defects (±PEO)*

Refsum syndrome:
    autosomal recessive inheritance, peripheral polyneuropathy, elevated spinal fluid protein, elevated serum phytanic acid levels, 'onion bulb' changes in peripheral nerves, lipid granules in central nervous system and other tissues (+PEO, ichthyosis)

Ocular myopathy:
    pharyngeal weakness, hearing loss, vestibular dysfunction, spasticity, ataxia, delayed sexual development (PEO and retinitis pigmentosa constant features)

Abiotrophic ophthalmoplegia externa (Cogan syndrome):
    CSF protein elevation, cardiac conduction defects, cervical muscle weakness (±PEO, retinal degeneration)

Cockayne syndrome:
    mental retardation, dwarfism (±PEO)

Hallgren syndrome:
    deafness (±PEO)

Secondary retinitis pigmentosa:
    congenital lues, congenital rubella, other maternal virus infections, traumatic or non-specific vascular lesions (PEO not usual)

Laurence-Moon-Biedl syndrome:
    mental retardation, hypogonadism, polydactyly, obesity, retinal changes. Usually associated with sex-linked recessive mode of inheritance. Female carriers often have diffuse chorioretinal atrophy (PEO uncommon)

Other conditions:
    primary retinal dystrophy

---

*PEO = progressive external ophthalmoplegia.

---

mentosa is one type of retinal degenerative disorder and an electroretinogram (ERG) can facilitate classification into primary or secondary. In the primary disease the ERG is usually subnormal or absent before subjective visual loss or marked funduscopic changes are evident. In the secondary disorder, marked abnormalities may occur clinically before alterations are detected in the ERG.

In Tay-Sachs disease, the deposition of ganglioside in the ganglion cells of the retina gives it a whitish appearance, most conspicuous around the macula, which then appears as a cherry-red spot. In other types of cerebromacular degeneration (Bielchowsky, Spielmeyer-Vogt and Kufs) a cherry-red spot does not appear because the ganglioside is deposited chiefly in the inner and outer nuclear layers. Pigmentary degeneration of the macula appears relatively later. Cherry-red spots also occur in some cases of Niemann-Pick disease, and they have been described in metachromatic leukodystrophy.

Retinal hemorrhages occur in hypertensive retinopathy, with hemorrhagic diatheses such as leukemia, and in the presence of subdural hematoma and other head injuries. Retinal hemorrhages may also be evidence of child abuse.

The optic disc

The appearance and size of each optic disc are important. In both children and

TABLE VI

Causes of visual impairment

Congenital malformations: congenital hydrocephalus, encephalocele, hydranencephaly, microcephaly, optic-nerve hypoplasia, porencephaly	*Other systemic disorders:* leukemia, collagen vascular, vascular abnormalities including intracranial hemorrhage, metabolic disorders (hypernatremia, galactosemia, diabetes mellitus, etc.)
Tumors: cerebral glioma, craniopharyngioma, intracranial tumors associated with hydrocephalus, optic glioma, perioptic meningioma, retinoblastoma	*Neurodegenerative disorders:* cerebral storage, leukodystrophies, demyelinating, retinal degeneration, optic atrophies
Neuroectodermoses: Sturge-Weber, tuberous sclerosis, neurofibromatosis, von Hippel-Lindau	*Trauma:* contusions, concussions, laceractions; subdural, epidural, intracerebral and intraventricular hemorrhages
Infections: rubella, cytomegalovirus, toxoplasma, T. pallidum (maternal); gonococcal (perinatal); optic neuritis (presumed virus), chorioretinitus, meningoencephalitis (various causes) (postnatal)	*Drugs and toxins:* lead encephalopathy, idiosyncratic drug reactions, methanol ingestion

adults, papilloedema is one of the valuable indications of increased intracranial pressure. It may not be present if the increased pressure is very recent, and may not occur if the pressure is relieved by an open fontanelle, or, in a young child, by very prompt separation of the sutures. Usually blurring of the nasal and superior borders of the disc is the first sign of papilloedema. The temporal border is the last to become elevated, with protrusion of the papilla into the globe of the eye. The disc initially is hyperaemic, which leads to dilatation of the veins, disappearance of normal venous pulsations, increasing tortuosity of the veins and contraction of the arteries, and the appearance of hemorrhages. The hemorrhages are evident earliest in the areas around the disc, are frequently linear or flame-shaped, and radiate out from the disc. Papilloedema must be distinguished from a congenitally blurred and somewhat elevated disc, without a physiological cup. This is seen especially in hypermetropic eyes, in which the disc is actually raised only a little, there is no dilatation of the veins and no hyperemia. A venous pulsation at the disc usually indicates normal intra-cranial pressure at that instant. Sometimes elevation of the optic disc is caused by harmless hyaline bodies (*drüsen*) deep in the optic nerve. Papilloedema must also be distinguished from harmless persistence of embryonal myelinated nerve-fibers radiating out from the disc, from infiltration about the optic-nerve head in leukemia and from optic neuritis. In doubtful cases one may need to examine the eyes after a short interval, or seek an ophthalmologist's opinion.

Optic neuritis is difficult to distinguish from papilloedema, but usually there is greater exudation over the disc; while the physiological cup may be lost or the disc even elevated a few diopters, usually the degree of actual edema is not proportionate to the other changes (congestion, infiltration, exudation and hemorrhages). In optic neuritis there is marked loss of visual acuity (this is slight in early papilloedema), and usually there is pronounced loss of the central visual field.

Optic atrophy is the other major abnormality of the optic disc. The principal feature is excessive pallor, but experience is required to evaluate this in infants, who normally have a paler disc than do adults. The hypoplastic optic-nerve head is small and in most cases has a peripapillary halo, which corresponds to the size of the disc. In optic atrophy the disc margins stand out in depth and diameter and the lamina cribosa may be increased in prominence and extend to the edge of the disc. The capillaries supplying the disc are fewer and less prominent than normal and the retinal arteries may also be narrowed. Often it is possible to count the number of vessels on the optic disc (as they cross its margin). In optic atrophy the number of visible vessels is decreased from about the 20 normally present to less than five. Initially rising venous pressure, which accompanies increased intracranial pressure, distends the vessels and makes a larger number visible. Primary optic atrophy may have a wide variety of causes, infectious, genetic or demyelinating (retrobulbar neuritis). Bilateral small, pale, optic-nerve heads signify severe congenital malformations, such as hydranencephaly. The appearance of secondary optic atropy is similar, but as it usually follows papilloedema or optic neuritis, more often than not there are residual signs of these conditions. The disc margins may be blurred or the lamina cribosa may be hidden by connective tissue or proliferation of glia. Generally, optic atrophy is associated with considerable loss of visual acuity and with concentric contraction of the visual fields (tunnel vision).

Causes of visual impairment are summarized in Table VI.

TESTING VISUAL ACUITY

Any assessment of visual acuity made during a basic neurological examination is at best a screening test, done within the limits of the time and equipment available. It is essential that, where it is indicated, further expert examination be carried out by an ophthalmologist. Referral should be made when there is doubt as to the child's serviceable vision, when the child has a major handicap, and particularly when the parents have queried their child's visual ability. It is essential to realise that very often it is parents rather than professionals who are the first to detect visual problems in their children, and, as with hearing loss, when parents state an anxiety about their children's ability to see it must be taken seriously.

Sophisticated techniques using evoked responses have now demonstrated that adult visual acuity occurs as early as six months of age, though it is difficult to demonstrate this by behavioral methods. At present the best clinical tests for screening vision in infants and young children are the STYCAR vision tests (Sheridan 1976*a*), used extensively in Great Britain but somewhat difficult to obtain and therefore not commonly used in the United States*. For older children the Snellen chart*, either miniature hand-held or standard, is a good and accurate test of visual acuity.

*See p. 4 for suppliers' addresses.

Directions

A gross estimate of the child's vision is made by watching the ability to follow a face, respond to facial expression, reach for a small toy, and follow a moving object such as a colored ball or finger-puppet.

The test chosen for formal vision screening will depend on the age of the child. At six weeks a baby should follow a suspended colored ball in an arc through 180° at a distance of 30-45cm (12-18in) while lying on his back. Similarly, he should follow a face at this distance and should be seen to watch his mother's face when held in her arms. From six months to 2½ years the STYCAR balls (rolling and fixed) are a useful test of distance vision at 3m (10ft). The commonly-used Snellen E test is a far less satisfactory test of vision.

The STYCAR equipment consists of a graded series of white balls ranging in diameter from 63 mm (2½ in) down to 3mm (⅛ in). They may be used free or mounted on thin black metal rods. The child is seated comfortably on his mother's knee or, if older, on a low chair, and the balls are rolled in decreasing size across a dark cloth (green baize is ideal) at a distance of 3m (10ft) from the child. The child can be observed to track the moving ball and fixate on it when stationary. At six months the child should be able to follow down to the 5mm (³⁄₁₆ in) sized ball and at one year to the 3mm (⅛ in) ball. Sometimes the younger child becomes so fixated on the examiner's face that it is hard to get him interested in the balls. One way of overcoming this is to use an upright screen with a narrow viewing slit, behind which the examiner sits. The balls are then used mounted on the metal rods and held out one at a time in decreasing size beyond either edge of the screen, whereupon the infant can be observed to fixate and track the ball as it is moved.

As Sheridan emphasized, these techniques test the child's minimal observable distance rather than his minimum discriminatory distance, and cannot be translated into visual acuities. Ideally, each eye should be tested separately, but this may be difficult because many small children resist a patch being put over one eye.

Miniature toys test

This test is useful between the ages of two and three years, although the STYCAR letter-matching tests are preferable and can be used with many 2½-year-olds. The original test contains four miniature toys (car, airplane, doll, chair) and a set of miniature cutlery (knife, fork and spoon). The latter measure 5.5cm in length, and the child is required to name the toys and cutlery held by the examiner at a distance of 3m, having previously been shown the objects and asked to name them. Discrimination between the knife, fork and spoon at 3m requires good visual acuity. A child who cannot name the toys or cutlery can be asked to match them with his own set on a table in front of him.

Letter-matching tasks

These tasks can be used with many children at 2½ years, and regularly with most three-year-olds. They depend on the child's ability to match the shapes of letters long before he can name them. For the illiterate child the advantage over the E test is that he has more choice to make than simply distinguishing which way the prongs of the E are pointing: therefore it is a more attractive task and easier to administer.

52

One of the problems in testing vision in young children is the difficulty of holding their attention at a distance as great at 6m (20ft), particularly in a cluttered room not intended for vision testing. This is why tests for younger children have been devised which can be used to give an accurate assessment of vision at three metres. Preschool children are given a card with five, seven or nine letters on it and the examiner has a flip-pack of the same letters, with a single letter on each page, becoming progressively smaller. After teaching the child the matching task while sitting across the small table from him, the examiner then retires to a distance of 3m and tests distant vision by showing the child one letter at a time and asking him to find it on the card in front of him. The letters were selected by Dr. Sheridan as those which young children find most easy to discriminate. The five-letter card has the letters VTOHX, and the seven-letter card AHOTUVX. Ability to match the smallest letters on the cards is equivalent to a visual acuity of 6/6 at 3m.

For older children of 4½ years and more, it is possible to use a mount of a series of letters, as in the Snellen test card, and to point to one letter at a time and ask the child to match it on his own card (or alternatively to name the letter). This is done with the examiner either at a distance of 6m or sitting beside the child and using a mirror sited at a distance of 3m.

These tasks should be repeated, and each eye should be tested separately by encouraging the child to wear a patch or having the parent cover one eye at a time.

Snellen charts can be used for older children who can recognize letters and numbers, starting with the largest letters on the top line and going down the chart line by line. Again, each eye should be tested separately.

Color vision

Recognition of color can be tested by asking questions about familiar objects and the child's own clothes: 'Is this car red?'; 'Can you find me something blue?'. Small colored cubes are useful for color-matching which does not rely on the child's ability to name colors. Give the child a few small cubes of various colors, select a green one and ask him to find any others which are of the same color, and so on. This test will detect the child who cannot discriminate between primary colors.

A child with normal visual acuity and normal recognition of numbers can be tested more formally with the Ishihara color chart*. The first number in the Ishihara is '12'. Cover the '1' with a card and ask for the other number, and vice versa. The next number is an '8'. If, as often happens, the child sees it as a '3', be careful to go back to Figure 1 in order to make sure that the child understands. Use the '69' number by holding a card over the '6' or the '9'. Hold the card upside-down to check results. Other numbers will confirm the presence of red-green or partial red-green deficiency.

Discussion

Clues about possible visual impairment may have been gained from questioning the parents about the child's reading and television-viewing habits. (For example, a

*See p. 4 for suppliers' addresses. (H-R-R plates from the American Optical Co. can also be used.)

child's insistence on always sitting very close to the set might be the result of poor vision.) Parents are usually right if they say the child cannot see properly, although they may be unaware of the degree of visual impairment, especially if only one eye is involved.

True loss of vision is associated with absent pupillary light-reflex, so it is important *not* to be too hasty about putting in mydriatic drops to get a better look at the fundus. A poor pupillary light-response may last for several days after drops.

Congenital absence of vision, whether ocular or cortical, or blindness acquired in early life, probably always is associated with some abnormal eye-movement at rest. Roving, large-scale and frequently disconjugate eye-movements, not organized into a regular nystagmus, are typical of blindness acquired before the age of fixation. Nystagmus or roving movements are useful in providing clues to visual deficits or blindness, and in documenting early onset of visual deficit in older children or adults. Uniocular blindness acquired at any age usually results in lateral deviation of the blind eye in the position of rest, but this must be distinguished from strabismus, whether or not in conjunction with amblyopis ex anopsia. Poor or absent visual acuity in an infant who is otherwise normal and whom examination shows to have 'normal' fundi may be a sign of the congenital form of Leber optic atrophy. Ophthalmological consultation may confirm this condition by characteristic findings on an electroretinogram.

Unilateral blindness or severe visual defect is very difficult to demonstrate in children who are too young to test with standard charts, but sometimes may be suspected if a child objects violently to having one eye covered but not the other. Evoked responses to visual stimuli (see Chapter 11) can also be used to distinguish 20/20 from 20/200 vision.

Psychogenic blindness is a common school-problem in the United States, usually among girls. These children appear to be unconcerned (*'la belle indifférence'*), in spite of a history of marked visual loss. They may be unable to recognize letters on the 20/400 line, but, smiling, may be able to pick up small objects with ease. A normal response to the test for stereoscopic vision is a good indication that the child is not blind in one eye. A red-lens cover test can also be useful in revealing psychogenic uniocular blindness. The red lens allows the black letters on a chart to be read, while obscuring the red letters. The spurious blindness is revealed if the allegedly normal eye is covered with a red lens, the 'blind' eye is left uncovered and the child reads out both red and black letters.

Some degree of color blindness, usually a partial defect of red-green discrimination, occurs in 5 to 6 per cent of the male population but in only 0.3 per cent of females. Many learning-disabled children become confused with figure and background on the tests and can be shown to be not color blind, but neurologically immature in their responses. However, 'color-coding' is often used as a teaching tool for the learning disabled, and the status of their color vision should be established in order to avoid additional problems in the classroom. Usually a parent will know whether color blindness is present once the possibility has been raised.

TESTING AUDITORY ACUITY: CRANIAL NERVE 8

Directions

A great deal of important information about the child's ability to hear will have been gathered from the history and the indirect observation. Obviously, if a hearing impairment is suspected, formal definitive audiometric testing should be done, but preferably on a separate visit. Testing of hearing during the basic neurological examination seeks to establish whether or not the child has functional hearing. The parents should always be asked whether they think their child hears normally; usually they will be the first to suspect any abnormality.

Directions for testing the hearing of infants and young children are given in Chapter 8.

Over the age of three years it is important to check that the child has functional hearing to soft voice, and various sets of picture cards have been devised for this purpose (STYCAR, Reed) (see Chapter 1). Sets of directions, which may be simple or complicated according to the age of the child, can also be given: 'Give the block to me'; 'Give the block to me when I drop my pencil but not before'.

Test for conduction deafness in an older, co-operative child by vibrating a tuning fork (256 frequency) and asking whether it is louder when held 2-3cm (1in) away from the ear to be tested, or when the tip is pressed against the mastoid process (the Rinne test). Vibrate the tuning fork again and place the tip on the child's forehead. Ask him to indicate in which ear, if any, the sound is louder (the Weber test). Do an otoscopic examination.

Discussion

Proper lateralization of sound indicates that functional hearing is present. The child's inability to follow verbal directions accurately may be the only indication of significant hearing loss. Hearing loss in children may be overlooked during a clinical examination, even by an experienced examiner, because children become adept at imitating and guessing correctly the expected response. They may appear to turn to sound, while in fact responding to visual cues. An examination consisting of systematic observation of a child's response to selected sounds and to a consistent set of verbal instructions decreases the chance for error.

A positive response to the percussion made by a loud noise might obscure a hearing loss. In the Rinne test, normally a tuning fork is heard longer by air conduction than by bone conduction. Both are diminished proportionately with nerve deafness, but bone conduction is retained and may be better than air conduction in cases of hearing impairment associated with disease of the middle ear or abnormality of the external auditory canal. In the Weber test, the vibrating tuning fork should be heard equally well in each ear. When there is conduction deafness the Weber test is lateralized to the abnormal side, with nerve deafness toward the normal side.

Hyperacusis, an exaggerated or unpleasant perception of loud sounds, often is attributed to paralysis of the facial nerve's motor branch to the stapedius. The exaggerated startle response found in Tay-Sachs or other degenerative diseases is caused by a central rather than a peripheral disorder. The apparent increased sensitivity of blind children to sound probably is attributable to surprise rather than to neurophysiological phenomena. There is no evidence that loss of either hearing or vision alters the child's ability to respond with the unaffected faculty.

TESTING THE VESTIBULAR PORTION OF CRANIAL NERVE 8

Caloric and rotational stimuli may be used to test vestibular function. These stimuli produce changes in the endolymph current in the semicircular canals and, secondarily, test the vestibular apparatus. Rapid changes in position may elicit nystagmus and dizziness in normal infants and children. Because rapid and slow components of eye movements occur after horizontal movement, correct interpretation of results often depends upon careful observations and comparisons of movements, first in one direction and then in the other. Care must be taken to control both acceleration and rate.

Abnormal findings or symptoms directly related to the vestibular system suggest the need for electronystagmograms (see Chapter 11) or other more sophisticated procedures. Caloric testing (stimulation of the vestibular canals by injections of cold or warm water into the auditory canal) is a relatively simple procedure but requires patience and experience for reproducible results.

Normal vestibular function of an infant or a child small enough to hold at arm's length may be determined during the routine neurological examination. Routine examination of vestibular function of an older child who is too heavy to lift may be done by caloric testing or by using a specially designed chair. However, these tests require considerable additional time and much co-operation on the part of the child, so the examiner must decide whether the anticipated results justify the procedure.

Testing vestibular function of infants and young children
Directions

Hold the infant or child under the arms, facing you at eye-level (holding neck and head steady if necessary), at a distance of about 40-45cm (15-18in). Turn full-circle and observe the direction of quick and slow movement of the eyes. Vertical gaze can be tested by lifting the infant up and down.

Discussion

Normal infants show full and obligate deviation of the eyes in the direction toward which the examiner is rotating, with the quick phase of nystagmus when rotated in the opposite direction. The direction of the movement is reversed when the rotation stops. With older children, the nystagmus is more prominent than deviation of the eyes in the horizontal plane.

A normal response indicates intact brain-stem function between the vestibular system and the oculomotor nuclei. Movement of the eyes in response to rotation is a primitive response and usually is well preserved. However, the fact that responses almost always are within normal limits reduces the value of this test.

Testing vestibular function of older children: caloric testing
Directions
Examine the ears for possible perforation of the eardrum (which would contra-indicate the test) or obstruction of the external auditory canals (which would need cleaning). Have the child lie supine with the head elevated on a pillow about 30° above the horizontal. Using a syringe with a short length of tubing, inject 10ml of cold (30°C) or warm (44°C) water slowly and steadily against the tympanic membrane over a period of one minute. After a short rest-interval, repeat the test with the other ear. Assistance may be needed to keep the child's head in the proper position. Nystagmus usually begins shortly before or shortly after the end of irrigation, but the test should be repeated at least twice before concluding that there is no reaction.

Discussion
    Irrigation with cold water produces deviation of the eyes towards the side of the irrigation, with the quick phase of the nystagmus away from it. If the right ear is stimulated the quick phase of the nystagmus is to the left; past-pointing is towards the right and if the patient gets up from the bed he tends to fall to the right and to have vertigo (the feeling of whirling) toward the left.

Use of the 'Barany' chair
Directions
    Have the child sit erect in a standard 'Barany' chair. Tilt the child's head forward about 30° (to place the horizontal semicircular canals in the horizontal plane). The pupil of the eye and the external auditory meatus should lie in a plane parallel to the floor. Ask the child to close his eyes, and rotate the chair 10 times over a 20-second period.

Discussion
    An older child, seated in a chair designed specially for the purpose and rotated to the right, will show past-pointing and postural deviation to the right, with vertigo toward the left. If the child's eyes are opened or the eye movements are recorded, nystagmus is seen with the quick component to the right (the direction of rotation) and the slow component to the left. The response of the older children in the chair appears to be opposite to that of the infant being held. However, this is not contra-dictory because in a chair the child is in the center of the rotating axis, but if the infant is being held the examiner is in the center of the axis and the infant is rotating about the examiner.

                    TESTING SMELL: CRANIAL NERVE 1

Directions
    With a child over five or six years of age, test his ability to smell by asking him to occlude one nostril, close his eyes and identify several common odors, such as tooth-paste, oranges or cinnamon.

Discussion

Anosmia in children may occur after head injury: apart from this, it is seldom significant and should not be taken as evidence of abnormality unless accompanied by other signs. Usually, apparent anosmia is due to a common cold, sinusitis, allergic or other rhinitis or nasal obstruction by a polyp or deviated septum. Children with Kallman syndrome (hypogonadotropic hypogonadism and anosmia) cannot smell and also have cryptorchidism, congenital deafness and cleft palate, and in some instances renal anomalies. The gonadotropic defect is hypothalamic; probably the anosmia is due to hypoplasia of the olfactory lobes.

EXAMINATION OF FACIAL MUSCLES; NOSE, MOUTH AND PHARYNX: FACIAL NERVES 5, 7 ,9, 10, 12

Directions

Observe the face for asymmetry, grimacing, tics, involuntary movements or drooling. Listen to the child's speech for evidence of a hypernasal quality or dysarthria. Note the presence or absence of tears. Ask the child to drink from a cup (or bottle) and notice how he swallows. Ask the child to imitate you as you close your eyes for a moment, smile, whistle and put out your tongue. Ask the child to keep his eyelids closed as you try to open them against gentle pressure. Ask him to open his jaw wide and move it from side to side against the resistance of your hand. Test the jaw-jerk reflex by asking the child to open his mouth slightly, then place your finger on the mid-point of his chin and tap it with a finger of the other hand, or a reflex hammer. Look for a sudden elevation of the chin. Ask the child to open his mouth again so that you can inspect the tongue in its resting position, noting symmetry, size, size in relation to the oral cavity and mandible, and unusual characteristics of its surface. Look for fasciculations (small furrow-like depressions which appear and disappear irregularly) and involuntary movements.

Inspect the palate for shape of the arch, presence of a cleft palate, bifid (cleft) uvula, and symmetry of the palatal arch at rest. Look at the teeth, noting their general appearance, hygiene, eruption in relation to age, discoloration and abnormalities of formation. Inspect the gums for evidence of disease, hypertrophy or a lead-line.

Test the child's ability to taste by using different droppers containing salt, sugar, vinegar and quinine solutions placed on the protruded tongue.

Test the gag reflex at the end of this part of the examination by moving a tongue blade from side to side by 1-2cm over the tongue and gradually moving the blade further back until the gag reflex is elicited. Look for absent, minimal or asymmetric activity of the soft palate, or displacement forward during gagging.

Discussion

Cranial nerves

The motor division of the fifth cranial nerve, the trigeminal (Fig. 24), supplies the muscles of mastication—the temporalis, the masseter and the pterygoid. The

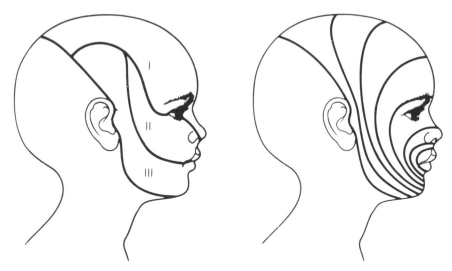

Fig. 24. *(Left)* Sensory innervation of the face by the first, second and third divisions of the trigeminal nerve. *(Right)* Segmental arrangement of the representation of pain and temperature from the face in the spinal tract of the fifth nerve and in its nucleus. The arrangement has been compared to onion peel. The area around the mouth, which is the most rostral, has the highest representation. The more posterior and inferior regions are lowest in the upper segments of the cervical cord.

sensory portion supplies the skin of the face, the eyeball, the paranasal sinuses, the nasal cavity, the mucous membranes of the hard and soft palate (except the posterior border), the nasopharynx, the buccal mucous membranes, the gums, the teeth, the lips and the tongue (for sensations other than taste).

A unilateral lesion of the trigeminal nerve results in a deviation of the jaw to the paretic side. The jaw-jerk is absent in the presence of a nuclear or peripheral trigeminal-nerve lesion, and it is exaggerated if a supranuclear lesion exists. Experience is needed to decide whether a jaw-jerk is normal, depressed or exaggerated: there is some variation from one individual to another, and an exaggerated response may be elicited in normal babies.

The sensory function of the fifth cranial nerve is extremely difficult to test in children. The corneal reflex (p. 36) remains the most reliable test.

Cranial nerve 7

The anatomy of the facial nerve is extremely complicated and is shown in Fig. 25.

Lesions of various types located at different levels in the course of the facial nerve produce various combinations of impairment of its functions (Table VII). Interpretation of these signs and the various pathological bases of facial paralysis are reviewed in standard textbooks of neurology and in the medical literature (*e.g.* Paine 1957). Partially recovered facial palsies are particularly difficult to evaluate because of the possibility of associated contractures and because in peripheral facial palsy the upper face may recover first, thereby giving the impression of a supranuclear lesion, which theoretically would spare the upper part of the face. Also, while the upper part

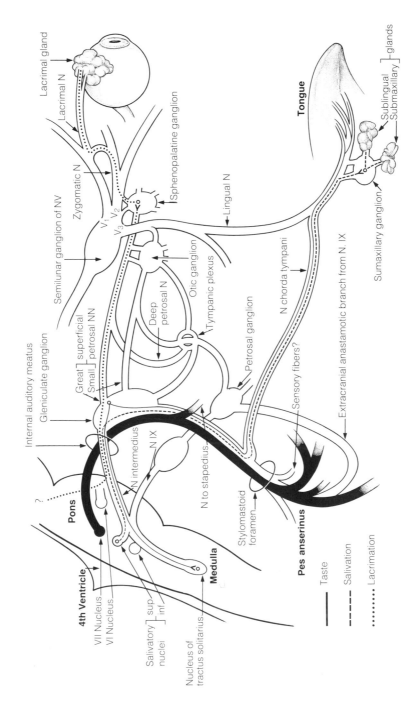

Fig. 25. Anatomical arrangement of the facial nerve. The course of the motor fibers is shown in black. Relative sizes have been somewhat distorted for clarity and to allow labeling. Minor anastomotic connections and possible secondary sensory pathways have been omitted.

Lacrimal gland

Lacrimal N

Tongue

Sublingual
Submaxillary glands

Semilunar ganglion of NV

Zygomatic N

Sphenopalatine ganglion

V₁ V₂
V₃

Lingual N

Sumaxillary ganglion

Internal auditory meatus

Geniculate ganglion

Great superficial
Small petrosal NN

Deep petrosal N

Otic ganglion

Tympanic plexus

Petrosal ganglion

N chorda tympani

Sensory fibers?

Extracranial anastamotic branch from N. IX

N intermedius

N IX

Pons

N to stapedius

Stylomastoid foramen

Pes anserinus

4th Ventricle

Medulla

VII Nucleus
VI Nucleus

Salivatory sup.
nuclei inf.

Nucleus of
tractus solitarius

Taste

Salivation

Lacrimation

60

TABLE VII
Clinical findings in facial paralyses due to lesions at various anatomical locations*

Location of lesion	Voluntary movements Upper face	Lower face	Emotional movements	Lacrimation	Salivation, submaxillary and sublingual	Taste, anterior 2/3 of tongue	Hyperacusis
Supranuclear	Retained	Lost	Retained	Retained	Retained	Retained	Absent
Nuclear	Lost	Lost	Lost	Retained	Retained	Retained	Present
Intracranial (between pons and int. aud. meatus)	Lost	Lost	Lost	Usually lost	Usually lost	Usually lost	Present
In canal at or above geniculate ganglion	Lost	Lost	Lost	Lost	Lost	Lost	Present
Between ganglion and nerve to stapedius	Lost	Lost	Lost	Retained	Lost	Lost	Present
Between stapedius and chorda tympani	Lost	Lost	Lost	Retained	Lost	Lost	Absent
Between chorda tympani and branching on face	Lost	Lost	Lost	Retained	Retained	Retained	Absent
In pes auserinus	Variable	Variable	Partly lost	Retained	Retained	Retained	Absent

From Paine and Oppé (1966).

of the face usually has a more bilateral supranuclear innervation than the lower, it is not always spared in unilateral supranuclear facial paresis.

A lesion involving the upper-motor neuron of the seventh facial cranial nerve is characterized by the child's inability to move the corner of his mouth on the affected side when crying or smiling, or to wrinkle his forehead and close his eyes on that side. In the case of a very mild unilateral paralysis which includes the upper face, there may be only a wider palpebral fissure on the affected side.

Bell's palsy (Fig. 26) is a syndrome consisting of sudden onset of unilateral facial paralysis of unknown etiology. It is rare in infancy. An immune response to a viral infection may be one explanation. The facial muscles contract on the normal side, the nasolabial fold on the affected side is flattened, and the child cannot close his eye on that side. Attempted closure causes upward deviation of the eye (Bell's sign). Contracture from an old facial paralysis may lead the examiner at first to believe that the weakness is on the opposite side. Young children, and particularly newborns, with a congenital anomaly of absence of the depressor anguli oris muscle on one side (Hufnagel's palsy) fail to draw down that corner of the mouth during crying, as is usual in babies (Fig. 27). Distinguishing this from facial paresis depends on there being no other area of weakness, and on the relative thinness of the cheek just below the angle of the mouth. The latter is appraised by palpation, with one finger in the child's mouth and one on the cheek.

Impairment of emotional facial movements, particularly smiling or crying, if voluntary movements are retained, is thought to be associated with disease of the

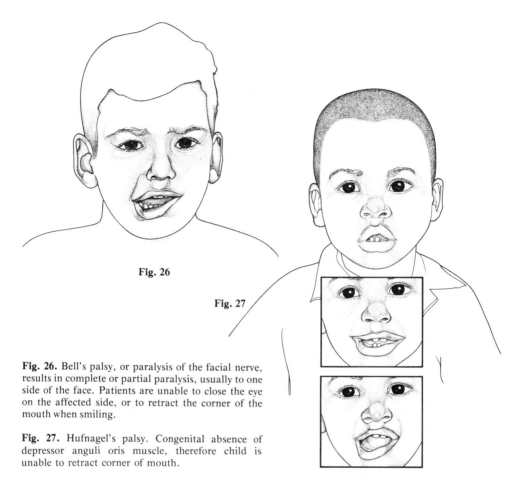

Fig. 26

Fig. 27

Fig. 26. Bell's palsy, or paralysis of the facial nerve, results in complete or partial paralysis, usually to one side of the face. Patients are unable to close the eye on the affected side, or to retract the corner of the mouth when smiling.

Fig. 27. Hufnagel's palsy. Congenital absence of depressor anguli oris muscle, therefore child is unable to retract corner of mouth.

extrapyramidal cortical projections, the basal ganglia or thalamus, or possibly the reticular part of the pons superior to the facial nucleus. In children, a mask-like face may reflect a postencephalitic state of suprabulbar paresis.

A bilaterally expressionless and hypotonic face may be a congenital defect, especially if combined with impaired abduction of the eye in Moebius syndrome (see Fig. 23, p. 43). Acquired bilateral paralysis of the facial nerve should raise the question of Guillain-Barré syndrome.

Facial myokymia, or continuous undulating movement of the facial-muscle fibers, is a rare clinical finding and is most frequently associated with multiple sclerosis. Usually only one side of the face is affected. Facial paralysis in children which is not associated with poliomyelitis or Guillain-Barré syndrome usually indicates a pontine lesion or posterior fossa malignancy. Facial myokymia can be a presenting feature of medulloblastoma (Korobkin *et al.* 1975).

There are several useful reflexes referrable to motor function of the facial nerve. The response to percussing either the upper or lower lip may spread to involve contraction of the orbicularis oris, with protrusion of the lips, referred to as the 'snout reflex'. This occurs with bilateral supranuclear lesions and with a variety of degenerative cerebral diseases. There may also be a sucking reflex. The palmomental reflex is elicited by scratching the thenar surface of the hand: the response is ipsi-lateral elevation and retraction of the angle of the mouth. This reflex is normal in infancy, but at later ages suggests disease of the pyramidal tract in the opposite frontal lobe. An easily elicited palmomental reflex is associated with postencepha-litic syndromes or degenerative disorders.

The facial nerve conveys the sense of taste from the anterior two-thirds of the tongue. It is well known that sensation of taste is based to a large extent on smell, so children with anosmia may complain instead of being unable to taste their food.

There have been reports of lacrimation on the side of an injury to the facial nerve. Like other autonomic phenomena (skin temperature, skin resistance), this response is variable and depends on the extent of the insult and the duration of other symptoms.

The tongue and cranial nerve 12

Examination of the tongue can reveal other limitations, such as facial weakness, inability to cope with secretions and difficulty in swallowing.

Diminished tongue-mass occasionally may represent congenital hypoplasia but more often reflects atrophy and implies a lesion of the lower motor unit, because atrophy is minimal with supranuclear lesions. The bulk of the tongue may be increased by hypothyroidism, amyloid disease and glycogen storage disease. A tongue which is large in proportion to the mandible and the oral cavity may contribute to mechanical obstruction, as in the Pierre-Robin syndrome and in sleep apnea.

There are a wide variety of abnormalities in the appearance of the surface of the tongue in many systemic diseases and in nutritional deficiencies. Deficiences of B-group vitamins may also affect the nervous system, and inspection of the tongue (which would be smooth and red) may provide a valuable clue. The tongue is smooth in familial dysautonomia. Fasciculations must be distinguished from the synchron-ous, tremulous movements during a child's normal crying and from the adder-like movement of the tongue of a child who is at a decerebrate stage. Bilateral weakness, atrophy and fasciculation in infants is pathognomonic of progressive spinal muscular atrophy (Werdnig-Hoffmann disease). In adults, and rarely in older children, such a combination may suggest motor neuron disease (amyotrophic lateral sclerosis or progressive bulbar palsy) or syringobulbia.

Injury to the 12th cranial nerve (the hypoglossal nerve) on one side causes unilateral lingual paralysis and hemiatrophy of the tongue. The tongue protrudes to the paralysed side ('the tongue points to the side of the lesion'). On retraction, the wasted and paralysed side rises higher than the other. The larynx deviates to the normal side because of paralysis of the depressors of the hyoid bone. In bilateral hypoglossal paralysis the tongue is motionless and swallowing is difficult, but taste and tactile sense in the tongue are normal.

Hypertonus and loss of voluntary control of movement of the tongue to command or to imitation may be conspicuous in cerebral tetraparesis, as well as in suprabulbar paresis. Patients with athetosis and dystonia frequently have comparable unwanted movement of the tongue, which is most obvious when they are asked to move it and when speech, chewing or swallowing are attempted. This loss of supranuclear control of movements of the tongue and oral musculature can be a major handicap in both spastic and athetoid cerebral palsy, is of major importance in relation to speech and eating, and is a social handicap as well.

Pseudobulbar palsy

Pseudobulbar palsy, or more accurately suprabulbar paresis (Worster-Drought 1974), is an isolated paresis or weakness caused by bilateral lesions in the cerebral hemispheres of the muscle structures which derive their nerve supply mainly through the 10th and 12th cranial nerves. The clinical symptoms include dysarthria, impaired swallowing, restricted tongue protrusion (although it may be moved passively) and restricted movement of the palate, with preservation of the gag reflex. The congenital form is considered to be a developmental defect, with bilateral involvement of the corticobulbar fibers. If only the corticobulbar fibers are involved, there is no paresis of the extremities. Suprabulbar paresis may be found in association with tetraplegic cerebral palsy; it may also be acquired after cerebrovascular accidents, encephalitis or trauma. If the corticothalamic fibers are interrupted, the syndrome may also include loss of emotional control and unprovoked outbursts of laughing or crying.

The palate and cranial nerve 9

The presence of a high palatal arch is non-specific. It may be found in several genetically determined conditions such as Friedreich's ataxia, Charcot-Marie-Tooth disease, familial spastic paraplegia and myotonia dystrophica. It is also a frequent finding in the group of conditions comprising the first arch syndrome. A cleft palate often is associated with hearing loss, so any child with a cleft palate is a good candidate for thorough audiometric testing. A cleft uvula may be a normal variant, but a bifid or cleft uvula may also suggest the presence of a submucous cleft palate. A cleft uvula is a frequent finding in the Noonan syndrome (XY Turner phenotype).

Paralysis of the ninth cranial nerve may be evidenced by only a slight drooping of the palatal arch at rest, although both sides elevate equally when saying 'aah'. Motor fibers of the vagus supply all of the striated muscles of the soft palate, pharynx and larynx, except the stylopharyngeus and the tensor veli palatini. Unilateral vagal paralysis produces drooping of the palatal arch on the affected side, while uvula and medial raphe deviate toward the normal side. Phonation increases retraction of the uvula toward the normal side. In some instances in which fifth-nerve function is normal, contraction of the tensor veli palatini will prevent obvious drooping of the palate. If the vagal paralysis is bilateral the palate cannot elevate on phonation, although again it may not droop markedly.

Cranial nerve 10

Vagal lesions produce surprisingly little difficulty in articulation or swallowing, although with acute lesions there may be dysphagia, especially of liquids, and some regurgitation of fluids into the nose when swallowing. Acute unilateral lesions may give speech a nasal quality and this effect is accentuated with bilateral vagal paralysis.

Phonemes such as 'b', 'd' and 'k' tend to become 'm', 'n' and 'ng', respectively. The effect is very similar to that of a cleft palate.

Incomplete oropharyngeal closure

Some children have insufficient velopalatine tissue to close the oropharynx properly. Feeding difficulty and poor oral control may be early symptoms. Because there is no true paralysis, the condition may be difficult to recognize. Speech may be difficult to understand and have a muffled nasal quality, the greatest difficulty being in the pronunciation of consonants. This type of inadequate closure leads to the diagnosis of 'cleft-palate' speech, even though the palate is anatomically closed. In some cases adenoid tissue helps to close the space, so its removal by surgery or its decrease at the time of adolescence leads to further deterioration of speech. There may be associated, non-specific neurological symptoms (Pollack *et al.* 1979).

The teeth and gums

The condition and hygiene of the teeth and gums give a good indication of the child's general health and care. However, dental hygiene can be very difficult for cerebral-palsied children, particularly with athetosis. If parents have not been advised about this there may be severe dental caries, which do not necessarily reflect parental neglect. Irregularities of eruption, malformations of the teeth and discolorations are valuable indicators of the child's development. In ectodermal dysplasia, teeth do not develop properly, if at all, and alveolar processes are partially or totally absent since alveolar bone does not develop in the absence of teeth. If teeth are present, they are small and conical. There is over-closure of the mandible and protrusion of the lips. Hypoplasia of the primary teeth may be associated with intra-uterine stress. The effect of congenital syphilis on the formation of permanent teeth results in central notching of the incisive edges, known as Hutchinson incisors. Hypothyroidism results in prolonged retention of the deciduous teeth. In cleidocranial dysostosis the eruption of the teeth is delayed and the teeth are poorly formed. Brown-yellow discoloration of deciduous teeth may be a consequence of tetracycline therapy.

Gum hypertrophy is a common finding among individuals who take diphenyl-hydantoin. Such hypertrophy also may be idiopathic or, rarely, caused by fibromata. It may be a finding in some of the lipoid storage diseases. A lead-line, consisting of a dark blue or black line on the gingival margin, indicates exposure to lead over a long period of time.

EXAMINATION OF THE NECK: CRANIAL NERVE 11

Directions

Observe the head and neck to see if there is any evidence of turning (rotation to one side about a vertical axis) or tilting (the chin elevated toward the side to which the face is turned, with slight depression of the occiput). Inspect the neck for webbing and abnormal shortness. Palpate the thyroid. Palpate the sternocleidomastoids and test their power (innervated by the 11th cranial nerve) by asking the child to rotate his head to one side and then the other against the resistance of your hand. Ask him to touch his chin to his chest and then to each shoulder and finally to look up at the ceiling.

Discussion

Klippel-Feil syndrome

Individuals with Klippel-Feil syndrome have a short neck, a low hair-line and limitations of active and passive movement. They may have associated kyphosis, scoliosis, torticollis and facial asymmetry. There is fusion or a reduction in the number of cervical vertebrae, and there may be hemivertebrae and atlanto-occipital or cervical-thoracic fusion. Children with this syndrome may have neurological soft signs, learning defects and mirror-writing. The syndrome may also be associated with spina bifida, syringomyelia, congenital deafness and congenital heart-disease. The reasons for these findings are not clear.

Platybasia

A short neck and restricted movement are also found in platybasia, a congenital bony abnormality in the occipito-cervical region, usually in the position of the atlas and the odontoid process. The clinical symptoms, compression of the medulla and pons, usually do not begin until adolescence. There may be an Arnold Chiari malformation—herniation of an abnormal medulla and cerebellum through the foramen magnum.

Webbing

Webbing of the neck suggests the syndromes of Turner, Bonnevie-Ullrich and Noonan and chromosomal aberrations—trisomy 18 and deletion of part of 18.

Stiffness

If accompanied by a tendency to retract, and pain and resistance to flexion, stiffness of the neck usually is associated with meningitis or other meningeal irritation. However, subarachnoid hemorrhage can produce a neck equally as stiff as in meningitis. With or without tenderness to pressure over some region of the cervical spine, a stiff neck can also be due to a bony lesion or an intraspinal tumor.

Torticollis

Maintained torticollis in children most often is neonatal torticollis, the physiological basis for which is doubtful. Distinction should be made between this and the effects of tender lymph-nodes, retropharyngeal abscess and other actute processes. Paralytic torticollis results from a lesion of either the upper or lower motor neuron. Head-tilting without actual tightness of the sternocleidomastoid muscle is often termed torticollis, but it may have other causes. For example, the head may be tilted to compensate for and prevent diplopia associated with paralysis of the extra-ocular muscles. However, head-tilting in children should suggest a tumor in the posterior fossa: such tumors may produce tilting to suppress diplopia, but the phenomenon occurs in other cases without diplopia, and in some obscure way may alter the fluid dynamics within the posterior fossa to reduce headaches.

CHAPTER 5

Assessment of Movement, Power, Tone and Reflexes

Directions

If the child is young, help him undress, noting in passing apparent muscle strength and range of motion as the clothes are removed. Help him remove shoes and socks and inspect the shoes carefully for unusual patterns of wear. Some shy children may prefer to undress a little at a time or to stay partially clothed, and will need reassurance and encouragement. Observe the child's sitting posture and whether he sits erect without needing support from his arms. Note any abnormal position of the head in relation to the trunk.

Look at the hands for symmetry, size, development and abnormalities. Look at the shape and position of the thumbs and fingers and inspect the nails. Look for tremor at rest, and hand preference. Test the grip of each hand by asking the child to squeeze your fingers hard. Note any abnormal movements.

Look at the lower limb, noting the posture and position of the feet in relation to the legs. Look for evidence of asymmetry or wasting, and check the pedal pulses. Note any abnormal movements.

Discussion

The development of the hand should be appropriate for the child's stature and condition. The hands should be equal in size, strength and tone. Any discrepancy should be carefully evaluated when the child is undressed. Congenital anomalies of the fingers (syndactyly, webbing, absence, nail dysplasia) often are manifestations of birth defects. Distal displacement of the thumb is one of the manifestations of trisomy 18, and a proximally displaced thumb occurs in the Cornelia De Lange syndrome. (The detection of abnormal palmar creases and the study of dermatoglyphics are specialized techniques which can help identify chromosomal abnormalities.) A child with trisomy 21 (Down syndrome) has a broad palm, with dysplasia of the middle phalanx of the fifth finger. Long slender fingers may indicate arachnodactyly (Marfan syndrome) and short stubby fingers pseudohypoparathyroidism or achondroplasia. Dystrophic nails are found in chondro-ectodermal and ectodermal dysplasia. Peri-ungal fibromata are associated with tuberous sclerosis (Fig. 28). In the Lesch-Nyhan syndrome there is evidence of self-mutilation of the hands and fingers. Bitten nails and cold sweaty palms are often significant signs of tension and anxiety in a mature, well-behaved child who is trying very hard to please.

Some conditions or diseases involving the muscles which control the foot can produce talipes equinovarus (heel up, ball of foot externally rotated) and pes cavus (a foot with an unusually high longitudinal arch) (Fig. 29). Pes cavus may also be a benign condition, dominantly inherited, in which case there is no muscle imbalance.

It is usually stated that a cavus foot results from weakness of the intrinsic muscu-lature of the foot, but an important co-factor is probably greater preservation of

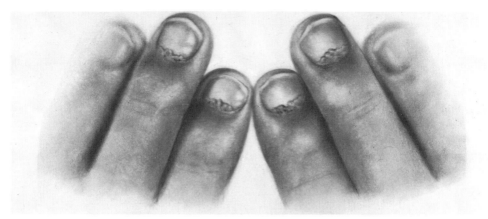

Fig. 28. Neurofibromata: soft nodules (tumors) on the nails.

power in the tibialis posterior muscle than in the tibialis anterior or peronei (Tyrer and Sutherland 1961). A cavus foot is seen not only in Charcot-Marie-Tooth disease, but also in Friedreich's ataxia, some myelodyplasias, and in some tumors or other acquired lesions of the lower spinal-cord. Basically pes cavus is a forefoot equinus, with secondary posterior subluxation and clawing of the toes, producing active dorsiflexion at the end of the swing phase of gait. Spasticity in the lower extremity, of whatever cause, may be associated with a foot which resembles the cavus deformity, but the posture of the spastic foot depends chiefly on tightness of the Achilles tendon, and the degree of inversion, forefoot adduction and heel-to-toe shortening is very much less. Unless familial pes cavus, a true cavus foot should always suggest a spinal origin.

Inability to dorsiflex the child's foot 20° above the horizontal plane indicates some shortening of the heel cord. Equinovarus feet may also be seen in peroneal muscular atrophy (Charcot-Marie-Tooth disease). In that condition the shortening of the Achilles tendon is secondary to foot-drop resulting from involvement of the peroneal nerve. Myotonic dystrophy, arthrogryposis and myelodysplasia are other conditions which can result in an equinovarus foot.

Abnormal movements

Abnormal movements are characteristic of extrapyramidal disease and are present in a wide variety of clinical manifestations. There is a great deal of overlap, and often it is difficult to distinguish a tic from a choreiform movement or a myoclonic jerk. One can broadly classify all these syndromes as dyskinesias, either hyperkinetic (chorea, hemiballismus, tics) or hypokinetic (*e.g.* Parkinsonism). Their causes, based on clinical presentation, are listed in Table VIII.

Myoclonus

Myoclonus is a quick, non-rhythmic contraction of single muscles or small muscle groups, sometimes resulting in a sudden jerky movement of the limb. The sudden involuntary jerk of a limb experienced while dropping off to sleep is one type of myoclonic jerk; it is a benign condition, usually termed a 'sleep startle'. Myoclonus

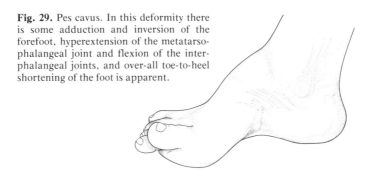

Fig. 29. Pes cavus. In this deformity there is some adduction and inversion of the forefoot, hyperextension of the metatarso-phalangeal joint and flexion of the inter-phalangeal joints, and over-all toe-to-heel shortening of the foot is apparent.

TABLE VIII

Causes of dyskinesias

Chronic non-progressive:	*Acute:*
asphyxia, hyperbilirubinemia, familial non-progressive, autosomal recessive non-progressive (dominant), familial striato-nigral dysplasias	carbon monoxide poisoning, cardiac bypass surgery, *H. influenzae* meningitis, encephalitis lethargica, mumps encephalitis, familial paroxysmal choreoathetosis, post-dialysis dyskinesia, burns encephalopathy, scalds, hypernatremic dehydration, heavy-metal poisoning (*e.g.* manganese, thallium), drug-induced dyskinesias, extrapyramidal epilepsy, tumors of the third ventricle convulsive tics, Gilles de la Tourette syndrome, familial striatal necrosis, Leigh encephalopathy, intermittent maple-syrup urine disease, subacute sclerosing panencephalitis, Sydenham chorea, chorea gravidarum
Chronic progressive:	
Huntington chorea, Hallervorden-Spatz disease, Wilson disease, ataxia telangiectasia, Fahr syndrome, Pelizaeus-Merzbacher disease, encephalitis lethargica, Jakob-Creutzfeld disease, subacute sclerosing panencephalitis, striato-nigral degeneration, Hunt disease, juvenile Parkinsonism, Hunt pallido cerebellar degeneration, Lesch-Nyhan syndrome, late infantile or juvenile Leigh disease, glutamic aciduria, dystonia, musculorum deformans, piloid astrocytoma basal ganglia, sulphite oxidase deficiency, familial striatal necrosis	

can be classified by its level of origin as spinal, cerebellar, basal ganglia or cortical. Cortical myoclonus may be epileptic or the result of one of a variety of degenerative disorders.

Myoclonus usually moves from one area to another, but may be rhythmical in the same area, as in myoclonus of the palatal or pharyngeal muscles. It may be enhanced by attempted voluntary activity, emotional stress or, often, by a wide variety of sensory stimuli.

Myoclonic jerks occur quite commonly in young babies, possibly associated with the organization of sleep state, and usually do not prove to be of any clinical significance. Their appearance as a new phenomenon in older infants (after the age of three months) and children should always be taken seriously and investigated, although sometimes no cause will be found.

Tremor

Tremor is an involuntary trembling or quivering. Although it is often associated

69

with other evidence of motor dysfunction, it may be found alone and unexplained. It can appear after infection, trauma or cerebral insult, or it may be familial. It may be a mild non-progressive condition or the harbinger of a more serious disorder such as Huntington's chorea. A static tremor (tremor at rest) can be seen best while the examiner supports and holds the child's wrists in a neutral position, with the child sitting comfortably. The extent of the tremor can be estimated by observing first the fingers, then the upper extremities and eyelids. Fine or medium rapid tremor (nine or ten per second) most often is familial or constitutional but may be due to hyperthyroidism or hypoglycemia. Medium or coarse slower tremor usually reflects abnormality in the basal ganglia, and is at first relatively suppressed when activity is attempted, but later breaks through in greater amplitude. Observation of the legs and feet may show involvement which has been unnoticed previously. An intention tremor is not present at rest, but is induced by attempted voluntary activity; for example, it is exaggerated by the finger-to-finger, finger-to-nose and heel-to-knee tests. In otherwise normal individuals, tremor may be brought on by stress, fatigue or excitement. Benign essential tremor is a familial condition. Titubation, a term used to describe nodding of the head to and fro or from side to side, may be associated with essential tremor. The term is also used to describe a more generalized shaking of the head and trunk accompanied by an ataxic gait.

Chorea

Chorea is defined as rapid involuntary jerks or fragments of movement occurring unexpectedly and irregularly. Any muscle or muscle-group may be involved, but the localization and intensity are extremely variable and unpredictable. Each movement is of short duration and separated in time from other episodes. The child exhibits poor co-ordination and lack of static support, and frequently finds it impossible to maintain uniform posture. Usually muscle tone is diminished. Chorea, like athetosis, is increased by attempted activity, emotional stress or sensory stimuli. In severe cases of Sydenham's chorea the intensity of the involuntary movement may prevent sleep, or it may continue during sleep and cause the child to fall out of bed. Chorea and athetosis can occur in the same individual and are common components of dyskinetic cerebral palsy (see Chapter 7). A slight degree of choreoathetotic movement of the fingers with the arm extended indicates mild disturbance of motor function, commonly encountered in children with minimal cerebral dysfunction.

Athetosis

Athetosis and chorea co-exist in many children, the word 'athetosis' literally meaning 'not fixed', or 'without posture'. The posture is constantly changing and the movements are relatively slow, worm-like and repetitious, chiefly involving the peripheral musculature of the limbs and face. The movements of the athetoid child are slower than those of a child with pure chorea and they involve gradual changes in posture which are secondary to changes in muscle tone. There are certain characteristic postures, such as hyperextension of joints, particularly the fingers; the arm also extends, abducts and internally rotates into the extended position. There is a positive Babinski-like posture of the feet and toes. Often the mouth is held tonically open, the tongue protrudes and there are exaggerated facial expressions.

Feeding is difficult, particularly chewing, and speech is always affected. The muscles are usually hypotonic at rest, but show exaggerated tone during the unwanted movements. Grimacing, crying and inappropriate emotional responses can accompany the fluctuating muscle tone. In children suffering from syndromes of brain damage, it is rare for athetosis to appear in the first year of life, although athetosis of the hands, dilatation of the alae nasae and fanning of the toes is often seen in normal infants at birth, and may be very obvious after relatively mild asphyxia. Many patients with so-called athetoid cerebral palsies have movements which are more appropriately described as dystonic.

Dystonic movements

These movements are involuntary. They are characterizeed by sudden muscular spasms, chiefly involving the muscles of the neck and trunk, although proximal musculature of the limbs also may be involved. Strange postures and slow spasmodic rotations (torsions) are characteristic. Muscle tone, appraised by palpation during passive manipulation, is at times below and at times above normal. Attempted movement precipitates contractions of muscle groups opposing the original movement. Dystonia usually ceases during sleep but in severe cases may persist, possibly in response to minor sensory stimuli, and may even prevent sleep. Dystonia is used here in its limited sense as a particular type of unwanted movement, not in the general sense of a persistent disturbance of muscle tone, nor as being diagnostic of the disease dystonia musculorum deformans.

Ballismus is a term used to describe large-scale, violent tossing or flinging movements which begin suddenly in the proximal muscle groups of a limb and spread to involve the whole limb or the major part of it. They may be either single or repeated. These movements are irregular both in location and in lack of rhythmicity. The face may also be involved. The movements are so violent and unexpected that the patient may injure himself or fall down. Conventionally, a diagnosis of hemiballismus implies a lesion in the contralateral subthalamic nucleus.

If the dyskinetic movements are of recent onset, the ingestion of a drug (usually phenothiazine or haloperidol) should be considered. Tardive dyskinesia, a syndrome characterized by choreiform movements of the head, legs and trunk and bizarre posturing, has its onset after prolonged ingestion of neuroleptic drugs, so it is rare in early childhood.

Habit spasm

A tic or habit spasm is a rhythmical, but usually repeated and stereotyped, movement of restricted muscle groups which resembles voluntary movement much more than it does myoclonus. In children the tic often affects the musculature of the face, neck and upper extremities. Tics are common, especially among young school-children (seven to 12 years of age), and it is estimated that up to 25 per cent of normal children have some form of tic (Weingarten 1968). Boys are more often affected than girls (in a ratio of approximately 3:1). The pattern of tics often changes from month to month, even though they are stereotyped at any single time. The tic may consist of

71

head-nodding, head-turning, blinking, winking, grimacing, mouth-opening, clucking, grunting, throat-clearing, tongue protrusion, shoulder-jerking or arm-flinging. Whether or not a yelp or other noise is uttered may need to be determined by history. Characteristically, tics do not distort or interfere with voluntary movement, and invariably cease during sleep or with sedation. Even more than other types of unwanted movement, tics are variable and may increase or decrease in severity while the child is being watched, or while he is tense or concentrating. Anxiety is likely to make a tic more obvious, but there is no good evidence that tiqueurs are any more psychiatrically disturbed than other children. Habit spasms frequently are confused with movement disorders that are 'organic' in origin. Habit spasms include the 'blindisms' of visually impaired children (eye-rubbing, rocking, hand-flapping), grinding teeth (bruxism), and head-banging and rocking, which may be seen in normal but deprived children under the age of two. These spasms often are seen in retarded children, particularly when they are bored and unstimulated. There is evidence for genetic predisposition for tics, which is inherited in a dominant fashion (Abe and Oda 1980).

A common form of severe habit-spasm is the Gilles de la Tourette syndrome (or *'maladie de tics'*), which includes grimacing, stretching the back and neck, compulsive barking, or shouting obscene words. Severe psychopathology may be present in some instances. The condition usually presents in childhood, commonly as early as five years of age; it should be regarded as serious if a 'tic-like' movement is accompanied by a sound. Shapiro *et al.* (1978) believe that the Tourette syndrome has an organic cause. There is often a familial incidence.

Spasmus nutans is a condition of unknown cause which consists of the triad of head-nodding, nystagmus and head-tilt. The nodding is rhythmic and involuntary, and the nystagmus may be horizontal, vertical, rotatory or mixed. The condition disappears during sleep and may be altered by voluntary action. Onset usually is around the age of six months, and the condition disappears one to two years later. The condition is benign and affected infants are physically and developmentally normal.

The 'bobble-head doll' syndrome

This syndrome is commonly associated with third-ventricular cysts. It may precede hydrocephalus and other signs of increased intracranial pressure. Onset has been reported between four months and nine years of age. Characteristically the movements are rhythmic to-and-fro head bobbing, or, less often, side-to-side, and appear to be most obvious when the child is upright, occurring at the rate of two to four per second. Rarely, the shoulders and trunk may be involved. It can be alleviated by distraction, by activity and by volitional control.

In contrast to spasmus nutans, the bobble-head doll movements tend to be more dysrhythmic, less constant and to occur later in life. Spasmus nutans often decreases if the child's eyes are covered or if fixation of vision occurs. Congenital nystagmus, with or without spasmus nutans, usually can be confirmed by history. It is unusual for children with ocular albinism to exhibit head movements, other than compensatory ones. Benign essential tremor usually does not disappear with activity. In contrast to the bobble-head doll syndrome, tic-like movements in children are arrhythmic and tend to change in character over several weeks of observation. Postural tremor almost never involves only the head.

Continuous jerky movements

These are characteristic of the Angelman ('happy puppet') syndrome, a condition also characterized by severe mental retardation, microcephaly and seizures (Mayo *et al.* 1973).

'Hyperkinesis'

Fidgeting is normal in most preschoolers and can be expected in older children who are tired, anxious or bored. The movements should cease when the child is diverted or asked to perform a specific task. The bugaboo of 'hyperkinesis' is often raised when a child 'cannot sit still'. The truly hyperkinetic child is in constant motion and over-reacts to new environmental stimuli (see Chapter 9).

TESTING MUSCLE POWER AND TONE

Directions

With the child sitting on the table with legs dangling (if this is a position of comfort), test for muscle power and tone by testing the power of the child to move groups of muscles against resistance (kinetic power) and his power to keep a joint fixed in order to withstand an attempt to move it (static power). Test each joint for range of motion, noting whether any limitation is caused by bony defects or contractures of muscles or tendons. Passively move each extremity to determine the degree of resistance and to evaluate the tone of the muscle*.

Begin with the shoulder. If possible, judge the strength of the shoulder girdle by lifting the child under the arms. He should not slip through your hands. Ask the child to try to raise each shoulder while you press down. Look for winging of the scapula, which could signify weakness of the trapezius. Ask him to hold each shoulder steady while you try to depress it. Ask the child to extend each arm; you then raise it and test for range of motion.

Ask the child to shake hands, then to pronate and supinate each hand against your resisting hand. Have the child extend his arm and point toward you. Attempt to

---

*The system generally used for recording gradations of muscle power is that of the Medical Research Council Manual (1963). Degrees of paresis are graded as follows: 5 = normal; 4 = active movement of joint against gravity and against resistance simultaneously; 3 = active movement against gravity but not against resistance; 2 = active movement with gravity eliminated by appropriate positioning of the limb; 1 = visible or palpable flicker of contraction but no movement of joint; 0 (paralysis) = no detectable contraction. These grades (5-0) correspond closely to the grades N, G, F, P, Tr and O of the Harvard Infantile Paralysis Commission.
Because more than one muscle is involved in certain movements of the joints, and because a muscle may have more than one possible action, depending on the position of the joints, the examiner must know the appropriate posture of the body and the position of the limb for the testing of each of the major muscles. An admirably short and simple outline, with excellent photographs, is published by the Medical Research Council (1963). Similar instruction and pictures are contained in *The Neurologic Examination* (De Jong 1958).
Tables IX and X summarize the innervation of the upper and lower extremities.

73

TABLE IX
Movements of upper extremity
(Only the most important muscles are listed, although others participate)

Movement	Muscles involved	Innervation	Spinal segment
Shoulder girdle (scapula)			
Elevation	Trapezius	Spinal accessory, C3,4	Cr 11; C3,4
	Levator anguli scapulae	Dorsal scapular, nn. to levator	C3,4,5
Depression	Lower fibres of trapezius	Cervical 3 and 4	C3,4
	Pectoralis minor	Medial anterior thoracic	C7, T1
	Subclavius	n. to subclavius	C5,6
Protraction	Serratus anterior	Long thoracic	C5-8
(abduction)	Pectoralis minor	Medial anterior thoracic	C7, T1
	Upper part of pectoralis major	Lat. and med. anterior thoracic	C5-T1
Retraction	Rhomboidei major and minor	Dorsal scapular	C4,5
(adduction)	Middle part of trapezius	Spinal accessory	Cr 11
Shoulder joint			
Elevation	Deltoid	Axillary	C5,6
(abduction)	Supraspinatus	Suprascapular	C5,6
Adduction	Pectoralis major	Lat. and med. ant. thoracic	C5-T1
	Latissimus dorsi	Thoracodorsal	C6-8
Flexion (forward	Subscapularis	Subscapular	C5,6
elevation)	Coracobrachialis	Musculocutaneous	C6,7
	Biceps (+ ant. fibres of deltoid and pectoralis major)	Musculocutaneous	C5,6
Extension (back-	Latissimus dorsi	Thoracodorsal	C6-8
ward elevation)	Triceps	Radial (musculospiral)	C6-8
	Teres major (+ post. fibres of deltoid and subscapularis)	Lower subscapular	C5, 6
Internal rotation	Subscapularis	Subscapular	C5,6
	Teres major (+ ant. deltoid, latissimus, pectoralis major)	Lower subscapular	C5,6
External rotation	Infraspinatus	Suprascapular	C5,6
	Teres minor	Axillary	C5,6
Elbow			
Flexion	Biceps	Musculocutaneous	C5,6
	Brachialis	Musculocutaneous	C5,6
Extension	Triceps	Radial	C6-8
Radio-ulnar joint			
Pronation	Pronator teres	Median	C6,7
	Pronator quadratus	Median	C7, T1
Supination	Biceps	Musculocutaneous	C5,6
	Brachioradialis	Radial	C5,6
	Supinator brevis	Radial	C5-7

74

Table IX *(continued)*

Movement	Muscles involved	Innervation	Spinal segment
Wrist			
Flexion	Flexor carpi radialis	Median	C6-8
	Flexor carpi ulnaris	Ulnar	C7-T1
Extension	Extensor carpi radialis	Radial	C6-8
(dorsiflexion)	Extensor carpi ulnaris	Radial	C6-8
	Extensor digitorum communis	Radial	C6-8
Abduction (radial	Flexor carpi radialis	Median	C6-8
deviation)	Extensores carpi radialis longus and brevis	Radial	C6-8
Adduction (ulnar	Flexor carpi ulnaris	Ulnar	C7-T1
deviation)	Extensor carpi ulnaris	Radial	C6-8
Thumb			
Radial abduction	Abductor pollicis longus	Radial	C6-8
	Extensor pollicis brevis	Radial	C6-8
Palmar abduction	Abductor pollicis brevis	Median	C6-7
	Abductor pollicis longus	Radial	C6-8
	Flexor pollicis brevis	Median + ulnar	C6-8
Ulnar adduction	Adductor pollicis	Ulnar	C8, T1
Palmar adduction	Flexores pollicis longus and brevis	Median + ulnar	C6-T1
	Extensor pollicis longus	Radial	C6-8
	1st Volar interosseus	Ulnar	C8-T1
Opposition (to	Opponens pollicis	Median	C6,7
5th finger)	Opponens digiti quinti	Ulnar	C8, T1
Fingers			
Flexion of	Flexor digitorum sublimis	Median	C7-T1
proximal joints			
	Flexor digiti quinti brevis	Ulnar	C8, T1
	Interossei	Ulnar	C8, T1
	Lumbricales	Median + ulnar	C6-T1
Extension of	Extensor digitorum communis	Radial	C6-8
proximal joints			
	Extensor indicis proprius	Radial	C6-8
	Extensor digiti quinti proprius	Radial	C6-8
Flexion of distal joints	Flexor digitorum profundus	Median + ulnar	C7-T1
Extension of distal	Interossei	Ulnar	C8, T1
joints	Lumbricales	Median + ulnar	C6-T1
Adduction	Volar interossei	Ulnar	C8, T1
Abduction	Dorsal interossei	Ulnar	C8, T1
	Abductor digiti quinti	Ulnar	C8, T1

From Paine and Oppé (1966).

TABLE X

Movements of lower extremity

(Only the most important muscles are listed, although others participate)

Movement	Muscles involved	Innervation	Spinal segment
Hip joint			
Flexion	Psoas major (+ minor if present)	nn. to Psoas muscles	L1-4
	Iliacus	Femoral	L2-4
Extension	Gluteus maximus	Inferior gluteal	L5-S2
(abduction)	Glutei medius and minimus	Superior gluteal	L4-S1
	Piriformis	Sacral 1 and 2	S1,2
	Tensor fasciae latae	Superior gluteal	L4-S1
	Sartorius	Femoral	L2-4
Adduction	Adductores magnus, longus, brevis	Obturator	L2-4
	Pectineus	Femoral	L2-4
	Gracilis	Obturator	L2-4
Internal rotation	Ant. parts of glutei medius and minimus	Superior gluteal	L4-S1
	Tensor fasciae latae	Superior gluteal	L4-S1
External rotation	Gluteus maximus	Inferior gluteal	L5-S2
	Obturatores internus and externus	Obturator (+ n. to obturator int.)	L2-S3
	Gemelli superior and inferior	nn. to Obturator int. and quadratus femoris	L4-S3
	Tensor fasciae latae	Superior gluteal	L4-S1
Knee			
Flexion	Biceps femoris	Tibial and common peroneal	L5-S3
	Semimembranosus and semitendinosus	Tibial	L4-S2
	Popliteus (also gracilis, sartorius, gastrocnemius)	Tibial	L5-S1
Extension	Quadriceps femoris	Femoral	L2-4
Ankle			
Plantar flexion	Gastrocnemius and soleus	Tibial	S1,2
Dorsiflexion	Tibialis anterior	Deep peroneal	L4-S1
	Peroneus tertius	Deep peroneal	L4-S1
	Extensores dig. longus and hallucis longus	Deep peroneal	L4-S1
Tarsal joints			
Inversion of foot	Tibialis posterior	Tibial	L4-S1
Eversion of foot	Peronei	Superficial and deep peroneal	L4-S1
	Extensor digitorum longus	Deep peroneal	
Great toe			
Plantar flexion	Flexor hallucis longus	Tibial	L4-S1
	Flexor hallucis brevis	Medial plantar	L4
Dorsiflexion	Extensores hallucis longus and brevis	Deep peroneal	L4-S1
Abduction	Abductor hallucis	Medial plantar	L4-S1
Adduction	Adductor hallucis	Lateral plantar	L5-S2

76

Table X *(continued)*

Movement	*Muscles involved*	*Innervation*	*Spinal segment*
Other toes			
Plantar flexion	Flexor digitorum longus	Tibial	L5, S1
	Flexor digitorum brevis	Medial plantar	L4-S1
	Flexor digiti quinti brevis	Lateral plantar	S2
Dorsiflexion	Extensores digitorum longus and brevis	Deep peroneal	L4-S1
Abduction	Dorsal interossei	Lateral plantar	S1,2
	Abductor digiti quinti	Lateral plantar	S1,2
Adduction	Plantar interossei	Lateral plantar	S1,2

From Paine and Oppé (1966).

TABLE XI
Causes of hypotonia without accompanying weakness

Central nervous system
  Mental retardation: non-specific primary mental retardation, trisomy 21 (Down syndrome), Prader-Willi syndrome

  Cerebral palsy: hypotonia, dyskinesia, early stages of spasticity

  Diseases of the basal ganglia: Wilson disease, cerebral dysgenesis, anoxic or traumatic encephalopathies, familial dysautonomia

General
  Hypothyroidism and other endocrine disorders
  Prematurity
  Malnutrition
  Environmental deprivation
  Rickets
  Chronic renal disease
  Electrolyte imbalance
  Metabolic, *e.g.* glycogen storage disease
  Ehlers-Danlos syndrome

TABLE XII
Causes of hypotonia accompanied by weakness; classified by level of abnormality

Anterior horn cell
  Progressive spinal muscular atrophy (Werdnig-Hoffman disease, Kugelberg-Welander disease)
  Spinal-cord injury
  Tumors, vascular anomalies, malformations
  Poliomyelitis

Nerve fiber
  Infectious polyneuritis (Guillain-Barré syndrome)
  Diphtheria
  Poisoning: lead, mercury, thallium, arsenic
  Drug toxicity
  Acute intermittent porphyria, hereditary motor sensory neuropathies: peroneal muscular atrophy (Charcot-Marie-Tooth disease), hypertrophic interstitial neuritis (Déjérine-Sottas disease)

Neuromuscular junction
  Myasthenia gravis
  Infantile botulism

Muscle
  Muscular dystrophy
  Myotonic dystrophy
  Congenital non-progressive myopathies (central core disease, nemaline myopathy)
  Familial periodic paralyses
  Dermatomyositis
  Endocrine and metabolic myopathy (hyperthyroid myopathy, McArdle disease)
  Steroid myopathy

77

raise and lower the upper arm against his resistance, then have him attempt to raise and lower against the resistance of your hand placed on his upper arm. Repeat with the arm extended laterally at shoulder height. Have the child flex his arm and ask him to attempt to flex and extend his forearm against your resisting hand, then have him try to withstand your attempts to flex and extend it.

Hold the child's elbow with one hand and flex and extend the forearm. Note any resistance or limitation of motion. If resistance is present, determine whether it is (a) rigid, with very little movement; (b) plastic, with the same degree of resistance to passive movement throughout the range of motion; (c) the 'clasp-knife' type, beginning with resistance to passive movement then suddenly giving way; or (d) jerky ('cog-wheel'). Test for a positive stretch reflex by holding the elbow and irregularly altering the speed of passive flexion. Spastic muscles are slow to respond. A normal child may resist, but the resistance is voluntary. (A positive stretch reflex may be likened to the sensation felt on opening a door which is equipped with a pneumatic spring-closing device. The initial movement is smooth when it is opened, but marked resistance is felt if it is closed quickly (Mac Keith 1959).

Test each wrist, knee and ankle in a similar manner for stretch, tone and limitation of motion. In testing the knee, stabilize the hip-joint by holding the thigh with one hand. The hips and thigh muscles are tested later, when the patient is lying down.

Diminished muscle power

If the examination discloses reduced muscle power, the physician must determine whether the infant or child has weakness with normal muscle tone, has hypotonia without weakness, or has both weakness and hypotonia. Weakness (the inability to move an arm or leg against gravity) accompanied by normal muscle tone could be caused by a systemic illness or fatigue. Hypotonia without true weakness is commonly associated with mental retardation, some forms of cerebral palsy and certain biochemical disorders such as hypothyroidism. Hypotonia accompanied by weakness indicates a neurological lesion below the level of the anterior-horn cells. Correct identification of the abnormality depends on associated findings about muscle mass and tone, reflexes and sensory function, or on the presence of certain abnormal movements such as fasciculation. The causes of hypotonia are listed in Tables XI and XII.

Hysteria and malingering

The differential diagnosis of true muscular weakness from that simulated by hysteria or malingering is notoriously difficult. True conscious malingering is much less common among children than adults, and every apparent case of malingering probably has in it an element of hysteria or some other psychological causation. Perhaps the best method of differentiating genuine from simulated paralysis is by observing the child's spontaneous movements in ordinary activities, particularly movements against gravity, when he is not aware that he is being observed. (Hysteria is much closer to genuine paralysis in its manifestations than malingering, so this test by observation is not always reliable.)

When examining muscle power, the examiner may gain the impression that the child is making little effort to execute the movements requested, and in some instances strong contraction of the opposing muscle group may be seen or palpated. (For example, it may be possible to palpate a contraction of the triceps as an antagonist to the biceps when the child is asked to flex the elbow.) Particularly characteristic is a tendency for a reasonable degree of muscle power to manifest itself before suddenly falling off. Another clue lies in the failure of the limb to 'follow through' by movement in the direction of action of the contracted muscle when the resistance of the examiner's hand is withdrawn. If the paralysis is hypotonic in nature, lifting a limb and suddenly dropping it will result in a completely limp fall of a flaccid extremity. Hysteria may be comparable, but in malingering the limb is dropped rather more slowly to avoid painful contact with the examination table or furniture. Certain muscles may be found to contract normally in reflex movement when they appear to be paralysed in voluntary action (for example, an apparently paralysed latissimus dorsi may contract during coughing). In hysterical hemiplegia, Hoover's sign may be helpful: the child lies on his back and the examiner places one hand under each of the patient's heels. The child is then asked to elevate the apparently paralysed lower extremity, keeping the knees extended. A child with a genuine hemiplegia is unable to do so, whereas the normal child will exert a strong counter-pressure with his heel against the examiner's hand. In the case of malingering, and in some examples of hysteria, there is no counter-pressure from the normal side, while downward pressure may be felt on the supposedly paralysed side. Though absence of the muscular wasting which accompanies profound paralysis may suggest malingering, there are several exceptions: acute paralysis produces wasting only after a period of a few weeks and hysterical paralysis can produce considerable muscular wasting if the limb is not used for a sufficient period of time. Alternatively, immobilization of a limb may lead to slight enlargement of the extremity with oedema, and trophic changes in the skin and nails.

Fasciculation

Fasciculation is defined as a rapid involuntary contraction of one or more motor units of a muscle, usually insufficient to produce movement of a joint but visible as a transient furrow in the skin overlying the muscle. It is presumed to be due to involuntary discharge of one or more motor units. Fasciculation is difficult to see in skeletal muscle if there is much subcutaneous fat. Coarse fasciculations are often repetitive in the same neurons. These may occur in normal muscle at times, especially with fatigue; similar coarse fasciculations may be encountered with imitative lesions of nerve roots.

Muscular weakness of localized or patchy distribution may point to an affection of some peripheral nerve, to a plexus lesion, or to involvement of some segment of spinal innervation (myotome). The manifestations of a brachial palsy depend on the level of injury to the brachial plexus. The most common cause of injury is traction at birth. In Erb's palsy (Fig. 30) there is injury to the upper trunk of the plexus, resulting in paralysis of the upper arm. The humerus is adducted and internally rotated; the elbow is extended, the forearm pronated and the wrist flexed. Injury to

79

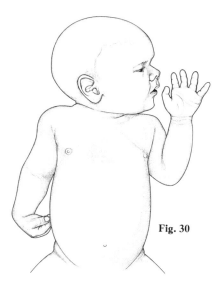

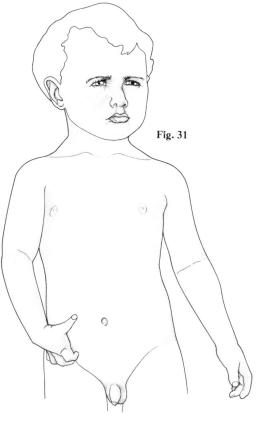

Fig. 31

Fig. 30. Erb's palsy. The arm is extended and adducted at the elbow, with the humerus internally rotated. The forearm is pronated and the wrist is flexed.

Fig. 30

Fig. 31. Klumpke paralysis associated with Horner syndrome. The typical Klumpke posture is for the elbow to be flexed, the forearm supinated and the wrist extended, with a clawlike deformity of the hand. The metacarpo-phalangeal joints are hyperextended. In Horner syndrome the pupil on the affected side is contracted.

the lower trunk of the plexus occurs rarely and causes Klumpke's paralysis (Fig. 31), a weakness of the extensors of the forearm and the flexors of the wrists and fingers. Involvement of sympathetic fibers in the injury may be shown by a Horner syndrome on the same side. A miotic pupil, mild ptosis and defective sweating on the affected side constitute the syndrome.

Muscular bulk

Clinical appraisal of muscular bulk inevitably is subjective and must be carried out by inspection and palpation, bearing in mind the normal standard expected for the patient's size, constitution and build. Estimation of muscle mass is especially difficult in obese children or in babies, who normally have thicker layers of sub-cutaneous fat. It is usually wise to confirm an impression of asymmetry by actual measurements of the circumference of the limbs. In the case of the calves, the largest circumferential measurement obtainable may be taken as a basis for comparison, but for the thighs, upper arms and forearms one should record the circumference at a measured distance from some bony landmark (the anterior superior iliac spine and the olecranon are suggested).

Atrophy and hemiatrophy

Atrophy or wasting may result from any affection of the lower motor unit, whether myopathy, abnormality of the neuromyal junction, peripheral neuropathy or disease of the anterior-horn cells. Wasting also occurs as a consequence of lesions of the upper motor neurons: in these circumstances it is usually less extreme, but the differences are relative and cannot be used on their own for differential diagnosis. Distinction rests rather on other observations, such as changes or asymmetry in tone and reflexes, associated sensory changes, the presence of fasciculations (which imply an irritative lesion of the lower motor unit), and often on electrical tests. Other possible causes of atrophy are disuse or immobilization, an effect of arthritis or other joint disease, and various nutritional and endocrine disturbances.

Hemiatrophy almost always is accompanied by neurological abnormality. Underdevelopment of bone, as well as muscle, is seen in many longstanding deficits of motor function acquired early in life. Unequal development of the legs, a shortening of one leg or reduction of muscle bulk in the calf or the thigh may be the first presenting sign of spinal dysraphism.

Hypertrophy, hemihypertrophy and pseudohypertrophy

Muscular hypertrophy is much less frequent than atrophy. True muscular hypertrophy may be functional in the case of children who are unusually athletic. Genuine muscular hypertrophy also is associated with myotonia congenita, but not with muscular dystrophy. Hypothyroidism also may cause muscle enlargement, but usually with reduced power and slowed contraction and relaxation.

Congenital hemihypertrophy, the counterpart of hemiatrophy, includes hypertrophy of other tissues as well as muscle in the affected areas (Table XIII, p. 97). Hemihypertrophy may be hemangiomatosis or lymphangiomatosis. It may involve a single digit, a single limb, unilateral face or half the body. Usually it affects more than one system, and is generally present from birth. Hemihypertrophy may have associated CNS findings of cerebral-hemisphere enlargement, mental retardation and seizure disorder. It is associated with a number of other anomalies in the Silver syndrome, and is more appropriately termed an asymmetry. Malignancy, especially a Wilms tumor, may be associated with hemihypertrophy. Other conditions occasionally associated are dizygous twinning and chromosomal anomalies.

Pseudohypertrophy often accompanies muscular dystrophy and especially affects the calves and the muscles of the shoulder girdle. It is not true hypertrophy (although biopsy shows some muscle fibres to be enlarged in diameter) but is the result of infiltration and replacement of muscular tissue by fat, giving an abnormally firm, rubbery feel on palpation. Pseudohypertrophy is most characteristic of the sex-linked recessive type of dystrophy beginning in early childhood (the Duchenne type), but a certain degree also occurs in other varieties of dystrophy, which probably explains the occasional reports of females with pseudohypertrophic muscular dystrophy. The 'miniature wrestler' syndrome describes a child with symmetrical hypertrophy of the muscles of the extremities, without appropriate muscle power. The condition is unusual and should be distinguished from storage disease and from muscle hypertrophy secondary to hypothyroidism.

81

Muscle tone

The word 'tone' is used by different authors in different ways. Thus, French authors who use the word 'tonus' mean something rather different from the word 'tone' used by English-language authors. For a discussion of this see *Locomotion from Pre- to Postnatal Life* (André-Thomas and Autgaerden 1966). In English, people refer to the hypertonic child, including in this description a stretch reflex which they have elicited, usually by using a patellar hammer to obtain a brisk reflex. It is better to restrict the use of 'tone' to the resistance felt by the examiner on passive movement of the limbs. The examiner assesses the resistance, and from his clinical experience builds up an idea of normal tone, as distinct from 'hypertonicity' or 'hypotonicity'. Recently it has become possible to measure this phenomenon more scientifically, but in clinical practice this is not yet commonly done (see Otis *et al.* 1983). The resistance of a limb to passive movement is affected not only by the muscles' state of reactivity but also by tendon and fascial connections which lie between the joints. In resting muscle no motor units may be firing, and following slow passive stretch no activity may be detected electromyographically, so presumably in these circumstances the resistance felt is simply a manifestation of the mechanical properties of the muscles and tendon alone. With more rapid movement, however, motor units are active, and actual contractural activity of the muscles affects the tone.

The ligaments of young children and infants are more relaxed than they become later, and in consequence the tone is lower than it is in older children and adults. Children respond differently than do adults to an examination, and the tone of infants below toddler-age has to be examined without their co-operation. However, the infant may also tolerate movements which would lead to muscle activity in an older child: thus one can flap the hand of an infant and observe that there is no development of increased tone in the flexors and extensors of the forearm.

Muscle tone is most easily assessed in the limbs, to which the examiner frequently restricts his examination. Tone may be assessed 'across' any movable joint or joints. It is relatively easy to move an infant's neck or to move a baby around the spinal axis, but obviously this becomes increasingly difficult as the child gets older and bigger. The limb should be moved slowly and then more rapidly, since types of movement yield several different responses (which have descriptive names). These include: *lead pipe* (rigidity) to slow and fast movement; *clasp knife* to fast movement; *cogwheel* to fast movement; *waxy* to slow and fast movement.

In general, slow, smooth, passive motion will produce less resistance in a spastic extremity than will fast movement. The response in a child with normal muscle tone is consistent, regardless of speed, unless resistance is voluntary.

Tone may vary over a short or longer period of time. Classically the child with athetoid cerebral palsy has fluctuating tone which varies from moment to moment. In other conditions tone changes much more slowly; a small baby may be floppy, but over the first two years tone may increase to such an extent that spastic diplegia is recognized. Abnormal tone may be generalized throughout the body or limited to one portion only.

Muscle tone is strikingly diminished if afferent proprioceptive input to the spinal cord is interrupted by involvement of the peripheral nerves, dorsal-root ganglia, dorsal roots or root zones and posterior columns. This interruption of the afferent arc of the stretch reflex is a major component of the hypotonicity of peripheral neuropathy and is the chief explanation in such conditions as tabes dorsalis and Friedreich's ataxia.

Lesions of the basal ganglia or at other extrapyramidal levels may be associated with hypotonicity or with hypertonicity of the rigid type. The 'cog-wheel' phenomenon seen in adults with Parkinsonism also occurs occasionally in postencephalitic states in children. Rigid hypertonus may be accompanied by limitation of range of motion, but usually the characteristic contractures of long-standing spasticity are lacking. However, positionally induced contractures are common among non-walking individuals who spend all their time in a sitting or recumbent posture. General slowing of movement or loss of associated movements are also characteristic of extrapyramidal hypertonus, but tendon reflexes are scarcely (if at all) exaggerated and may be suppressed by the hypertonicity.

Voluntary and hysterical rigidity are difficult to distinguish from pathological organic rigidity. The hypertonus may be bizarre in character or distribution, or may simulate any other recognized type of hypertonus. Opisthotonus (*arc de cercle*) was considered to be a major feature of classical hysteria. Apprehension (with resultant muscular tension and a constant or variable reinforcement maneuver) may produce exaggerated tendon reflexes, even though the rigidity is voluntary or hysterical.

Catatonic rigidity resembles extrapyramidal rigidity in some ways, and manipulation of the limbs gives a feeling of resistance of the 'lead-pipe' or 'waxy' type (*flexibilitas cerea*) described above. In catalepsy, episodic suspension of voluntary movement and generalized rigidity may be paroxysmal. More prolonged catatonia, with the limbs staying in whatever position they are placed by the examiner, may occur following administration of certain drugs, notably the fluorinated phenothiazines.

Reflex rigidity is a spasm of skeletal muscle induced by sensory irritation, usually by pain. The muscles are shortened and hypertonic, and usually tender. The signs of meningeal irritation fall into this category.

Myotonia is a type of hypertonicity of peripheral origin, associated either with hyperexcitability of the motor endplate, with abnormal neuromuscular transmission and a defect of the normal phase of relaxation, or perhaps with abnormality in the muscle itself, with continued contraction of myofibrils once depolarization has taken place.

Myotonia is increased by anxiety, cold or forced effort and is diminished by procaine amide or quinine. If accompanied by muscular hypertrophy and good muscle power it suggests myotonia congenita, whereas in myotonic dystrophy there is muscular wasting and weakness (as well as other associated findings). It should be mentioned that the myotatic response to percussion is also exaggerated in tetany, tetanus and myxedema.

Juvenile myasthenia gravis
The juvenile form of myasthenia gravis can occur as early as one year of age, but commonly it is not identified before the age of seven. The presenting symptoms are

generalized weakness, fatigue, muscular fatiguability, unilateral or bilateral ptosis, and ocular, facial and limb weakness. Dysarthria may be present in the oropharyngeal form. Deep tendon reflexes are intact. Usually the weakness is least obvious in the morning, but it can vary from hour to hour and day to day. A respiratory illness may exacerbate the symptoms, which generally are progressive over several weeks. Often the change in the child's facial expression is apparent to the family and may have been documented in photographs, so inspection of photographs taken in earlier years would eliminate congenital ptosis and pre-existing facial weakness. Ocular symptoms alone are unusual in children. The degree of weakness is out of proportion to the child's previous skills and mental abilities.

A careful baseline assessment of the child's muscle power should be made before the first administration of intravenous edrophonium chloride ('Tensilon')*. The response is never as dramatic if the test is repeated the same day. The length of time the child is able to stand with outstretched arms and the duration of unblinking upward gaze should be recorded before and after edrophonium chloride has been given. In addition, if the equipment is available it is advisable to measure peak expiratory flow-rate and the lungs' vital capacity. A child with myasthenia gravis will show improvement in muscle power, including disappearance of ptosis, within 30 to 60 seconds (Fig. 32).

Muscular dystrophy

Muscular dystrophy is a cause of hypotonia and muscle weakness in childhood. The term includes various types of muscle weakness which are inherited and which are characterized by progressive degeneration of skeletal muscle, without evidence of structural abnormality in the peripheral nerves or the central nervous system. The most common form, inherited as a sex-linked recessive trait, is the severe, progressive, pelvi-femoral weakness known as the Duchenne type. The diagnosis of Duchenne muscular dystrophy is rarely made before the age of 2½ years, unless there is already an affected child in the family.

A boy with early signs of progressive muscular dystrophy will appear to be clumsy and will fall suddenly and frequently. His activity will be more circumscribed than is normal for his age. Although deterioration in motor skills may not occur until mid or late childhood, new skills are not acquired. He may learn to ride a tricycle, for example, but he will never be able to master a bicycle. Very early signs may be hard to evaluate unless there is a positive family history, and more than one visit may be necessary to judge the progress of symptoms and make a definite diagnosis.

The boy may look muscular, but his diminished strength is not in proportion to muscle bulk. Pseudohypertrophy of the calves is a common finding. There is a lumbar lordosis and a tendency toward spontaneous equinus posture of the feet. Eventually, shortening of the Achilles tendon develops. Because the weakness affects the gluteal muscles, the boy has much greater difficulty in going up steps or rising from the floor than he does in walking. When getting up from the floor, he has difficulty in extending the pelvis on the femora, and may give a push on one knee with a hand, or

*For details of administration, see Chapter 11.

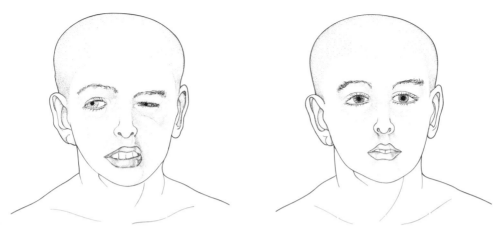

Fig. 32. Myasthenia gravis, before and after drug treatment. Before treatment the child cannot open his eyes when trying to follow the examiner's hand moving in front of him.

get the trunk erect by a series of movements of the hands up the thighs—'climbing up the legs', or the Gower sign (Fig. 33). This last-mentioned phenomenon is by no means specific for muscular dystrophy: it can also be seen in children with polymyositis, old poliomyelitis, Guillain-Barré syndrome or any other condition which produces considerable weakness of the gluteal muscles.

Weakness always occurs in the proximal muscles before the distal ones, and the muscle of the pelvic girdle are affected more than the scapulohumeral group. The knee-jerk and upper-arm reflexes disappear early in the disease but the ankle jerk persists. Often mental retardation is an incidental finding, but the exact relationship between it and muscular dystrophy is unclear (see Leibowitz and Dubowitz 1981).

After the clinical examination has shown that muscle weakness and clinical findings are compatible with the Duchenne type of muscular dystrophy rather than any of the other causes of muscle weakness and hypotonia (see Tables XI and XII), special studies must be done, preferably in a medical center where expert interpretation is available. Progressive spinal muscular atrophy, some of the congenital myopathies and dermatomyositis may resemble muscular dystrophy in its early stage. Serum creatinine phosphokinase (CPK) is markedly elevated in the early stages of Duchenne muscular dystrophy. A diagnosis can be established in a child at risk (belonging to a family known to have the disease) by the finding of a very high level of CPK in cord blood. A two- to five-fold increase in CPK levels is found in 70 per cent of known carriers (Moosa 1974). Electromyograms show the small, splintered, polyphasic action potential characteristic of all myopathies. Nerve conduction velocities usually are within the normal range. Muscle biopsy is characteristic and shows a random mixture of fibers of small and large diameters, and replacement of muscle tissue with fat.

Other milder forms of muscular dystrophy are the limb-girdle type and the rare scapulohumeral type, both of which have milder symptoms, slower progress and are inherited as autosomal recessive traits. One symptom of facioscapulohumeral

85

dystrophy is facial weakness, which may precede the scapulohumeral involvement. It is inherited as a dominant trait, produces minimal disability, and is compatible with a normal life-span.

Myotonic dystrophy

This condition used to be thought to have an onset in late childhood or adult life, but it is now recognized that it may occur in infancy and early childhood. It is a cause of weakness in childhood which may go unrecognized unless another member of the family is affected. The first presenting sign may be inability to release a grasp, and facial weakness, ptosis and sternocleidomastoid weakness are consistent early features. There is generalized hypotonia and muscle weakness and a characteristic myopathic facial expression, with a triangular-shaped mouth. Developmental delay and mental retardation are common.

One means of diagnosis is through observation of the mother or father, who may have the characteristic facies or some subclinical evidence of myotonia, such as the inability to close the eyes completely or the 'slow release' of hand grasp. Myotonic dystrophy is inherited as an autosomal dominant trait.

EXAMINATION OF THE REFLEXES

Directions

The standard deep tendon reflexes (biceps jerk, triceps jerk, knee jerk, ankle jerk) should be tested when the child is relaxed and comfortable and sitting symmetrically with the head in midline. Percuss the tendon in the proper place and note the speed, vigor and amplitude of the response, the range of movement produced and the duration of the contraction. Any duplication of the movement or clonus should also be noted. The response is conveniently graded as follows: 0 = absent; ± or Tr

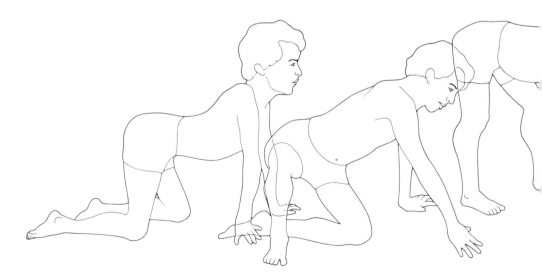

(trace) = very faint visible or palpable contraction but no movement; 1+ = hypo-active; 2+ = normal; 3+ = hyperactive; 4+ = hyperactive and reduplicated, inducing clonus.

Palpate the reacting muscle, since some reflexes normally produce a muscular contraction which can only be felt, with little or no visible joint movement. Hypoactive reflexes may also produce palpable contraction, even though no movement of the joint is elicited.

If reflexes in the lower extremity are hypoactive or absent, attempt to 'reinforce' them by having the child execute the Jendrassik maneuver—gripping the flexed tips of the fingers of each hand with those of the opposite hand and pulling with one hand against the other. If the child does not understand this, a comparable result can be achieved by having him make a vigorous fist with each hand.

Have the child place his arms comfortably on his lap in a semi-pronated position. Test the biceps jerk by tapping a reflex hammer against your finger or thumb placed on the insertion of the biceps tendon. Take the child's wrist in one hand, gently flex his arm, and tap the triceps tendon just above the olecranon. Test the knee jerk by tapping the semi-flexed knee just below the patella in the midline. Test the ankle jerk

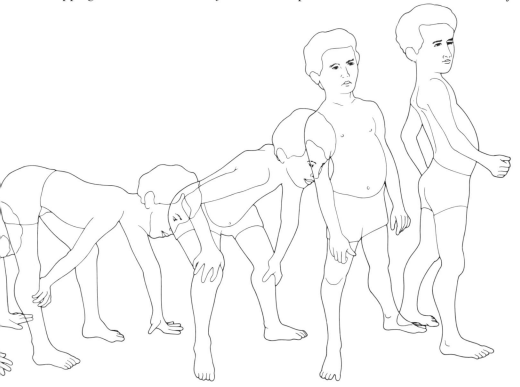

Fig. 33. Gower sign, a maneuver indicating weakness of the pelvic girdle, lumbosacral spine and shoulder girdle, used in getting up from the floor. The child positions his knees so he can put his hands on them and push himself up with his arms, keeping his legs wide apart to maintain balance because of lordosis and pelvic girdle weakness. The calves are enlarged because of pseudohypertrophy.

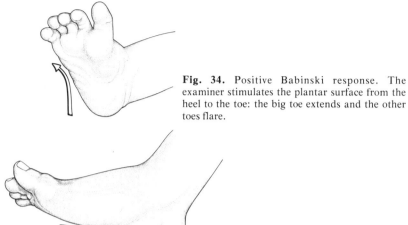

Fig. 34. Positive Babinski response. The examiner stimulates the plantar surface from the heel to the toe: the big toe extends and the other toes flare.

by holding the child's foot in a neutral position and tapping the Achilles tendon above its insertion at the calcaneus. This may be done with the child kneeling on a chair (Paine and Oppé 1966). Test for ankle clonus (regular jerky contractions of the calf muscles) by holding the child's lower leg with one hand and dorsiflexing the child's foot abruptly with the other.

Test for the presence of the Babinski sign by applying forward pressure with your thumbnail, the edge of a knitting needle, or a key along the lateral border of the sole, crossing over the distal ends of the metatarsals toward the base of the great toe. A clear, consistent, isolated dorsiflexion of the great toe is a positive response (Fig. 34).

Discussion

Tendon reflexes

In order to classify reflexes as normal, exaggerated or depressed, the examiner must be familiar with the standard of normal for the different reflexes, some of which require livelier action than others in order to be classified as normal. For example, the biceps jerk is often more vigorous than the triceps, but each would be graded 2+ if considered normal for itself. There is also variation with age. In infants under a month of age the predominant flexor tone of early infancy almost invariably suppresses the triceps jerk entirely, and the ankle jerk may be feeble and difficult to obtain. The strong flexor tone of the upper extremity may also suppress the biceps jerk unless it is repeatedly and patiently tested. Young children often are relatively hypotonic and their reflexes may be depressed in comparison with adult standards. If all the reflexes are proportionately hypoactive, yet present and symmetrical, one would record the findings as seen (1+ but not 2+) but accept them as normal in the absence of indications to the contrary. Other children, chiefly older ones, may have universal and symmetrical hyperactive reflexes, which again should be regarded as normal if there are no other findings and if the superficial reflexes and plantar responses are also normal. Hyperreflexia assumes greater significance in the presence of pathological reflexes which are referrable to pyramidal abnormality.

The deep tendon reflexes may be somewhat increased in diseases of the extra-pyramidal systems, but it is with pyramidal involvement (or with the clinically consistent combination of pyramidal and extrapyramidal affection which produces spasticity) that hyperreflexia is most striking. The reflexes may be exaggerated, and additional evidence is provided by their being obtainable from a larger than normal afferent zone or by their spread to include other muscles, such as spread of the knee jerk to include contraction of the adductors of the hip. The knee jerk and adductor jerk may both show a crossed spread to the opposite side up to the age of eight months, or possibly a year. After that age the crossed adductor response (a reflex adduction of the opposite thigh) indicates spastic cerebral palsy.

Affections of the upper motor neurons typically produce hyperreflexia, but pure pyramidal lesions or the mysterious group of hypotonic cerebral palsies may be associated with depressed or absent reflexes. Lesions of the anterior lobe of the cerebellum produce hypotonia and hyporeflexia, and certain reflexes are pendulous if elicitable. Sometimes reflexes also are absent in cerebellar disease, but this may be because the extreme hypotonia makes it difficult to get the tendon sufficiently tense to stretch it by tapping it with a hammer.

The Babinski sign

In 1896 Joseph Babinski described events which follow stimulation of the sole of an adult's foot. Ordinarily there are reflex movements consisting of flexion of the toes, foot and thigh. If a normal adult stays immobile, stimulation of the sole of the foot is not associated with movements of the toes towards extension. In certain pathological states, however, stimulation of the sole evokes extension of the toes, particularly of the great toe. The abnormal extensor response is executed more slowly than the normal flexion response and is most pronounced in the great and second toes. Flexion is stronger if the inner part of the sole of the normal adult is stimulated than if the same stimulus is applied to the outer part. The opposite is true of the extensor response. Babinski also observed that the response is best elicited when the leg is slightly flexed and the stimulus is applied after the muscles appear well relaxed. A positive response occurs in both the adult and infantile forms of hemiplegia and is associated with an organic lesion of the central nervous system. It can be observed in some subjects with hemiplegia, following stimulation of the toes of the unaffected side. Babinski reported its occurrence in cases of acute myelomeningoencephalitis, immediately after a grand mal seizure, in various forms of spinal paralysis, and in Friedreich's disease. He noted too that it did not occur in cases of hysteria, pro-gressive myopathy or poliomyelitis. He associated the phenomena of the toes with disturbances of the pyramidal tract, which were unrelated to the duration, intensity or extent of the paralysis or injury.

These observations have been variously described as the Babinski phenomenon, response or reflex. From quite early it was recognized that an extensor response was normally present before an infant learned to walk independently. A fetus as early as four to six months can show similar extensor responses. Transecting the cord during fetal life, however, converts the extensor plantar response into the flexor form. In the immediate neonatal period it is possible to obtain both extensor and flexor responses of the toes. After about 10 days of age the responses usually are symmetrical and extensor in nature. A bilateral response of the toes can be obtained by stimulation of either thigh, the abdomen or the upper chest (Brain and Wilkinson 1959). The response may be either extensor or flexor if it is elicited from these higher levels. After three weeks of age the receptive field shrinks progressively and after eight months of age tends to be limited only to the side stimulated. (Observe Botticelli's *Madonna and Child with Angels, c.*1468: Cone and Khoshbin 1970.)

The effects of supraspinal centers on the Babinski sign remain poorly understood. For example, a child who is known to have hemiplegia and a positive Babinski may not have this evidence of a pyramidal-tract injury during recovery from anesthesia or during a serious systemic illness. During natural non-REM sleep the Babinski response persists in patients with lesions affecting the pyramidal tracts, and during REM sleep the reponse is less consistent. It is now believed that the Babinski sign is mediated by the extensor hallucis longus (not the brevis) and can be demonstrated by electromyography.

If the pyramidal tract has been injured, the rising movement of the great toe and fanning of the other toes may be elicited in the following ways (the name of the 'sign' is shown in parentheses): (1) percussion of the great toe or stroking the plantar surface of the great toe (Rossolimo); (2) flexion of one of the outer toes (Gonda); (3) stimulation of the medial aspect of the distal tibia (Oppenheim); (4) stimulation of the dorsum of the foot with a pin (Bing); (5) kneading the gastrocnemius (Gordon); (6) squeezing the achilles tendon (Schaefer); (7) stroking the lateral side of the ankle (Chaddock); (8) plantar flexion of the foot at the ankle (Moniz); (9) stimulation of the metatarsophalangeal region (Throckmorton); (10) single percussion of the plantar surface about the middle of the sole (Zhakovski, also Jonkovski); and many others.

In interpreting an apparent Babinski sign it must also be noted that the response is closely mimicked by one phase of athetosis of the foot. A child with what is thought to be clear extrapyramidal disease should not be said to have a Babinski sign unless the examiner is confident that stimulation in the conventional manner will produce a more dramatically abnormal response than that which the child produces spontaneously in his writhing or as a result of cutaneous stimulation almost anywhere on the body.

A Babinski sign is seen in a significant minority of patients with muscular dystrophy, a fact which is not easy to explain. It may be attributable to weakness of plantar flexors of the great toe in comparison with dorsiflexors, in view of the greater involvement of the muscles of the calf in pseudohypertrophic dystrophy. The available power for plantar flexion and dorsiflexion of the great toe should always be tested objectively in the case of patients who 'ought to have a Babinski but do not', or who present the response as an unexpected or inconsistent finding.

TESTING SENSATION

Testing the hands, feet and the three divisions of the trigeminal nerve for sensory response to touch is satisfactory for screening purposes. Although response to pin-prick is easier to interpret, the procedure might destroy a rapport which has been carefully established, and the examiner must judge whether it is warranted. Testing for sense of vibration and position should also be done.

Complete sensory examination of the entire body is rarely indicated unless the history or other physical findings particularly suggest sensory deficit, lesions of the peripheral nerves or a spinal condition. Routine sensory examination of young children is unrewarding, however. If sensory mapping is indicated, a separate examination should be scheduled. (See next section for details.)

Directions

Demonstrate testing for touch and pain (if appropriate) while the child has his eyes open. For touch, use a piece of cotton and ask the child to say 'Now' whenever his skin is touched. Test pain by using a safety-pin, using the sharp and blunt ends in random sequence and asking the child to distinguish between 'sharp' and 'dull'. After the demonstration ask the child to close his eyes, and then test the hands, feet, cheekbones and mandibles.

Test for sense of vibration by using a tuning fork. Ask the child to tell you if the tuning fork is vibrating or still when the stem end is applied to the finger joints. Repeat the procedure, applying the fork to the great toe and then the lateral and medial malleoli. He may keep his eyes open, but obviously he should not look at the fork.

Test for sense of position by asking the child to close his eyes and to indicate whether a finger or toe is moved up or down.

Discussion

Appreciation of pain is more easily demonstrated than perception of touch. Proper identification of the sharp or dull end of a pin enables the examiner to tell whether the child is sensitive to pain or touch. This requires cortical discrimination and tests additional functions, but success in sharp-dull discrimination does at least require intact perception of pain.

Since the tests outlined for sense of vibration and position require for the most part a discriminative answer by the child, they depend on integrity of the entire proprioceptive pathway, including some cortical function in the parietal lobes. It is not surprising, therefore, that children with signs and symptoms associated with the parietal lobes sometimes show defective perception of passive movement or position. The majority of such children probably suffer from a deficit of cerebral integration and gnosis rather than from actual impaired proprioception. Children with spastic hemiparesis frequently have defects of cerebral sensory function in the affected hand, but stereognosis is affected far more frequently than position or passive movement, and the proprioceptive functions are probably never abnormal if these are intact.

An isolated abnormal response to the testing of sense of position means very little, except that the child may be tired or confused. However, if there are other suspicious clinical findings, a degenerative condition involving the posterior columns, such as Friedreich's ataxia, must be considered. In these degenerative conditions of the posterior columns, sense of position and passive movement is diminished in the toes earlier than in the fingers. The examiner may need to use quite small increments of movement in order to avoid missing a subtle deficit. If sense of position or vibration appears to be absent in the fingers or toes, these sensations should then be tested at the wrist and ankle, or elbow and knee, in order to follow the progress of the condition in serial examinations. However, the earliest involvement of these modalities is always distal.

SENSORY MAPPING

Description

Sensory mapping is a systematic, detailed search for areas of analgesia which correspond to the distribution of the peripheral nerves or segmented sensory levels. Complete sensory mapping requires obtaining responses to pain, touch and temperature, but with infants and young children, response to pain may be the only one that can be measured.

Principal uses

Sensory mapping is difficult and time-consuming, and several evaluations may be necessary, but it should be attempted for all children with a myelomeningocele, and when a spinal lesion or a peripheral neuropathy are suspected.

Method

Pain (by pin-prick), and if possible touch and temperature, are tested by applying stimuli at intervals of about an inch along imaginary lines drawn down the anterior, posterior, lateral and medial axes of the limbs (and in the case of larger children, down four additional axes placed midway between those). The points used for examining the trunk may be more widely spaced. Any area of hypasthesia or hypalgesia (or of hyperasthesia if there is exaggerated reaction to sensory stimulation) should be mapped out as completely as possible by marking its boundary on the skin with a pen. Because of the effect of spatial or temporal summation, errors and misinterpretation inevitably arise. Successive stimulations should be made from the hypasthetic area toward the normal area, but the approach should also be reversed in order to evaluate the possible effects of summation.

Results

The result of sensory mapping should be compared with the known distribution of cutaneous nerves and with the arrangement of the spinal dermatomes (Fig. 35 and 36) in order to try to localize the lesion responsible. However, caution is necessary since there is considerable anatomical variation among normal individuals in the location of the boundaries of peripheral nerve-supply and spinal dermatomes. For example, the ulnar nerve may supply only the palmar aspect of the fifth finger and ulnar border of the hand, or it may supply half or more of the fourth finger, with a correspondingly greater extension over the dorsal and palmar surface of the hand. The cutaneous dermatomes also show some variation.

The dermatomes overlap to a considerable degree, possibly so much so that the distribution of T4 might be completely duplicated between the inferior distribution of T3 and the superior T5. Overlapping is less extensive in the case of the peripheral nerves, but as one approaches the boundary of an area of sensory deficit it is common to find a gradual shading off of anesthesia into hypasthesia.

In a search for spinal lesions, segmental sensory levels should be compared with the segmental innervation of any paralysed or paretic muscles and with any localizing signs referrable to the autonomic nervous system. If these coincide, one's attention is directed to a particular spinal level, but it must be recognized that in the presence of extensive lesions such as myelomeningoceles, often the motor and sensory findings are irregular and inconsistent. In attempting to localize lesions along the vertebral column, it is important to remember that the cord is higher than the bones. In adults and in children above eight years of age, the first cervical spinal segment is at the level of the body of the first cervical vertebra, the first thoracic segment is slightly above the upper margin of the first thoracic vertebra, the first lumbar spinal segment is opposite the top of the body of the 10th thoracic vertebra, and the first sacral segment is opposite the body of the 12th thoracic vertebra, the cord ending at the lower margin of the first lumbar vertebra. The position of the spinal cord is relatively lower in infants and young children, but even in the newborn the tip of the cord is no farther down than the third lumbar vertebra. Thus, one might reasonably make a downward adjustment of two vertebrae in infants up to six months of age, and of one-and-a-half or one vertebrae between that age and five years.

Discordant or dissociated deficits with respect to pain, temperature and touch are also important. If loss of appreciation of pain and temperature in an area of the upper extremity is accompanied by retention of sense of touch, it suggests syringomyelia, in which the pathways for pain and temperature are interrupted at their decussation in the ventral cord. Some dissociation of sensory deficit may also occur with insults to peripheral nerves.

Limitations

Inconsistency between one examination and another is normal to a much greater degree in children than in adults, and even greater inconsistency must be anticipated if the examination has had to be carred out by pin-prick, using crying as a criterion of sensation. Peripheral neuropathies often chiefly involve the more distal distribution of the nerves and there may be 'glove and stocking' distribution of analgesia or anesthesia, which fades through an area of hypasthesia into normality without a sharply definable border. This distribution is just as characteristic of polyneuropathy as it is of hysteria, although the latter is likely to be suspected first by the inexperienced examiner. Highly inconsistent findings from one examination to another indeed are typical of hysterical anesthesia, although the borders of the anesthetic zone are likely to be sharply defined on each individual test. Apparent hemianesthesia ending precisely at the midline (organic anesthesia ends a bit short of this line), or a

93

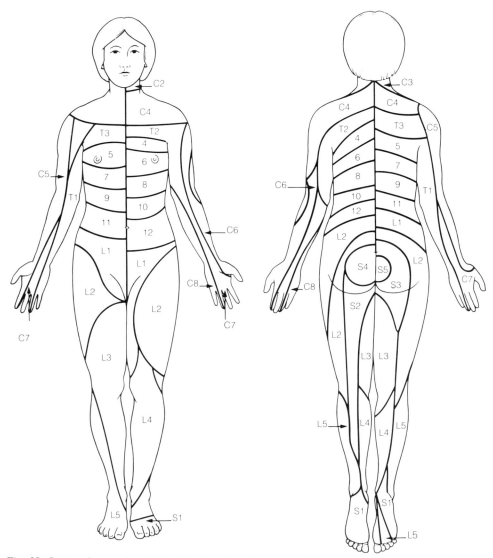

Fig. 35. Sensory innervation of the skin by spinal dermatomes. The usual maximal areas of the odd-numbered segments are shown on the right side of the body, the even-numbered on the left. There is some variation from person to person, and considerable overlapping of dermatomes is normal; *e.g.* the area of T8 is almost completely duplicated by the lower part of T7 and the upper part of T9.

sharp level for absence of sense of vibration in the middle of a bone, may suggest that the sensory deficit is feigned or hysterical. However, children are more guileless than adults and usually it is easy for an experienced examiner to detect a malingering child. However, frank malingering is rare among children, and hysteria often resembles organic disease much more closely than it does malingering. Study of the galvanic skin-response and other procedures for assessing autonomic function of the nerves may help in evaluating sensory neuropathies.

94

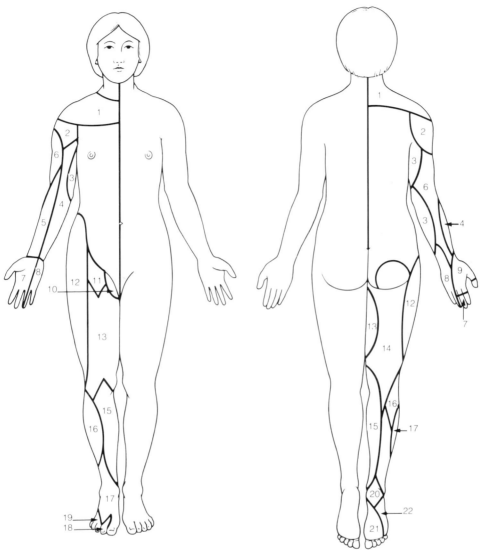

Fig. 36. Sensory innervation of the skin of the upper and lower extremities. 1 = supraclavicular; 2 = axillary; 3 = medial brachial cutaneous; 4 = medial antibrachial cutaneous; 5 = lateral antibrachial cutaneous; 6 = dorsal antibrachial cutaneous; 7 = median; 8 = ulnar; 9 = radial; 10 = ilioinguinal; 11 = lumboinguinal; 12 = lateral femoral cutaneous; 13 = anterior femoral cutaneous; 14 = posterior femoral cutaneous; 15 = saphenous; 16 = common peroneal; 17 = superficial peroneal; 18 = deep peroneal; 19 = sural; 20 = tibial; 21 = medial plantar; 22 = lateral plantar.

CHAPTER 6

Examination of the Trunk, Posture and Gait

Directions

Ask the child to lie down, to roll onto his stomach and try to relax. Look carefully at the body proportions and for any asymmetry. Inspect the skin for unusual pigmentation, nevi, or evidence of injuries (see Chapter 4). Inspect the spine for scoliosis at rest, and for obvious meningoceles, myelomeningoceles or operative scars which could indicate their removal. In the case of unoperated lesions, illumination with a flashlight may help to estimate the extent to which nervous tissue is involved in the sac. Examine carefully any cutaneous dimples, tufts of hair or openings of sinus tracts overlying the spine, since often these are accompanied by intraspinal abnormalities. (Low sacral pilonidal dimples or sinuses are usually benign.) Palpate the spine for missing or malformed vertebrae and for localized tenderness. Put one hand on the child's pelvis and lift each leg, estimating power, resistance, and symmetry of response. Ask the child to raise each leg above the level of the table.

Ask the child then to roll onto his back. Look again for evidence of asymmetry or unusual body proportions. Test the superficial abdominal reflexes while the child is relaxed, by lightly scratching the abdominal wall on each side above, level with and below the umbilicus. Palpate the abdomen in the usual manner. Place one hand under the child's occiput, flex the neck and let the head drop back into the other hand. Slowing of the reaction could indicate flexor hypertonus in the musculature of the neck. Flex, extend and rotate the neck, looking for limitation of motion.

Mark each iliac crest and medial malleolus symmetrically. Measure the length of each leg from the iliac crest to the medial malleolus. Flex and extend the upper leg. Evaluate the child's hip-joint by placing one hand on the joint to fix the pelvis and the other under the child's flexed knee. Test abduction, adduction and rotation. Have the child rest comfortably with his arms at his sides, and ask him to slide his right heel down his left shin from the knee to the ankle. Repeat with the left heel down the right shin.

Discussion

Midline spinal defects

Various overlapping terminologies are used to describe midline defects in the spine. The term spinal dysraphism describes malformations of any or all tissues in the midline of the back, including diastematomyelia, dermal sinus, dermal cysts and lipoma formation, but excludes meningocele and myelomeningocele (Till 1968). Spina bifida occulta is the proper term for missing spinous processes. These may be accompanied by hair or dermal sinus but have no nervous-system involvement. If nerve roots are involved, as in diastematomyelia or intraspinal lipoma, the appropriate term is myelodysplasia with spina bifida. The term myelodysplasia

TABLE XIII
Differential diagnosis of hemihypertrophy

Beckwith-Wiedemann syndrome	Russell-Silver syndrome
Klippel-Trenaunay-Weber syndrome	A-V aneurysm
Langer-Giedion syndrome	Congenital lymphemia
Maffucci syndrome	Facial tumors
McCune-Albright syndrome	Multiple exostoses
Ollier syndrome	Neurofibromatosis

includes myelomeningocele but excludes meningoceles, which do not have nervous tissues. A subcutaneous lipoma with a dimple usually indicates spinal-cord involvement.

Scoliosis in the prone position

Scoliosis, present in the prone position as well as when the child bends forward and during standing, is always structural in origin.

Asymmetry of the limbs

Hemiplegia is the most likely cause of asymmetry of the limbs of a child referred for neurological examination. The tendency for one lower limb to fall into external rotation at the hip in the supine position, with the foot pointing laterally, is a sensitive sign of hemiparesis. Inequality of leg length or reduction of muscle bulk can be caused by myelodysplasia. (See Chapter 5 for a discussion of the causes of asymmetry and hemihypertrophy, and see Table XIII.)

Abdominal reflexes

Depression of the superficial abdominal reflexes, in association with exaggerated deep tendon reflexes, is an important sign of pyramidal-tract lesions. Exaggeration of the superficial reflexes usually is not significant; often it is merely the result of extreme ticklishness, but it can also occur with psychogenic disorders. It is unusual for superficial reflexes to be affected in cerebellar disease. The abdominal reflexes may be depressed for other reasons, including poor relaxation of the abdominal muscles, acute surgical abdominal problems, distension of the bladder or nearness to the site of an old surgical incision. They may also be missing in the very obese child, and even when the abdominal wall is relaxed, as, for example, in a child who has had nephrosis and ascites. Occasionally, retention of the upper abdominal reflexes and absent lower reflexes may indicate the level of a spinal lesion. Abdominal reflexes become symmetrical again soon after most infantile hemiplegias and are of less diagnostic value than in young or middle-aged adults.

The knee-heel test

The knee-heel test should be performed smoothly by a child over six years of age. A child with a minor neurological dysfunction often has difficulty performing the test at first, but will improve considerably with practice. However, a child with a degenerative disease of the nervous system or a cerebellar lesion usually continues to have difficulty.

EXAMINATION OF THE CHILD STANDING

Directions

Ask the child to sit up, without using his hands if possible. Have him get up, unassisted if possible, and stand. Observe the posture and look carefully for indications of unsteadiness, scoliosis, kyphosis and lordosis. Test the flexibility of the spine in flexion and extension and laterally. Have the child bend over and relax, with the arms dangling. Stand at the child's head and look for a straight spine, without lateral curvature or rotation. Look at the bending child from the side and make sure there is smooth curvature of the spine from the neck to the buttocks. Kyphosis would show up as a sharp angulation.

Ask the child to straighten up, place his feet together and extend his arms, palms down, while you count to 10. Look for a tendency for him to sway or fall and be aware of any consistent direction of the fall. If possible, have the child repeat the test with his eyes closed. Ask him to open his eyes and stand first on one foot and then on the other for 10 seconds each. Have him repeat the test with his eyes closed. Ask him to walk along a previously marked line on the floor (preferably the line should be at least 2.5m (8ft) in length). Have him walk the line again, this time putting the heel of one foot in front of the toes of the other. Ask him to walk backwards along the line. Have him hop a short distance forward on one leg and hop back on the other. During all these tests look for ease of performance and be aware of any unusual abnormal associated movements. (Age norms are given in Table XIV.)

If the child is old enough to do so, ask him to dress or undress himself, and observe the independence, co-ordination and skill exhibited. If the history and examination done thus far indicate the need, observe the child as he climbs stairs or walks a longer distance.

Discussion

Station and posture

The term 'station' refers to the child's posture when standing. 'Posture' describes the position or attitude of the body erect, sitting or recumbent.

Whatever the cause and whether primarily neuromuscular or not, muscular weakness may be sufficient in itself to cause an abnormality of station which closely resembles genuine ataxia. The picture can include swaying from side to side, trembling, some flexion of the hips and knees, and a tendency to seek support from furniture. Painful falls may also occur.

Although normal children from one to three or four years of age have a considerable tendency to exaggerated lumbar lordosis and a pot-bellied appearance, this stance is exaggerated by weakness of the muscles around the hip joints, as in muscular dystrophy. (The possibility of non-neurological causes should also be considered, such as bilateral dislocation of the hips, enlarged abdominal organs, ascites, coeliac syndrome, and so on.) The characteristic abnormal postures of the trunk and extremities in pyramidal and extrapyramidal syndromes may be detectable from observation of the standing child, but become more obvious during appraisal of gait.

98

TABLE XIV

Age at acquisition of motor skills

	Age (yrs)*
Stand with feet together, arms outstretched: eyes open	4
eyes closed	6
Stand on either foot, arms as desired: eyes open	5
eyes closed	9
(Examiner counts to 10)	
Finger-to-finger: eyes open	3
eyes closed	6
Three consecutive hops on either foot	5
Walk heel-to-toe for two meters	5

*The ages given are approximate. It is important to note *how* the task is done (symmetry, skill in performance, ability to follow directions and so on).

Scoliosis

Scoliosis can be both non-structural and structural. The non-structural type is secondary to posture, muscle spasm or inequality of leg length. There is no axial rotation. In structural scoliosis there is rotation which is visible on bending and on radiological examination. The bodies of the vertebral segments rotate toward the convexity of the curve, while the spines rotate toward the concavity of the curve.

If it begins in adolescence, scoliosis is very likely to be idiopathic. If present in a younger child, a bony anomaly should be suspected and roentgenograms obtained. Scoliosis may also result from poliomyelitis (recognized or unrecognized) or any other disease producing muscular weakening. Sooner or later it occurs in most cases of Friedreich's ataxia, and may be the earliest presenting sign. Its presence also indicates the possibility of neurofibromata of the intercostal nerves, or of intraspinal tumor. The latter more commonly causes tenderness and stiffness.

Kyphosis

Kyphosis may be a manifestation of vertebral anomalies such as platybasia or of certain birth-defects, including the mucolipidoses and the mucopolysaccharidoses. The term 'gibbus' is used to describe kyphosis with a lateral curve (*e.g.* kyphoscoliosis). Detection of a gibbous spine indicates the need to search for vertebral disease such as tuberculosis.

Sprengel deformity

Asymmetry of the scapulae, with one scapula higher than normal and accompanied on that side by impaired abduction and elevation of the shoulder, suggests the Sprengel deformity. Sometimes this abnormality is associated with scoliosis, torticollis and Klippel-Feil syndrome. It may be caused by an embryonic defect in the development of the scapular musculature.

Ataxia

Instability of standing posture which is not attributable to muscular weakness (proven by objective testing) is usually the result of ataxia. The term 'ataxia' implies an inco-ordination of cerebellar or sensory origin.

Sometimes it is difficult to distinguish true ataxia from mere clumsiness. The decision must be made with reference to the standard of normal gross-motor, fine-motor and visual-motor co-ordination for the child's age and mental ability (retarded children generally are clumsier than normal children), and to the range of normal, which is considerable.

Closing the eyes increases cerebellar ataxia to a mild degree, but the effect on sensory ataxia is much more marked because the inadequacy of the proprioceptive information becomes more apparent as visual cues are withdrawn. The first appearance of ataxia of station, or its marked exaggeration when the child closes his eyes while standing with the feet close together, is called the Romberg sign. Children with midline cerebellar lesions, and very typically with medulloblastomata, tend to fall forward or backward. The direction of swaying is more variable with lesions of the cerebellar hemispheres, but if these are unilateral the child tends to fall toward the affected side. Apparent ataxia when standing with the feet together, especially with eyes closed, may also be psychogenic (a 'false Romberg test'), but here there are several distinguishing cues. The hysteric sways from the hips instead of from the ankles, rarely falls, even though he may swing through a considerable arc, and does not injure himself if he does fall. Diverting his attention by asking him to execute the finger-to-nose test will sometimes diminish the ataxia, or at least not increase it, whereas true organic ataxia will increase during this maneuver. Children with organic ataxia often tend to steady themselves by touching the wall or pieces of furniture, but those with hysterical pseudoataxia do not.

The abnormal gait of a child whose pseudoataxia has emotional causes will disappear if the child walks with his eyes closed. Children with dystonia musculorum deformans walk better backward than forward, but those with an ataxic gait walk better forward. In younger children, ataxic movements of the upper extremities appear exaggerated and seem to be chaotic. Titubation, an elegantly descriptive word, signifies the shaking of the trunk and head commonly seen in cerebellar disorders and the staggering, reeling, stumbling gait of ataxia.

Ataxia may be insidious in onset and is usually found in conjunction with other signs or symptoms. These associated findings will provide clues to the reason for the ataxia. It may be associated with a motor defect, ataxic cerebral palsy (see Chapter 7), or with anatomical abnormalities such as the Arnold-Chiari malformation and posterior fossa cysts. Chronic cerebellar ataxia may be a manifestation of a metabolic disorder such as Refsum disease (phytanic acid storage disease), retinitis pigmentosa, peripheral neuropathy, anosmia, ichthyosis, maple-syrup urine disease or Hartnup disease. Progressive ataxia caused by a posterior fossa tumor almost always is associated with other evidence of intracranial neoplasm. Children who are later found to have pseudotumor cerebri may be ataxic, but the extent of the papilloedema is greater than would be expected in proportion to the other symptoms. The diagnosis of pseudotumor cerebri must be made by exclusion. Other causes of progressive ataxia are Friedreich's ataxia, ataxia telangiectasia, abetalipoproteinemia, metachromatic leukodystrophy, hydrocephalus, craniopharyngioma and neuroblastoma.

Cerebellar ataxia of rapid onset may be caused by the syndrome known as 'acute cerebellar ataxia', a condition marked by rapid onset of symptoms which often, but not always, are associated with a mild respiratory infection, probably caused by a virus. Alcohol or some drugs used on a chronic basis should be considered as a cause of ataxia of rapid onset. Phenytoin may also cause ataxia if administered improperly for seizure control: a chronic overdose can result from using the drug prescribed in the form of a suspension rather than a tablet or capsule. Nystagmus, gum hypertrophy and poor seizure-control would also be expected.

Ataxia caused by a vestibular disorder is uncommon in childhood and is usually brought to the attention of the physician by the child's complaint of vertigo.

Gross motor dysfunction

The tests described for assessing balance, walking and hopping are useful for ruling out gross motor dysfunction. Most five-year-olds can stand without support for 10 seconds with eyes closed and arms outstretched. Most also can stand on either foot briefly with the eyes closed. Ability to complete all these tests is strong evidence of unimpaired gross motor function. It is unlikely that a child with a significant movement disorder, cerebellar dysfunction or drug toxicity could do these simple tests.

It does not follow, however, that failure indicates significant disease, but it would be suspicious if hyperactive relfexes and a positive Babinski were found in a child who could stand unsupported on either foot for 10 seconds. Such a child would need to be re-examined.

Stair-climbing skills

Any history of muscle weakness, loss of motor skills or an unusual method of climbing or descending stairs indicates a need to watch the child's stair skills. It is important to assess a physically handicapped child's ability to negotiate stairs in evaluating daily-living skills, and it is a good guide to developmental maturity. The average child of three can climb stairs without holding on, and place alternate feet on alternate steps. The average child of five can descend without support, as an adult does. Of course one must take into account both the height of the step and the height of the child.

GAIT

A child who uses crutches or braces or who has an unusual gait should be observed carefully outside the confines of the examination room. If the history has brought out any difficulty with walking, it is important to determine whether the skill is delayed or whether it was once present and has been lost.

Development of gait

The time of achieving independent walking varies considerably, but normally occurs between 10 and 18 months of age. Population studies have demonstrated that 50 per cent of children walk independently by 12.1 months in Cardiff (Bryant *et al.*

1973) and by 12.5 months in Denver and Tokyo (Frankenberg and Dodds 1967, Ueda 1978).

A child who is not walking without support at 18 months may well be normal, but should be seen by a pediatrician since careful examination may reveal that some have cerebral palsy (Hardie and Macfarlane 1980). Children who are bottom-shufflers (commonly familial) are also likely to walk considerably later than average.

Initially a toddler's gait is wide-based and exaggerated: at first the hands are held up in a 'guard' position, but as the child develops confidence the position of the arms moves down, although they remain held out from the body for another one or two months. Reciprocal movement of the arms is clearly apparent by three years. At that age most children also can walk on tip-toe if asked to do so.

Acquisition of independent gait is one of the poorest guidelines for predicting intellectual abilities. *How* the child walks is as important as when he walked. The ability to walk presupposes standing balance, but some children may be able to walk once they have been assisted into the upright posture, even though unable to get up unaided. All of the reflexes and integrative mechanisms required for standing are used in walking, but walking also requires accurate integration and timing of a number of associated movements and synergisms. In walking, the two lower extremities alternately support the weight of the body and move forward. These phases of support and progression should be evaluated separately and their relative times estimated. One should look at the position of the body as a whole, the freedom of movement, the progressive movements of the lower extremities, the size and speed of the steps and the degree of separation of the feet, and at associated movements of the trunk, arms and head. The examiner should *listen* to the child walk; slapping, flopping, dragging or scraping noises may be heard. Asymmetrical footfall is typical of hemiparesis.

Sometimes a child with a motor handicap will tend to show off the walk he has been taught rather this his own genuine gait. Having the child walk around the examination room with his eyes closed or lightly blindfolded will reveal the true gait (Berenberg 1977).

Associated movement

The most important normal associated movement from the point of view of diagnostic examination is the pendular swinging of the arms during walking. Failure of one arm to swing normally, like its opposite, is a sensitive clue to hemparesis. Associated swinging of the arms is also characteristically suppressed in pyramidal disease, such as Parkinsonism or the dystonic cerebral palsies, but usually these disorders are obvious from other findings, and it is in the detection of mild degrees of hemiparesis that asymmetrical swinging is particularly helpful.

Abnormal gait

Different types of gait are characteristic of various neurological and orthopedic abnormalities. Only certain major variants with fairly typical clinical features can be considered here. Evaluation and interpretation of abnormal gait which does not follow any classical pattern, or includes combinations of difficulties, is a highly complex matter: it can be helpful to take motion pictures, particularly if they can be projected in slow-motion.

Ataxic gait

Ataxic gait is an unsteady, unco-ordinated walk with a wide base. The abnormal gait of cerebellar ataxia often is rather more pronounced with the eyes closed. The child walks on a wide base, staggering irregularly to either side, or swaying forward or backward. There may also be truncal tremor. Heel-to-toe walking and walking along a straight line are particularly difficult. Unilateral cerebellar disease produces swaying or deviation, predominantly toward the side of the lesion. A child with a tumor in the right cerebellar hemisphere will walk into a chair and stumble over it when walking around it clockwise, and will drift away from it when walking counter-clockwise. If asked to take a few steps alternately forward and backward, he may slowly drift to the right ('compass deviation'). Abnormal gait closely resembling that in cerebellar ataxia occurs with phenytoin or alcohol intoxication.

In some ways the gait of sensory ataxia also resembles that of cerebellar ataxia. However, it is much more abnormal when the eyes are closed than when they are open, whereas there is only a slight difference in cerebellar ataxia. There are several other distinguishing features: the heel is brought down on the floor first, followed by a slapping contact of the toes. The footfalls sound 'split' as the examiner listens to them: the phase of progression is prolonged because of difficulty in co-ordinating movements to place the feet on the floor. If the disability is symmetrical, the examiner will have difficulty in deciding whether the greater difficulty is in static support of the weight of the body or in forward displacement of the progressing limb. If a sensory ataxia is unilateral or much more severe on one side than on the other, greater time will be required for forward progression on the affected side, and the simultaneous phase of support will be prolonged on the less-affected side. Children with sensory ataxia tend to keep their eyes on the floor while walking in order to watch their feet. In adults, sensory ataxia is most often due to disseminated sclerosis, subacute combined degeneration of the spinal cord or tabes dorsalis, but in children more commonly it reflects a peripheral neuropathy of some type. Friedreich's ataxia produces a combined sensory and cerebellar ataxia.

Gait of spastic hemiparesis

The gait of children with spastic hemiparesis is highly characteristic. There is a tendency to an equinus posture of the foot, often with contracture of the Achilles tendon, which makes the lower extremity functionally longer on the paretic side. The child may compensate for this by circumducting the leg in an arc away from the hip, elevating the pelvic brim on the affected side and dragging the foot a little, scraping the toes against the floor. Another possible compensation for unequal length is slight flexion of the hip and knee, a posture which may also result from contracture of the hamstrings. The paretic lower extremity shows a prolonged phase of progression and a shorter phase of support. The scraping sound of the toe on the floor and the tendency to wear away the toe of the shoe, but not the heel, are highly characteristic. The examiner should observe the involvement of the upper extremity in evaluating the child's gait; there is a paucity of associated movement on the hemiparetic side, with abduction at the shoulders, flexion at the elbow, pronation in the forearm, and usually flexion of the wrist, perhaps with fisting of the hand.

Gait of spastic diplegia

Spastic diplegic gait is not merely a duplication of hemiparetic gait. In addition to the equinus position of the ankle, abductor spasm about the hips becomes a major problem. The child walks with a stiff, shuffling type of gait, often with some internal rotation, scraping the toes, but also abducting the lower extremities so that the knees bump against one another, or one foot crosses in front of the other in a scissors gait. If extensor hypertonus predominates, the child may walk on his toes with the lower extremities largely extended, but there is often flexion of the hips and knees (and tight hamstrings), resulting in a crouching manner of walking. Gait in spastic tetraplegia is similar, except that the upper extremities are also involved, in much the same way as with spastic hemiplegia.

Gait of spastic ataxia

The gait of patients with spastic ataxia varies according to the relative degrees of ataxia and spasticity. Subacute combined degeneration of the cord and disseminated sclerosis are the major causes of spastic ataxic gait in adults, but in children such gait suggests a mixed type of cerebral palsy or of various uncommon progressive spastic ataxias resulting from spinocerebellar degenerations (of other types than Friedreich's ataxia).

'Parkinsonian' gait

Gait closely resembling that of Parkinsonism in adults is sometimes seen in children with postencephalitic states or progressive diseases of the central grey-matter. The child's posture and gait are rigid, movements are slow, and there is a loss of associated movement. The posture is stooped, with the head projected forward. There is flexion at the shoulders, elbows and wrists, but the fingers are extended, in contrast to their posture in most cases of spasticity. The hips and knees are slightly flexed. The child takes small steps and leans forward over his centre of gravity, which leads to increasingly rapid steps as a means of maintaining balance ('festination').

Gait of dystonia and athetosis

The types of dystonic and athetotic gait are protean in their variety. Writhing contortions of the trunk and neck, a tendency to throw the head backward or from side to side, grimacing of the face, and grotesque (often writhing) movements of the extremities are characteristic of athetoid cerebral palsies or progressive disease of the basal ganglia in which dystonia is a significant component. Superimposed on this background one sees the choreic or athetotic movements in whatever form they take. During the phase of progression in walking, often there is a characteristic posturing of the lower extremity, with moderate flexion of the hip and knee, slight external rotation of the hip, an equinovarous foot. The rhythm of walking is uneven. There may be dorsiflexion of the toes or a Babinski-like posture. This type of prancing step, without other abnormality and physical signs to explain it, is often the mode of onset of progressive dystonia musculorum deformans. Patients with dystonic gait, especially at one stage in the evolution of dystonia musculorum deformans, may be able to walk backward more effectively than forward. A comparable superiority of backward gait also may be seen in hysteria and in the presence of weakness of the quadriceps muscles (as in femoral neuritis).

Gait of muscular dystrophy

In muscular dystrophy (the sex-linked recessive pseudohypertrophic or autosomal recessive femoral types), gait is chiefly characterized by weakness of musculature about the pelvis. Lumbar lordosis is marked and there is exaggerated rotation of the pelvis, throwing the hips from side to side with each step. The side-to-side pelvic movement is chiefly the result of weakness of the glutei medii (Sutherland *et al* 1981).

The gait of a normal child is characterized by momentary imbalance and prompt compensation: normal walking can be described as a 'controlled fall'. Before abnormalities of gait clearly occur, boys who later develop Duchenne muscular dystrophy usually have non-specific evidence of muscle weakness as they move from the supine to the standing position (Gower sign; see Fig. 33, p. 86). Lordosis secondary to weakness of the gluteus maximus occurs first. Longitudinal analysis of gait clearly shows increasing hip flexion, weakness of the quadriceps, decreased ankle dorsiflexion and decreased steps per minute. In contrast to the normal child, for whom the center of pressure of weight-bearing is first found in the heel before moving forward to the latent side of the foot, the boy who has muscular dystrophy compensates for loss of muscle strength by having the center of pressure move toward the center and to the medial aspect of the foot.

Gait of muscle weakness

Gait in which the foot drops is chiefly the result of weakness of the tibialis anterior muscle. The child may drag the foot, scraping the toe on the floor, or attempt to compensate for foot-drop by exaggerated lifting of the lower extremity (steppage gait), throwing the foot out and slapping the toe down before the heel strikes the floor (the footfall sounds 'split', as in sensory ataxia, but the sequence of placing the toe and heel is reversed). Generally walking is somewhat slowed, with a longer phase of progression and shorter phase of support. In addition to the anterior tibial, the peroneal muscles are often affected, in which case the foot tends to be inverted and the child walks on its lateral aspect. Foot-drop is the most frequent manifestation of the peripheral neuropathy of lead poisoning in children, who are less likely to develop the wrist-drop typical of adults.

Similar gait is to be expected with neuropathy of the common peroneal nerve, of traumatic or other origin, and may be seen in the early stage of progressive peroneal muscular atrophy (Charcot-Marie-Tooth disease).

Weakness of single muscles or of various combinations of muscles as a consequence of past acute anterior poliomyelitis or other causes may be associated with an enormous variety of abnormal gait patterns, which are very difficult for anyone other than an orthopedic surgeon to classify.

An antalgic gait is symmetrical, with a shortened phase of support to avoid the pain of weight-bearing on the affected side. It may be due to any painful lesion of the skin, soft tissues, bones or joints.

Psychic disturbances and abnormal gait

Psychic disturbances also may produce an almost infinite variety of disturbances of gait. Hysterical monoplegia, hemiplegia and paraplegia are all possible. Hysteria may produce inability to stand and walk (astasia abasia), even though muscle power is normal and no other organic disability is apparent. A tendency to walk on the toes or to go round and round in circles is typical of children with infantile autism, but it should be remembered that toe-walking can also be due to spasticity, even without contracture of the heelcord, if there is a strong stretch reflex. Many normal children also walk on their toes for a few weeks, or even months, at some stage of early childhood. The presence of wildly exaggerated, bizarre or unclassifiable abnormal movements of the limbs during walking may suggest an hysterical basis, but the possibility of Sydenham's chorea or dystonia musculorum deformans must also be considered.

Abnormal gait of orthopedic origin

Asymmetrical or otherwise abnormal types of gait due to orthopedic abnormalities are probably as frequent as those of neurological origin. Pediatricians will not need to be reminded of the possibilities of Legg-Perthes disease or other aseptic necroses, slipped femoral epiphyses, or the waddling gait of untreated congenital dislocation of the hip. If an abnormal gait is not readily classifiable or is not obviously explained by neurological disease or myopathy, diagnosis will be facilitated by roentgenograms of the extremity involved and orthopedic consultation. Further, neuromuscular disease involving unequal reduction of muscle power or unequal increase in muscle tone may result in orthopedic problems: an obvious example is the tendency to sublaxation of the hip if marked hypertonicity of the adductors accompanies spasticity of the lower extremity.

Descriptive terms for assisted walking

If crutches are used, several different kinds of gait can be recognized. 'Swing-through' gait occurs if the crutches are advanced and the legs are swung past them. In 'swing-to' gait, the crutches are advanced and the legs are swung to the same point. In 'four-point' gait, one crutch is moved, followed by the opposite leg, then the other crutch, followed by the other leg. In 'three-point' gait, the affected leg and both crutches are advanced together, followed by the normal leg. In 'two-point' gait the right foot and left crutch (or cane) are moved together, followed by the left foot and the right crutch (or cane). 'Drag-to' gait is the most primitive; it consists of the feet being dragged rather than lifted toward the crutches.

CHAPTER 7

Examination of the Child with a Specific Condition

THE CHILD WITH CEREBRAL PALSY

General comments

Evaluation of the child who is considered to have cerebral palsy must include a careful examination to define the motor handicap. Additional studies may be needed to be sure that the condition is indeed non-progressive. Other handicaps are likely to be present, and these must be identified. The general medical and health needs of the child must be ascertained, and an assessment must be made of the child's relationship to his environment: the home, school and community. Finally, the physician and the family (or agency) must agree on the long-range goals and on a list of priorities for their achievement.

The symptoms in cerebral palsy may change, but the child should continue to develop at a constant rate and there should be no loss of skills. A child who has a decrease or plateau in the rate of development is more likely to have a progressive condition than to have cerebral palsy. Mental retardation is a common finding in cerebral palsy, and the extent of retardation will affect habilitation and expectations. Cerebral palsy and developmental delay are closely associated, and the presence of one should always lead to a suspicion of the other. Approximately 50 per cent of children with cerebral palsy score below the educable level (Illingworth 1958, Nelson and Ellenberg 1978). Children with the dyskinetic forms of cerebral palsy are less likely to have intellectual impairment than those who have the spastic form. Spastic tetraplegia is often associated with severe intellectual deficits.

Although cerebral palsy is defined as a chronic, non-progressive condition, its symptoms change with age, and there is a constant need for medical care, advice, instruction and moral support as the child with a severe handicap progresses from infancy to adulthood. The physician who carries out an evaluation must consider it his duty to see that continuing care and support are provided as the child's needs change and the new problems arise (Osler 1889).

Classification of cerebral palsy

The classification presented in Table XV is especially useful in being primarily descriptive. It can be used simply as a reference to describe the clinical findings at the time of the examination; it has no deep taxonomic significance.

Clinical descriptions

The descriptions of clinical types of cerebral palsy indicate that the clinical entities are quite clearcut. Spasticity is considered to arise from a defect of the extra-pyramidal tract and the dyskinesias are believed to be caused by defects in the extra-pyramidal system. However, because there are probably pyramidal components in

TABLE XV

Classification of cerebral palsy

Spastic cerebral palsy	*Hypotonic cerebral palsy*
Hemiplegia	Atonic diplegia
Diplegia	Hypotonia and ataxia
Tetraplegia	Hypotonia and athetosis
Paraplegia	
Monoplegia	*Ataxic cerebral palsy*
Triplegia	
	Mixed
Dyskinetic cerebral palsy	Spasticity and ataxia
Athetosis	Spasticity and athetosis
Dystonia	

most extrapyramidal diseases, and extrapyramidal components in pyramidal tract diseases, often the clinical picture is mixed. Spasticity may be combined with ataxia or athetosis, and tremors and choreiform movements can occur in all forms of cerebral palsy. There may be truncal hypotonia and spasticity of the extremities, and hypotonia with ataxia. The clinical picture varies with age, and sometimes the variety of what is expected and acknowledged to be present in cerebral palsy can obscure the need to establish beyond doubt the absence of a progressive neurological condition such as Wilson's disease or the Lesch-Nyhan syndrome.

Spastic cerebral palsy

There is general agreement that the clinical findings in fully developed spastic cerebral palsy include the following:
(1) increased muscle tone of the 'clasp-knife' type, with give-way following build-up of resistance, accompanied by a positive stretch reflex;
(2) exaggerated deep tendon reflexes and possibly clonus at the ankle or other joints;
(3) positive Babinski reflex;
(4) depression of superficial reflexes (abdominal and cremasteric);
(5) loss of control and differentiation of finer voluntary movements;
(6) supression of normal associated movements;
(7) presence of certain abnormal associated movements;
(8) spasticity masking weakness.

Some authors use the term 'plegia' to indicate complete paralysis (usually of sudden onset) and 'paresis' to indicate weakness. The terms are used to describe spasticity of an arm and leg on one side. 'Diplegia' describes involvement of the arms and legs on both sides, the degree of involvement of the legs being greater than that of the arms. There is some disagreement as to whether congenital spastic diplegia is in fact a clinical entity rather than a form of tetraplegia. Little's monograph on cerebral palsy, published in 1861, uses the term to describe 'spastic rigidity of the limbs' of young infants and children and describes a definite clinical entity. 'Tetraplegia' describes equal involvement of both arms and legs, or deficits greater in the arms than in the legs. The term 'quadriplegia' is commonly used to describe the involvement of all four extremities, but it is an etymological bastard of both Greek and Latin derivation, and 'tetraplegia' is preferred. Cerebral monoplegia (brachial or crural) does exist, but it is rare that spasticity does not develop eventually in the other limb on the same side. Triplegia, also rare, has been described. 'Paraplegia' describes involvement of the legs only and is commonly used to describe a condition of spinal origin. A cerebral form does exist and must be differentiated from that originating from spinal-cord injury or disease.

Hypotonic cerebral palsy

The majority of children with cerebral palsy have the spastic form, characterized by increased muscle tone, increased deep tendon reflexes and a positive stretch reflex. A rare type of cerebral palsy is manifested by persisting hypotonia, mental retardation and microcephaly, and convulsive disorders are common. Yannet and Horton (1952) have described an atonic type involving all four extremities (also called 'atonic diplegia'), and ataxic and athetoid forms. The degree of hypotonia is out of proportion to the degree of mental retardation. Flexion contractures and positional deformities which occur in late childhood and adolescence may give the erroneous impression of muscle tightness and suggest a diagnosis of spastic cerebral palsy. Although a child with spastic cerebral palsy will be hypotonic in the early stages of the condition, hypertonicity eventually develops. In hypotonic cerebral palsy the hypotonia persists and mental retardation is always present.

Dyskinetic cerebral palsy (see also Chapter 5)

Athetosis is characterized by abnormal involuntary movements and postures. The movements are slow and worm-like. Characteristic postures are repeatedly assumed, such as hyperextension of joints, especially the fingers, and a Babinski-like extension of the toes. Movements may begin in a finger or toe and extend gradually in a writhing manner after a brief pause during which muscle tone increases. Gradually the writhing extends to the neck, head and face. Athetoid movements usually cease during sleep and decrease markedly with illness. They are increased by anxiety, tension and unfamiliar surroundings. Deep tendon reflexes may be normal or slightly increased. Children with athetosis exhibit different degrees of muscular tension, which are influenced by position and anxiety and can vary from hour to hour and from examiner to examiner. It is often very difficult to tell whether a child has 'pure' athetosis or whether there is accompanying rigidity to spasticity. Choreic movement—rapid, discrete, involuntary jerks which occur irregularly—may accompany athetosis, and there may also be a static tremor.

The rare dystonic form of cerebral palsy may be confused with athetosis. The dystonic movements primarily involve the neck, trunk and proximal portions of the extremities. Muscle tone fluctuates and the movements are slow, involuntary spasms resulting in unusual fixed postures. Dystonic cerebral palsy must also be distinguished from dystonic musculorum deformans, which is a specific progressive hereditary condition with usual onset in mid-childhood.

Ataxic cerebral palsy

Congenital ataxia is a rare form of cerebral palsy characterized by inco-ordination of voluntary movements, impaired balance, hypotonia with normal or slightly reduced deep tendon reflexes, and absent stretch reflexes. The hypotonia is noted in infancy, but the infants demonstrate more muscle strength than is commonly found in progressive spinal muscular atrophy, a condition with which congenital ataxia may be confused. The infants seem intellectually brighter than those with hypotonia associated with global developmental delay. The motor handicap becomes apparent when the child begins to sit upright or to stand. The condition may be associated with nystagmus and/or esotropia.

The term 'cerebellar ataxia', or more properly 'cerebellar palsy', is used to describe an ataxia, unaccompanied by any other findings, which is non-progressive and presumably present from birth. It is very rare.

Ataxia signifies difficulty with balance and co-ordination, manifested by walking on a wide base. Many forms of cerebral palsy (spastic, dyskinetic, hypotonic) will have an ataxic component. Ataxia may also be an ominous harbinger of a progressive disease such as Friedreich's ataxia, so the examiner must be sure that a child with the ataxic form of cerebral palsy indeed has just that and not an insidiously progressive condition.

The evaluation

The assessment of a child who is considered to have cerebral palsy includes the identification of the type and extent of the motor handicap, and other handicaps, and planning the best possible medical and social management. Once the motor disability and accompanying handicaps have been clarified and progressive conditions have been ruled out, the extent of the disability as it affects the child can be ascertained by determining four points of reference which can be used to monitor progress. These are: (1) the child's mental development; (2) the child's communication skills; (3) the child's ability in activities of daily living, and (4) the child's mobility. Progress in all these areas may be constrained by the actual physical limitations of cerebral palsy and by the environment, but the physician can discover whether or not the child is 'on schedule' for his expectations, and how the child is coping with his world. The four points of reference are established by a combination of history-taking, indirect observation and direct examination.

The history

History-taking is discussed in Chapter 2. When one assesses a child with cerebral palsy, it is important to pay particular attention to communication, activities of daily living and mobility.

The child's communication skills can be evaluated by observation and interaction and by the history. Receptive and expressive language skills should be analyzed. Is the communication adequate considering the child's mental ability? Is progress in language development satisfactory?

Activities of daily living include feeding, sleeping, dressing and toileting. The history should reveal whether constant attendance is required, whether the child's development has been hindered by lack of opportunity and whether the reported accomplishments match those observed.

Assessing mobility simply means finding out how a child gets from one place to another, whether on crutches, in a wheelchair, or by walking or crawling. What are the limits of the child's world? Room to room? Upstairs and down? Out of the house? Independent travel in the community? If the child can walk, the gait should be analyzed. If the child does not walk, the physician should assess whether independent walking can be expected by looking for the acquisition of landmarks necessary for its accomplishment: head and neck support, back stability and ability to co-ordinate movements of arms and legs. A child may be capable of walking, but only in special circumstances: for example, walking betweeen parallel bars in a therapy room with the support of a physical therapist may represent progress, but it is not true independent walking in the sense of going from one place to another. However, independent walking may not be the highest priority if maximum mobility by other means of locomotion is assured. What is important is the achievement of 'social' mobility.

The social portion of the history should find out how hard it is to care for the child and whether or not the care is satisfactory considering the realities of the environment. How are activities of daily living handled? Is the family coping to the best possible extent?

It is important to find out whether other physicians or agencies are involved in providing care and management. If too many people are involved, the family may be receiving conflicting advice.

Findings on examination
Hemiplegia
Congenital hemiplegia usually is not noted at birth. After a period of hypotonicity and hyporeflexia the deep tendon reflexes become hyperactive and muscle tone increases in the unused arm. Similar changes follow in the leg on the same side. There is preservation of the primitive grasp reflex, even before spasticity appears, and fisting of the involved hand. One of the earliest signs of spasticity in a child with hemiplegia is the presence of increased resistance on passive supination of the forearm on the affected side. However, full supination does not occur until the age of eight months in some normal babies. Another early clue may be a strong hand-preference, first noted when the infant begins to reach for things at about five to six months of age. Asymmetric hand-use may be signified by the difference in pincer grasp at eight or nine months of age, then in difficulty in piling blocks, characterized by dorsiflexion of the wrist. It should be noted that an asymmetric Moro response usually signifies brachial palsy or some local condition, rather than a central defect. Poor postural reflexes may be detected as early as four months of age in an infant with hemiplegia. Although asymmetries may be manifest this early, often it is not until six to eight months that they become obvious.

When the infant is supported on the weak side, the head, neck and trunk are not held in a normal position, the normal arm is not used as a counterbalance and the infant does not support himself as well as on the unaffected side. The involved arm does not extend (*i.e.* 'defend') when tested by the parachute reflex. If a child who is reported to have spasticity of a leg appears to have normal placing and normal parachute responses of the upper extremities, the etiology may be within the spinal cord, the hip or the leg itself. It can be very difficult to differentiate between myelodysplasia and monoplegia.

Mild hemiplegia may be overlooked until the child demonstrates a preference for one leg when beginning to walk. This results in an asymmetric gait and loss of associated movements. The characteristic posture of hemiplegia is adduction of the shoulder, slight flexion of the elbow, pronation of the forearm, flexion of the wrist and fingers, adduction and slight flexion of the hip, and adduction and inversion of the foot. Because the leg is functionally longer on the affected side, the child must circumduct the leg to compensate. Compensation may also occur by tightening of the hamstrings on that side. An affected upper limb may be under-developed, with sensory loss, most marked in the hand.

In acquired hemiplegia the hypotonic state is very brief and paresis quickly becomes apparent. There may be unilateral facial weakness, which is very rare in the congenital form, so its presence suggests that the condition was acquired.

The following specific findings are to be expected: increased muscle tone, hyperactive deep tendon reflexes, positive Babinski, positive stretch reflexes on the affected side, and asymmetric balance and righting reflexes. Strabismus and homonymous hemianopia are common, the latter appearing more often in acquired hemiplegia. Hearing should be checked. Asymmetry of hands, fingers and extremities should be noted. Palmar creases may be more marked on the affected side. A clue to under-development is a difference in the size of the thumbnails: ordinarily they are equal until the age of six years, after which the nail in the dominant hand becomes larger. A sensory loss on the affected side, especially in the hand, should be sought.

Muscle mass should be measured for future reference. Measurements should be taken at midpoints of the upper arm, forearm, calf and thigh. The leg length should be charted from the iliac crest to the medial malleolus.

Occasionally a hemisyndrome (hemihypertrophy or Silver syndrome: see Table XIII, p. 97) may be difficult to distinguish from hemiplegic asymmetry. Measurement of the cornea is useful: a difference in corneal size may be an indication of the presence of hemihypertrophy rather than of asymmetry as a result of cerebral palsy.

Diplegia

Spastic diplegia describes the clinical entity known as Little's disease. The infants often have a history of premature birth, with anoxia. The spasticity involves the legs more than the arms, and often an arm may be near-normal. The infant has strabimus, scissors the legs, and often stands on his toes. There is flexion of the arms and weakness of the trunk and neck.

Tetraplegia

The infant with spastic tetraplegia has all four extremities severely involved, although one side may be more involved than the other and sometimes the arms are more involved than the legs. Mental retardation, growth retardation and microcephaly occur. Muscle tone increases rapidly in all four extremities. Righting

112

responses are poor, as is later sitting posture. There is adduction of the shoulders, flexion of the elbows, pronation of the forearms, flexion of the wrists and fingers, flexion and adduction of the hips, scissoring of the legs and tight heel-cords. Constant or predominant extension, particularly if the ankles are kept closely together or scissored over one another (see Fig. 50, p. 152) is the most characteristic posture of spastic paraparesis or tetraparesis. This posture may make one suspect this type of spasticity several months before it manifests itself in other ways.

Damage to supranuclear connections of the lower cranial-nerves bilaterally affects the muscles of the lower part of the face. There is a history of poor feeding and swallowing difficulties. Drooling occurs, and there may be a lack of facial expression and speech defects.

Specific findings expected are increased muscle tone, hyperactive deep tendon reflexes, positive stretch reflexes in all four extremities and bilateral Babinski responses.

Dyskinetic cerebral palsy

The infant with dyskinetic cerebral palsy usually is referred because of delay in motor skills: for example, an 11-month-old infant is unable to sit. Often there is a history of clinical kernicterus or hyperbilirubinemia and feeding difficulties. The child is hypotonic and the deep tendon reflexes are normal or slightly increased. Control of the head, neck and limbs is poor. There is a persistent tonic neck reflex and neck-righting reflex (see p. 141 and p. 142). A tonic neck reflex in a one-year-old child with motor delay suggests dyskinetic cerebral palsy. However, there are other causes for a persistence of this reflex. These include dystonic phase of diplegia, transient dystonia of prematurity, and degenerative diseases. If the tonic neck reflex is absent at one year of age, dyskinetic cerebral palsy is not the cause of the motor delay. It is probably the result of mental retardation.

It is uncommon to find a child with no sitting balance, combined with spasticity and athetosis, who does not also have a tonic neck reflex. However, consistently imposable tonic neck reflexes in a presumed mentally retarded child usually imply some specific motor disability, with or without delayed development in all fields of activity, including the acquisition of balance. Persistent tonic neck and neck-righting reflexes lessen the chance of the child being able to sit or walk in the future (Crothers and Paine 1959).

Involuntary movements appear gradually, often not until three years of age, although minor manifestations (tremors, choreiform movements) may appear earlier in the fingers and toes. The movements may affect the trunk musculature as well as the extremities (Figs. 37 and 38). Involvement of the supranuclear connections of the lower cranial-nerves produces grimacing, drooling and dysarthria. Early hypotonia eventually gives way to tension, which may diminish or even disappear if the child is relaxed and posturally secure. If contractures and true hypertonus of the clasp-knife variety are present, dyskinetic cerebral palsy has a spastic component and can be considered a mixed form.

Mental development is often normal. However, although children with post-anoxic dyskinesia and familial dyskinesia often have mental retardation, the examiner

113

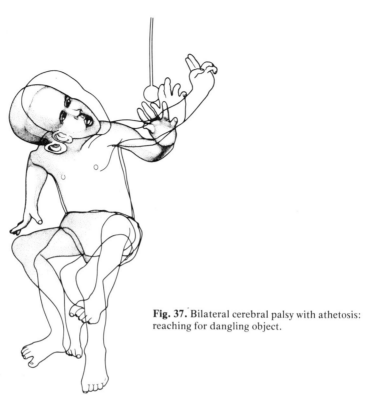

Fig. 37. Bilateral cerebral palsy with athetosis: reaching for dangling object.

should not be misled into thinking that retardation exists because of serious problems in communication. Dysarthria is caused by inability to control involuntary movement of the mouth and tongue and by inability to produce a constant flow of air because of truncal dystonia. Severe hearing-loss is a common finding in dyskinetic cerebral palsy.

Initial determination of the constancy and quality of the abnormal movements is best made by watching the child as he performs routine activities such as playing with toys, drinking from a cup and walking. During the formal test a more careful analysis can be made. Variable performance, variable responses during testing of reflexes, and variable muscle tone from one examination to the next all suggest a significant emotional component. Usually the clumsy, awkward, fidgety child who has difficulty in school can be distinguished from a child with athetoid movements by the inconsistency of his performance, especially if he is observed under optimal circumstances.

Children with dyskinesia became conspicuous because of their involuntary movements of the trunk and extremities, grimacing, drooling, dysarthria and difficulties in swallowing. Because they usually have normal intelligence, they are very conscious of their condition and of their relationships with their peers. Although all the activities of daily living can be performed, each one involves time and prodigious effort. The combination of a severe physical handicap with normal intelligence complicates proper school placement.

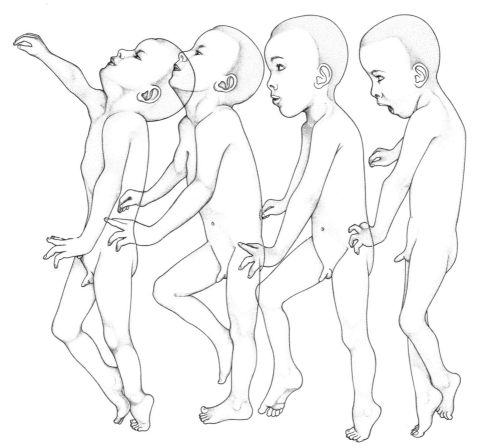

Fig. 38. Athetosis, characterized by abnormal involuntary movements and abnormal posture. The movements are irregular. Abnormalities include hyperextension of the fingers at the metacarpo-phalangeal joints, flexion or extension of the interphalangeal joints and of the wrist, flexion of the adducted elbow, pes planus or equinovarus and dorsiflexion of the big toe. (Same child as in Fig. 37.)

Consultations

Problems with visual acuity and strabismus are common in cerebral palsy, and referral to an ophthalmologist who has experience in working with developmentally disabled children may be necessary. A child with dyskinetic cerebral palsy is especially likely to need specific help from an otolaryngologist and audiologist, and from a speech and language pathologist.

An orthopedic surgeon may need to be consulted for long-range planning, even though surgery may not be performed until late childhood. The surgeon's goal is to preserve the function and integrity of the bones and joints to the best extent possible. He attempts to make maximum use of muscle strength by surgical intervention, bracing, casting, and directing the efforts of the physical and occupational therapists.

The surgeon should show good judgement in noting the child's mental limitations. A surgical procedure should not be carried out if the child does not have the capability of profiting by it. There is little need, for example, to correct a deformity in the ankle or knee if the child's mental development indicates that he will never walk. Occasionally a surgical procedure may be desirable simply to make it easier to care for the child. Relieving serious adductor spasm by tenotomies could make perineal care and toileting much easier, and relief of contractures around joints will give physical therapists' efforts more chance of success.

Planning

After the assessment is complete, the physician will know what needs to be done to maintain the health of the child and will have worked out a plan of medical management. In addition, he will have to help the family adjust to the condition. Realistic goals must be set and the family must be helped with the realities of having and caring for a child with cerebral palsy. The services of a social worker may be needed to work with the family, and to act as a bridge between the doctor and the family and the family and the community. A public-health nurse or home visitor may be needed to visit the home and to develop practical methods for and give instruction on coping with the disability.

Although cerebral palsy is defined as a chronic, non-progressive condition, its symptoms change with age, and there is a constant need for medical care, advice, instruction and moral support as the child with a severe handicap progresses from infancy to adulthood. The physician who does an evaluation must consider it his duty to see that continuing care and support are provided as the child's needs change and new problems arise.

THE INFANT OR CHILD WHO SEEMS FLOPPY

One of the common problems presenting to the pediatrician is the infant or child who appears weak or floppy. Sometimes this is the only abnormality detected in a small baby and will be cause of referral to a neurologist. Some aspects of the history and examination are considered here, together with diagnostic aspects of the more common conditions presenting with floppiness. For a comprehensive recent review of the subject, see Dubowitz (1980).

Floppiness is rarely a chief presenting complaint of the hypotonic infant. Usually the immediate problem which causes parents to seek medical advice is delayed development of motor skills. The 'floppy' baby is usually brought to the physician because of failure to sit or walk at the expected age, and hypotonia is then detected when physical examination is carried out. However, sometimes the parents mention in passing that the baby is excessively floppy. After hypotonia has been detected, the physician must decide whether it is non-specific; if it is related to a problem in the nervous system, further assessment is needed to determine whether the condition is suprasegmental or involves the lower motor neurons and muscles. The most common cause of hypotonia in infancy is mental retardation. Diseases involving the lower motor neurons are far less frequently encountered (see Tables XI and XII, p. 77, for causes of hypotonia).

The history

Evaluation of a floppy infant should include detailed questioning about prenatal events, the birth and the neonatal period, to determine whether anoxia may have occurred. Poor sucking, difficulty in swallowing, a weak cry and frequent respiratory infections might be clues to the presence of muscle weakness. Careful inquiry should be made about developmental milestones and the baby's general health, growth and habits. A family history is important in view of the hereditary nature of neuro-muscular diseases, and tactful questioning about the infant's environment and care should elicit any evidence of environmental and social deprivation.

The examination

The baby's position while supine may reveal evidence of asymmetry in muscle bulk, power and movement. The excessively relaxed 'pithed frog' posture does not point to any specific diagnosis, but often is to be found in spinal muscular atrophies (Fig. 39), myopathies, and occasionally scurvy (also characterized by tenderness of the bones and muscles). A similar posture may result from spinal lesions, although typically the posture of the arms is different in a child with injury of the spinal cord at birth.

The facial expression and eye movements should be examined carefully. Infants with progressive spinal muscular atrophy (Werdnig-Hoffmann disease) exhibit an alertness which is at odds with their obvious disability (Fig. 40). Careful measurements are important. A head circumference less than the third percentile suggests mental retardation as the cause of the hypotonia, and growth delay indicates that the cause is probably systemic or suprasegmental rather than stemming from the lower motor neuron. Inspection also should reveal any obvious congenital anomalies which could be associated with cerebral dysgenesis. A careful examination should look for evidence of systemic or metabolic disorder. The mobility of the joints should be determined, and the reflexes carefully tested. Clinical determination of weakness in a hypotonic infant or baby can be difficult and requires experience. If the baby can play with a toy while his arm is supported, but cannot raise his hand to his mouth spontaneously, the proximal rather than the distal muscles are involved. The power of the shoulder girdle can be estimated by supporting the baby in the erect position with a hand in each axilla: the weak infant will slip through. The tone of the anal sphincter should be checked by palpation.

Developmental analyses of motor, social and language skills are necessary to determine whether the infant's performance matches the achievements claimed by the parents, and whether the baby is 'on schedule'. An over-all delay suggests mental retardation. If motor skills are delayed it is important to know whether they were present earlier.

If a hypotonic infant with delayed development demonstrates brisk reflexes, with a positive Babinski sign, cerebral palsy is the likely cause. The hypotonia may be constant, as in hypotonic cerebral palsy, or it may precede the onset of spasticity. It can also be the manifestation of dyskinetic cerebral palsy. If the infant has hemiplegia the asymmetry develops later, as the first birthday approaches, so the initial hypotonia may have passed unnoticed. Infants with familial dysautonomia may show

117

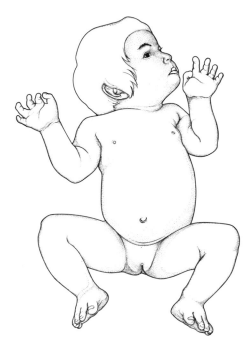

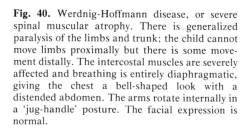

Fig. 39. 'Pithed frog' posture: in the supine position the child's limbs are spreadeagled because of hypotonia and the hands fall open.

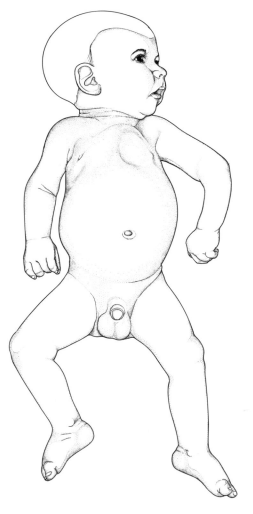

Fig. 40. Werdnig-Hoffmann disease, or severe spinal muscular atrophy. There is generalized paralysis of the limbs and trunk; the child cannot move limbs proximally but there is some movement distally. The intercostal muscles are severely affected and breathing is entirely diaphragmatic, giving the chest a bell-shaped look with a distended abdomen. The arms rotate internally in a 'jug-handle' posture. The facial expression is normal.

118

signs of hypotonia before the appearance of the other symptoms of disturbance of the autonomic system.

Clinical descriptions
Birth injury to the spinal cord
Although severe progressive spinal muscular atrophy (Werdnig-Hoffmann disease) is the condition most likely to be suffered by an infant who is hypotonic, weak and flaccid, birth injury to the spinal cord (possibly from a breech delivery) also must be considered.

Except for the automatic withdrawal responses demonstrable in the lower extremities, the clinical components of birth injury to the spinal cord may closely resemble those of Werdnig-Hoffmann progressive spinal muscular atrophy. The lower extremities are atonic and areflexic in many cases, and there is a paradoxical pattern of respiration, with bulging of the abdomen and retraction of the bell-shaped chest on inspiration because of intercostal paralysis (most of the lesions are lower cervical and upper thoracic in location). Analgesia to pin-prick below a particular sensory level is a distinguishing feature, and although obviously experiencing pain, the baby with Werdnig-Hoffmann disease can withdraw his legs only feebly, if at all, in response to pin-prick. If the lesion is in the lower cervical cord the arms may be in an abnormal position, with the shoulders abducted 90° and the elbows fully flexed from biceps spasm associated with a paralysed triceps.

The anocutaneous reflex is tested by lightly pricking the perianal skin, and the normal response is a visible contraction or 'winking' of the external anal sphincter. The pathway is in the inferior hemorrhoidal nerve and spinal segments S2-4 or 5. The infant with a spinal-cord injury has a weak anal sphincter, while the reflex is intact in spinal muscular atrophy.

Progressive spinal muscular atrophy
Progressive spinal muscular atrophy is a hereditary disease in which there is a decreased number of anterior-horn cells. The severity of the illness depends on the number of normally functioning cells in the anterior horn. Werdnig in 1981 and Hoffmann in 1893 first described a severe, infantile progressive form in which symptoms were evident at birth or shortly thereafter, with an inexorably progressive course leading to death from respiratory causes before the infant's first birthday. A less serious form, with later onset, a milder course and a better prognosis was described by Kugelberg and Welander in 1956. The severe and mild forms of spinal muscular atrophy can be considered as being the ends of a spectrum of symptoms. In general, the earlier the onset, the greater the disability and the poorer the prognosis. Onset of symptoms *in utero* or before six months of age usually indicates early death from respiratory complications. Later onset of symptoms can lead to a static condition, with survival into adult life. The condition is inherited as an autosomal recessive trait and empirically, at least, it breeds true. A family with an infant who has the severe form runs the risk of having another severely affected infant. A family in which one or more offspring have a mild form is at risk for the less serious type of spinal muscular atrophy, with later onset.

119

There may be a history of poor sucking and swallowing, and the mother may mention having been aware of decreased fetal movements. Occasionally the infant will seem normal after birth but there will be a sudden onset of symptoms during infancy. There is a paucity of movement in the arms and legs, and the arms may be internally rotated at the shoulder. The facial expression is alert. The infant can smile, understand and make his wants known. Eye movements are normal and the facial muscles are not involved. Bulbar weakness may produce pooling of secretions. Head and back control is poor. Weak intercostal muscles and diaphragmatic weakness produce abdominal breathing. Deep tendon reflexes are diminished or absent, but the anal sphincter has normal tone. Usually the legs are affected to a greater degree than the arms. There is surprisingly good use of the fingers if the arm is supported. If present, fasciculations of the tongue are diagnostic. Their positive indentification may be difficult, however, for in an infant they may be confused with tongue tremor.

Myasthenia gravis in infancy

Myasthenia gravis is a rare cause of hypotonia and weakness in infancy, but it is treatable and should not be missed. The symptoms of fatigue and muscle weakness are believed to be caused by a defect of neuromuscular transmission in the pre-synaptic area. An autoimmune action is believed to be at fault. Usually the transient neonatal form is associated with a mother who has the disorder or who is about to develop symptoms. The symptoms of the transient form can last two to four weeks. Rarely, symptoms in the newborn period persist throughout life, with no history of the disease in the mother.

THE CHILD WHO SEEMS BACKWARD

General comments

Backwardness, or retardation as it is more commonly called in the United States, is said to exist when a child fails to reach the developmental status appropriate to his or her chronological age. It may be presumed sooner when a child presents physical features or biochemical evidence of a disorder which is regularly associated with mental defect. Conventionally, 'backwardness' or 'retardation' are terms connoting delayed development of physical and intellectual skills. Physical growth-deficit is usually termed 'failure to thrive' or dwarfism, and delayed emotional development is categorized as 'immaturity'.

If an infant or child is suspected of being backward, the examiner must decide whether retardation indeed does exist, and if it does, how to evaluate it and how to help the family deal with the impact of the diagnosis.

Definition of mental retardation

The 'task force on classification and terminology' of the American Association on Mental Deficiency (AAMD) defined mental retardation as 'significantly subaverage general intellectual functioning (two standard deviations below the normal) existing concurrently with deficits in adaptive behavior, and manifested

TABLE XVI

Level of mental retardation according to IQ obtained

Level	IQ scale	
	Stanford-Binet	Wechsler
(Borderline)*	(69-84)	(70-84)
Mild	52-68	55-69
Moderate	36-51	40-54
Severe	20-35	25-39
Profound	$\leqslant 19$	$\leqslant 24$

*Borderline figures are given for comparison. Since the American Association on Mental Deficiency adopted its 1973 definition, persons scoring in this range are not considered mentally retarded (President's Committee on Mental Retardation 1976).

during the developmental period' (President's Committee on Mental Retardation 1976).

The normal values are based on standard IQ tests (Table XVI), and there are obvious criticisms of a definition based on standardized testing: a cultural bias certainly exists; there may be other handicaps which distort the results; or equally, the circumstances surrounding the testing may have an adverse effect on the results. Too often a single IQ value, useful for research and general classification, is attached to an individual and used arbitrarily as the sole basis for important administrative decisions concerning educational planning, vocational guidance and community living.

A different approach to the definition of retardation is based on function. An individual who could not function normally in his own social system and surroundings would be considered retarded. This functional definition is perhaps more valid for those children who, because they cannot do expected school-work, are identified as being mildly retarded and yet manage to master enough skills to enable them to become independent and self-sustaining adults.

Non-specific retardation

The proportion of backward children who have specific physical or metabolic findings to explain their condition is small, and most of them are in the moderate to severe range of retardation. For this reason a child with severe retardation should always be investigated, as an organic cause is likely. The physician is most often confronted with the need to detect and assess the retardation of children who have no associated abnormal physical features. Suspicion of backwardness therefore depends upon the familiarity of the parents or pediatrician with the developmental norms at various ages, and the extent to which the child deviates from them. Deviations become more apparent as increasing demands are made upon higher cerebral functioning, so moderate degrees of backwardness may not be suspected until schooling begins. Many retarded children who seem to be mildly dull in infancy appear to be much more backward when their difficulties in learning to read and write are exposed at school-age.

The evaluation

The physician who is asked to see a child who seems backward must first make sure that retardation exists. A premature diagnosis of mental retardation should be avoided at all costs. A dull-normal child may appear to be slow to his parents because his sibs are bright or because of a mistaken estimation of the slowness of the affected child in relation to his peers.

Adequate information about the child's past illnesses, recent admissions to hospital, evidence of environmental deprivation or recent changes in family life can be helpful in orienting the clinician. It is a common error to overlook evidence of mental retardation by making excessive allowances for a child's apparent fatigue, recent illness or immature behavior. A child who is fearful in a physician's presence makes diagnosis particularly difficult. Other factors which may be misleading include an unsuspected visual or auditory handicap, a systemic illness or a motor handicap.

The history

The developmental history shows either that there has been consistent and generalized delay from an early age or that development proceeded normally until a certain age, when abnormal development appeared. Essential information comprises the times at which the child passed the 'milestones' of development and the extent of his failure to reach the expected developmental level appropriate to his chronological age. The motor development of children with mental retardation is generally ahead of other aspects of development, whereas among those with cerebral palsy motor development alone may be delayed. There can be many reasons why some parents fail to give accurate information: they may be unfamiliar with the normal course of development, unobservant of the progress of their own child or they may have unconscious defenses which lead to delusions about their child's abilities. For this reason the testimony of others who know the child well, such as relatives or teachers, may be of great value.

However, experienced mothers are competent in comparing their own children and usually can state reliably whether a certain child was more 'forward' or 'backward' than his sibs. A complaint from a mother that one of her children is developing more slowly than his sibs or neighborhood contemporaries should always be taken seriously.

Questions should be asked about the general behavior and personality of the child, especially during the first year or so of life. Feeding problems, sleeping difficulties, undue irritability or placidity often are indicators of mental retardation, although by no means specific for it. If the history and examination support the probability of retardation, further historical information should be obtained in order to establish whether or not the disorder is progressive (Swaiman and Wright 1982).

The possibility of a progressive disorder should be considered if a child who was progressing at a regular (though slow) rate loses muscle tone, motor ability, ability to learn new words and, most importantly, affect: the child can no longer walk un-supported or hold a cup; newly acquired words are forgotten; the infant no longer recognizes his mother nor smiles in response to appropriate social stimuli. The occurrence of seizures, 'long-tract signs' and behavioral changes increase the

122

probability of a degenerative disorder.

Once a child has been categorized as retarded it is essential to try to determine the probable cause of the handicap, although most children with moderate to mild retardation will have no specific physical findings or ascertainable cause. Causal analysis is worthwhile, however, because it leads to possible treatment, better management of the child, comprehensive assessment of other handicaps and better parent counseling.

The examination

The examination may document causes suggested by the history and specific physical findings may suggest certain syndromes. The neurological examination must also produce an accurate appraisal of the child's physical and mental limitations, and associated handicaps must be sought.

The need for flexibility on the part of the examiner has already been stressed. It is particularly important for the child who may be mentally retarded to be given special encouragement and attention during the first few minutes of the examination. The child's eye contact or lack of it, awareness of a different person or change in environment and the ability to respond to a stranger are more easily assessed if the child is relaxed and comfortable.

The physician should look first for any obvious physical stigmata which suggest specific conditions or birth defects. There are over 150 defects which are associated with mental retardation, many of which are easily recognized. Others are so rare that the examiner will need to have recourse to a basic reference such as the *Birth Defects Atlas and Compendium* (Bergsma 1979).

Characteristic facies are seen in trisomy 21 (Down syndrome), hypothyroidism, gargoylism (Hurler syndrome, Fig. 41), the cri-du-chat' syndrome, the severe type of infantile hypercalcemia, Cornelia De Lange syndrome and some craniofacial disorders. It should be remembered that facial and midline anomalies are often associated with significant cerebral malformations. Examination of the skin may reveal a neurocutaneous syndrome which is sometimes associated with mental retardation.

A large head may be found with hydrocephalus and hydranencephaly, both of which may be associated with backwardness, but also in achondroplasia and cleido-cranial dysostosis, which are not. If suitable studies indicate no hydranencephalus, hydrocephalus, cysts or tumors, and the cranial vault has increased because the hemispheres are large, a storage disease is likely. Children with Tay-Sachs disease develop an enlarged head relatively late in the course of the disease. Primary macrocephaly, which can be familial, is rarely associated with retardation.

A small head may be indicative of primary microcephaly, but more often the restriction of cranial growth is the result of maldevelopment or damage to the underlying brain. Deformities of the skull due to premature fusion of the sutures (craniostenosis), which may be associated with retardation, should be distinguished from the postural plagiocephaly seen in infants who are slow to sit up or who were very immature at birth.

Eye signs of diagnostic importance in some forms of mental retardation include

123

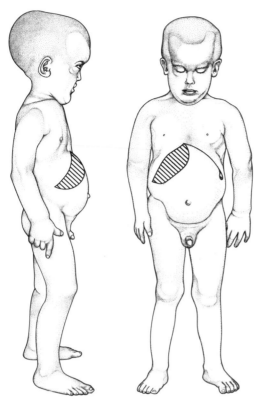

Fig. 41. Hurler syndrome. The head is large and the brow prominent; the bridge of the nose is flattened and the nostrils are wide. The lips are large and the neck short. The hands are broad and stubby, and there are contractures of the elbows and fingers. All patients have enlarged liver and spleen.

microphthalmia in congenital toxoplasmosis and trisomy 13-15, absence of tears in familial dysautonomia, and glaucoma in Lowe syndrome. (See also Chapter 4.) Conjunctival telangiectasia also occur eventually in the ataxia-telangiectasia syndrome; corneal clouding is a feature of gargoylism; and the Kayser-Fleischer ring is pathognomonic of Wilson's disease. Brushfield spots in the iris (see Fig. 21, p. 37) often occur with trisomy 21. Cataracts of the central type may be due to rubella syndrome or toxoplasmosis; lamellar cataracts are seen in galactosemia, hypoparathyroidism and in babies born extremely prematurely. Retinoscopy is of value in the diagnosis of toxoplasmosis (chorioretinitis), Laurence-Moon-Biedl syndrome (retinitis pigmentosa) and Tay-Sachs disease (cherry-red spot).

The trunk and limbs furnish less evidence of mental retardation syndromes than the head. As a group, the more severely mentally retarded grow poorly and frequently remain infantile. However, some syndromes are associated with obesity, such as the Laurence-Moon-Biedl syndrome and the Prader-Willi syndrome, in which there is obesity, infantilism and mental retardation. Growth failure of an extreme degree is a sign of hypothyroidism, and disproportionate dwarfism occurs in some forms of mucopolysaccharidosis. Short stature, a shield-shape chest, webbing of the neck and cubitus valgus are typical of gonadal agenesis (Turner syndrome).

Broad hands with a single transverse crease are characteristic of trisomy 21, as is the dystrophic middle phalanx of the fifth digit. Polydactyly is a component of the Laurence-Moon-Biedl syndrome and syndactyly is sometimes associated with craniostenosis (Apert syndrome).

'Rocker-bottom' feet, overlying fingers and involvement of other organ systems suggest significant developmental delay and indicate the need for chromosomal analysis.

General physical examination

A basic physical examination should pay careful attention to the child's skin, nutrition and oral hygiene, not only because these areas give an indication of his general health, but also may provide clues to the cause of the retardation.

Congenital heart-disease is associated with trisomy 21 (usually ventricular septal defect or persistent atrioventicular canal) and with gonadal agenesis (coarctation of the aorta). Hepatosplenomegaly is a feature of gargoylism, lipid histicytosis (Niemann-Pick disease) and cerebroside lipidosis (Gaucher disease).

Sexual maturation is delayed or imperfect in several of the syndromes caused by anomalies of the sex chromosomes, most of which are frequently associated with mental retardation.

Neurological examination

Details of the neurological evaluation are given in Chapters 4, 5 and 6. The greater the degree of retardation, the more the examiner must rely on observation and the more flexible must be the approach.

For unknown reasons, hypotonia is observed frequently among children who are moderately or severely mentally retarded. Deep tendon reflexes are present, equal and often slightly less brisk than one would expect for the child's mental or chronological age. This is often more than can be accounted for by estimated lack of use, size of muscle or thyroid function. Inconsistent responses to tests of postural reflexes, deep tendon reflexes and of visual, auditory and sensory functions are commonly found.

The extent to which hearing and vision are tested depends on the nature of the problem. In the case of a severely retarded child it should be sufficient to establish that hearing and vision are serviceable. A mildly retarded child who is having school problems deserves a thorough ophthalmological and audiological evaluation. Special techniques for assessing hearing and vision of retarded children have been developed by Sheridan (1976a, b). Impedance audiometry is an easily administered technique which is of value in detecting peripheral hearing-loss in young, unco-operative or retarded children (see p. 178).

Other handicaps may exist in children with the primary problem of backwardness. For example, an infant who is seen because of developmental delay may have retardation and early signs of cerebral palsy. Seizures are a common problem. Adolescents with trisomy 21 frequently develop myopia and conductive hearing-loss. The examiner must make a conscious effort to look for associated disabilities.

Developmental screening

An attempt should be made to gain a rough estimate of the child's developmental ability at the time of the assessment. Developmental or intellectual testing of an unco-operative child in unfamiliar surroundings is more often an exercise of the physician's intuition than of his scientific prowess. It has been shown, however, that the more-or-less intuitive estimates of experienced physicians correlate well with expert psychometry at the more extreme deviations from the normal range. Techniques for screening are discussed in Chapter 9.

THE CHILD WITH EPILEPSY

General comments

A child whose symptoms suggest epilepsy must be carefully evaluated to make sure that the attacks, if they are indeed true seizures, are recurrent and chronic rather than an indication of an acute process. If a chronic condition exists, idiopathic epilepsy should be differentiated from organic epilepsy, which has an identifiable cause (Table XVII).

The history

Whatever the cause, most cases of seizures in childhood are not associated with other abnormalities on neurological examination. The evaluation of an individual child therefore depends almost entirely on a careful history, together with electro-encephalographic evidence, unless the physician is fortunate enough to witness an actual seizure. In addition, often the description of the episodes by parents or other observers is inaccurate because of the fright and confusion the attacks generate.

It is wise to let the parents (or other observers) describe the episode in their own words, without interruption, but to follow this by carefully retracing the entire episode from beginning to end, being sure to get items in chronological order. The first important point is whether or not the child had any sort of aura or advance warning of impending seizures. Both child and parent should be asked about this, since their stories may differ. Frequently, the only evidence of an aura is that the child seemed frightened, 'looked funny', called out or ran to his mother immediately before the attack.

Next one wants to know whether the loss of consciousness or fall took place immediately or whether it followed the onset of abnormal movements. A minute description of the involuntary movements and of their evolution in time obviously is of the greatest importance, and particular attention should be directed to any focal features or suggestion of spread ('march') from one area to another, and the directions and sequences involved. A seizure which begins simultaneously in all the areas involved and does not spread should be differentiated from one beginning, for example, in the hand and then spreading up the arm. Whether a focal seizure eventually becomes generalized is an obvious point to determine, particularly in connection with the question of loss of consciousness. Focal seizures are consistent with retention of consciousness, but one should view with some suspicion the

TABLE XVII
Classification of epileptic seizures by clinical description*

1. **Partial seizures** (seizures beginning locally) *With elementary symptomatology* (generally without impairment of consciousness): with motor symptoms (includes Jacksonian seizures) with special sensory or somatosensory symptoms with autonomic symptoms compound forms (partial complex without loss of consciousness) *With complex symptomatology* (temporal lobe or psychomotor seizures, generally with impaired consciousness): with impairment of consciousness only with cognitive symptomatology with affective symptomatology with psychosensory symptomatology with psychomotor symptomatology (automatisms) compound forms[†] (variable descriptions from the same subject—'psychomotor seizures') *Secondarily generalized*	2. **Generalized seizures** (bilaterally symmetrical and without local onset) *Absences*[†] (petit mal) *Bilateral massive epileptic myoclonus*[†] (the Lennox-Gastaut seizures) *Infantile spasms*[†] (infantile myoclonic seizures) *Clonic seizures* *Tonic seizures* *Tonic-clonic seizures*[†] (grand mal) *Atonic seizures* *Akinetic seizures*[†] 3. **Unilateral seizures** (or predominantly) 4. **Unclassified epileptic seizures** (because of incomplete data)

*Abstracted from the international classification proposal by Gastaut (1969).
[†]Types most often recognized in infants and children. Older individuals often give better descriptions and therefore give more precise aid to classification.

description of a generalized seizure which was not accompanied by unconsciousness. It is important to obtain an exact description of the abnormal movements of the face, mouth, tongue or pharyngeal musculature, and to ascertain whether there were any repeated movements such as smacking the lips, gulping or swallowing. Seizures may terminate (less often begin) with a belch or with the passage of flatus, events sometimes resulting in the mother attributing the attack to 'gas on the stomach' or in the bowels.

The position of the head and eyes during the seizure is of special importance, since deviation to one side implies an irritative discharge in the contralateral cerebral hemisphere. Any late asymmetry of involuntary movements or any predominance of involvement of one side or one limb is also important information, even in the case of generalized seizures. With possible petit mal seizures, one also wants a careful description of the events involved. These attacks are sometimes unobserved or unrecognized by parents and in that circumstance it could be helpful if the physician attempted to imitate a petit mal attack and asked whether the child had ever done anything of the sort. The particular features to ask about are possible upward or other deviation of the eyes, a blank stare, rhythmic blinking, the degree of loss of contact with the environment and of course the duration of the seizure.

Valuable clues often may be gained by asking what happens when the child has an attack in the course of various daily activities. If he is engaged in a conversation, does he pick up where he left off or is there a lapse? Does he sway or even seem as if about to fall? If he is pouring milk from a pitcher into a dish of breakfast cereal, does he continue pouring so that the milk overflows, or does he drop the pitcher? In the case of akinetic ('drop') seizures, it is desirable, albeit difficult, to ascertain whether the attack is actually a sudden loss of muscle tone, causing the child to drop in his tracks, or whether it is a massive flexor spasm of the anterior musculature of the trunk, causing him to be thrown forward. In the latter case the history and perhaps inspection of the head are more likely to document recurrent injury.

The examiner should also ask about possible autonomic changes, particularly those which take place toward the end of a seizure. Traditional questions concern incontinence of urine or faeces, biting the tongue and retching or vomiting. Another highly important question is the presence or absence of sleep or drowsiness after the stage of involuntary movement and the apparent depth and duration of any sleep period. When the child 'came to', or at the end of the period of sleep, did he complain of headache, seem nauseated or confused, or have any apparent post-ictal weakness or aphasia, and how much, if anything, did he remember of each stage of the episode?

After getting as complete a description as possible of the initial suspected seizure, the physician will then go on to ask about subsequent attacks. If the seizures are nocturnal, occasional and irregular, bed-wetting may be a clue to an earlier time on onset or unrecognized subsequent spells. At the very least, information must be obtained on the frequency of the attacks, their variation in duration or character and their spacing in time; and on any trend to become more or less frequent, longer or shorter, or more or less severe. It is wise to get an accurate listing by dates, if that is possible.

It is customary to ask whether the episodes have tended to occur at a particular time of day, in any consistent relationship to times of meals, or on waking in the morning. Preprandial seizures may be suggestive of hypoglycemia, as may attacks occurring two hours or so after meals, if a glucose load is followed by an abnormal secondary depression of glucose in the blood. Early-morning seizures also may be hypoglycemic in nature, but this timing is also typical of many cases of idiopathic epilepsy or of epilepsy symptomatic of an organic cerebral lesion.

Possible precipitating factors must be inquired about and parental statements about these listened to with respect, even though frequently they may be inaccurate or even absurd. Fright, anxiety, fatigue, lack of sleep, over-exercise, apprehension or worry, pain or injury, and even such things as constipation or the intake of certain foods, deserve respectful consideration.

If the child has had prior medication for seizures, it is mandatory (but frequently difficult) to get a detailed chronology of what drugs and combinations of drugs have been given, in what dosages and for how long, together with any changes which took place in the seizures, any changes in behavior or personality, and any recognized side-effects.

Questions about the child's general medical history should cover areas which might have etiological importance, such as perinatal problems, injury, infections, immunization reactions and possible poisoning. The physician should also obtain information about the child's home, school and community, since satisfactory management of a seizure disorder depends as much on making the child's environment as problem-free as possible as it does on specific anticonvulsant therapy.

A seemingly disproportionate amount of time must be spent on history-taking in the evaluation of seizure problems. Repeated review, or even a renewed record, of the history may bore parents, child and physician alike, but it may reveal new information in obscure cases or in those not responding to treatment. It should not be necessary to point out (though it is frequently neglected) that accurate, detailed history-taking is more important in the evaluation and management of seizures than in any other common neurological problem.

The examination

Neurological examination is unlikely to reveal any specific findings. Nevertheless, the examination must be done carefully and any leads suggested by the history must be pursued. It is extremely important to determine whether the recurrent convulsions are a chronic problem or a manifestation of progressive disease. It is necessary to define any associated handicaps such as cerebral palsy or mental retardation.

There is the possibility of drug intoxication if a child who has been receiving therapy for seizures suddenly develops new neurological symptoms such as personality change, deterioration in performance, behavior change or difficulties with gait and balance. Physical findings suggestive of drug intoxication include nystagmus, gum hypertrophy, hiccoughs, slurred speech and rashes. The suspicion of intoxication can be confirmed by measuring levels of anticonvulsants in the blood by gas-liquid chromatography (see Chapter 11).

Clinical description of seizures

Although seizures are commonly classified by their clinical manifestations, the symptoms may overlap and electroencephalographic abnormalities are frequently non-specific. Diagnosis often depends on nothing more substantial than the clinical hunch of the examiner and the second-hand report of the parents. It may be very difficult, for example, to distinguish an akinetic seizure from a sudden episode of narcolepsy or from a postural collapse of a psychomotor seizure. The following descriptions of the common clinical forms of childhood epilepsy are intended only as a general guide for identification rather than as a presentation of strict diagnostic criteria.

Grand mal seizures

An aura is not a common symptom in a child with a grand mal seizure. There might be only localized spasm or twitching, but characteristically the onset is abrupt; the child becomes pale, stiffens and falls, the pupils dilate and the eyeballs roll up or to the side. The body goes into a tonic spasm (increased tone without visible movement), and the contraction of the diaphragm may force air up through the closed glottis, causing a peculiar shrill cry. Spasm of the masseter muscles may produce laceration of the tongue, and the contraction of the abdominal muscles may cause micturition and, rarely, defecation. The child's pallor gives way to suffusion, followed by cyanosis as the spasm involves the respiratory muscles. After an interval of between 10 and 30 seconds (which can seem an eternity to a parent), the clonic phase begins, respiration resumes and the cyanosis disappears. The duration of this phase is variable. Post-ictal symptoms may include headache, confusion, vomiting and somnolence.

Focal seizures

A unilateral, focal ('Jacksonian') motor seizure is typically clonic, although a brief tonic phase may occur first. Focal seizures usually involve the most highly specialized voluntary muscles, especially those of the hand, arm, face and tongue. More rarely, muscles of the leg and trunk are involved. The seizure may begin in one member, for example a thumb, then 'march' into a consistent pattern. More commonly, however, a focal seizure will begin simultaneously in all affected areas and will not 'march' or spread. If there is no spread the child may remain conscious. If the spread is rapid and consciousness is lost, it may be very difficult to distinguish widespread focal seizures from a generalized grand mal episode, especially if the seizure is reported rather than observed.

Petit mal seizures

A petit mal seizure is defined as a transient loss of consciousness lasting less than 30 seconds. The child stops whatever he is doing, the eyes roll up, the lids flicker and jerking movements of the body or arms may occur. The child rarely falls, but he might·drop what he is holding. A petit mal seizure sometimes can be brought on by hyperventilation or a blinking light. The frequency varies from one or two a month to several hundred a day. Girls are affected more than boys, and the onset of petit mal is rare before the age of three years.

Psychomotor seizures

A psychomotor seizure is traditionally described as a complicated but voluntary inappropriate motor act occurring in a state of altered consciousness. Its manifestations in childhood are quite variable, and the diagnosis may be difficult. The electroencephalogram is often normal between episodes. The child might cry out for help because he feels odd. There may be circumoral pallor. A typical childhood psychomotor seizure consists of gradual loss of postural tone. The child holds one arm out, makes a slow turn and crumples to the floor. After a few minutes he awakens and may be drowsy and confused about elapsed time, for example appearing at the lunch table and asking for breakfast.

Myoclonic seizures

An infantile myoclonic seizure ('lighting major' or 'jack-knife' epilepsy) consists of sudden flexion: the head may drop forward and the arms flex. A supine infant might suddenly flex his legs onto his abdomen, as if in pain, and thus be misdiagnosed as having 'colic'. The entire episode is over almost as soon as it starts, and could be missed by an inexperienced parent. The electroencephalogram (EEG) shows a typical pattern of hypsarrhythmia. Infantile myoclonic seizures usually occur before two years of age, in contrast to the later onset of petit mal. If the child has always shown developmental delay and if the onset is earlier than four months of age, the most likely cause is a congenital cerebral defect. If developmental progress has been normal up to about six months of age and the child then develops infantile myoclonic seizures and makes no further progress, the cause is probably an unrecognized encephalitis or a metabolic disorder such as Tay-Sachs disease or phenylketonuria.

Akinetic seizures

An akinetic seizure consists of a sudden loss of postural tone: the child stiffens suddenly and falls forward onto his hands and knees. Shaking and spasms do not occur and the episode lasts between 10 and 60 seconds. This type of seizure is often a sign of progressive central nervous system disease or of a congenital cerebral abnormality.

Reflex seizures

Reflex seizures are evoked by a sensory stimulus such as a blinking light or a touch or smell. The stimulus is consistent for an individual child.

Self-induced seizures

Some children learn to induce seizures voluntarily by a specific technique, such as hyperventilation, rapid blinking or watching a blinking light, television patterns or automobile headlights at night. Self-induced seizures are often an indication of a severe psychological problem.

Febrile seizures

Often a young child will be referred for assessment after several episodes of what are considered to be simple febrile seizures because the family and referring physician are concerned that epilepsy could develop. It is generally agreed that between 1 and 4 per cent of children who have febrile seizures go on to develop epilepsy. The results of a prospective study, based on a large number of children who developed febrile convulsions and were followed for at least three years, indicate that children who had abnormal neurological findings or development before the first episode, or whose first seizure was prolonged or complex, were more likely to develop epilepsy (Nelson and Ellenberg 1976). There is only a small risk that a normal child with a single uncomplicated febrile seizure will go on to develop epilepsy. Children who are potentially epileptic usually have an afebrile seizure within three years of the febrile seizure. More than five febrile seizures in a 12-month period and persisting EEG abnormalities are also strong predictors of epilepsy. It should be remembered that the EEG may remain abnormal for as long as two weeks after the febrile convulsion.

Centro-temporal epilepsy

'*Benign focal epilepsy*', or benign centro-temporal epilepsy of childhood with Rolandic foci, Sylvian seizures with mid-temporal EEG foci and the lingual syndrome occurs only in children and is a common type of 'partial' epilepsy. It is characterized by an onset between two and 12 years of age (usually between the seventh and 10th years), seizures which are most frequent during the times of awakening or going to sleep, and spikes or sharp waves (isolated complexes or groups) on the EEG in the area of the Rolandic fissure. Children who have this seizure during the day commonly exhibit head-turning (adversive movements), often accompanied by facial grimacing and perhaps rotation of the body away from the EEG focus. The child may fall and suffer brief loss of consciousness, but recovery is rapid. Striking features in some children are the feeling of suffocation and inability to speak (oropharyngeal phenomena).

Usually benign focal epilepsy is easily distinguished from psychomotor seizures by the fact that it begins as partial seizures and only secondarily becomes generalized. However, they may be confused if the history is inadequate. It is important to recognize benign focal epilepsy by its characteristic clinical symptoms and EEG findings. Note that the EEG abnormalities may be bilateral, but rarely involve the anterior temporal area, otherwise the child may be diagnosed incorrectly as having a tumor or be given inappropriate anticonvulsant therapy. Benign focal epilepsy should always be suspected if an otherwise normal child has nocturnal seizures. A common history in the United States is that a child between the ages of seven and 11 years, travelling by car, falls asleep and has a seizure. Daytime seizures are more difficult to diagnose unless the 'partial' nature of the seizure is recognized and the EEG pattern is correctly identified. The prognosis is excellent if proper management is obtained.

Seizure-like conditions

Although the symptoms of a typical seizure present no problem in diagnosis, some conditions have manifestations similar to those seen during an epileptic attack, and it is not always easy to differentiate them from a true attack. The diagnosis of epilepsy is fraught with such anxiety for a family that utmost care must be taken to be sure that the diagnosis is valid.

Syncope

A simple black-out involving nothing more than loss of consciousness and a fall is a possible form of seizure, but this problem requires very careful consideration of the differential diagnosis from other forms of syncopal attacks. Other forms include vasodepressor syncope, orthostatic hypotension, reflex heart-block, Stokes-Adams syndrome, cerebrovascular disease (less important in children than in adults), anoxia, hypoglycemia, paroxysmal tachycardia or other cardiac disease, and simple fainting (which, while heavily involving psychogenic factors, may be based on a fall in blood pressure).

Information about blood pressure is virtually never obtainable unless another physician examined the child at the time, and even information about the pulse rate is unlikely to be available unless a parent can be taught to check it accurately during an attack. Often it is merely said that the child's pulse was pounding or terribly fast, leaving one unable to decide whether the tachycardia was moderate and the consequence of the seizures, or extreme and possibly the immediate cause of syncope. A report of giddiness or light-headedness, or of feeling sick or weak, should not be equated with true vertigo, which is a hallucination of movement.

It is important to remember that vasodepressor and other forms of syncope may be associated with urinary incontinence, or even result in a few clonic movements if the child is maintained upright by a bystander in order to prevent the increased flow of blood to the brain which follows falling. If one is fortunate enough to obtain an EEG during a period in which an actual faint occurs, syncope can be differentiated from a seizure because in simple syncope there is no electroencephalographic change until the loss of consciousness; there is then generalized slowing, with prompt recovery when consciousness is regained. Aside from this means, the distinction between syncope and a seizure is difficult and rests entirely on an accurate history or the opportunity to witness an actual attack. The lack of post-ictal sleep is one of the best diagnostic points in favor of syncope, but the distinction is not absolute, and fainting may be followed by a certain amount of confusion or nausea.

Breath-holding

The difficulty in distinguishing breath-holding spells from seizures is compounded by the possibility that breath-holding may be followed by a seizure. In typical breath-holding, the child, usually between six months and four years of age, cries out, holds his breath in aspiration long enough to become cyanotic, then loses consciousness and falls limply to the floor. Consciousness returns promptly within a minute, and the child is then almost normal, lacking the headache, nausea, confusion or desire to sleep which characterize post-ictal states. Involuntary micturition may accompany either breath-holding or seizures, but clonic movements or rigidity suggest the latter diagnosis. There is probably a second type of breath-holding spell, in which the child holds his breath in inspiration and loses consciousness with a Valsalva maneuver, usually without a cry and without cyanosis. The first type of breath-holding may precipitate a seizure because of anoxia, but the second is less likely to do so. Typically, breath-holding is precipitated by frustration (with people or inanimate objects), but may follow sudden pain or fright (Stephenson 1980). Usually, but not invariably, it occurs in the presence of an audience. Breath-holding is a benign self-limiting condition, but a considerable amount of harm can be done if the family problems which underlie repeated attacks are ignored, and if the difficulties are compounded by confusing the breath-holding with epilepsy.

Migraine

The symptoms of classical migraine—an aura, visual symptoms, severe headache, vomiting followed by deep sleep—resemble a seizure disorder sufficiently closely to have provoked an as yet unresolved controversy about whether or not migraine is a form of epilepsy. The situation is complicated by the presence of abnormal EEGs in some children with migraine and the dramatic response of some instances of migraine to anticonvulsant drugs.

Vascular ring

In very young infants, brief periods of unconsciousness can result from the pressure of a vascular ring on the trachea. The apnea is considered a reflex response

133

to irritation from swallowing or coughing. The infants have swallowing problems, stridor or wheezing, and a typical brassy 'seal bark' cough.

Narcolepsy

Although narcolepsy is rare in childhood, it is a seizure-like disorder which must be distinguished from true akinetic or psychomotor seizures. A child with narcolepsy has an overpowering desire to sleep during the day. The onset can be abrupt: the child 'falls in a heap' into a light sleep, often during a purposeful activity such as walking or eating, or during an emotional upset. The child can be easily roused, and is alert rather than confused after the episode.

Pseudoseizures

Pseudoseizures are the most common neurological manifestations of conversion hysteria during childhood. The 'seizures' are realistically acted out and can be described in minute detail by the distraught parent, who is usually present to witness the attack. Administration of anticonvulsants by physicians who have been duped can complicate the diagnosis. Hysteria should be suspected when a normal EEG is obtained, in spite of 'uncontrolled' seizures.

THE CHILD WHO PRESENTS WITH HEADACHE

The history

Children whose complaint is primarily one of recurrent headache should be allowed to talk freely of their symptoms, with the minimum of direct questioning. When possible, the child's account should be compared with that of the parent: in the case of organic headache the histories generally are consistent, but with psychogenic headache there are often remarkable differences. By the time the child is brought to the physician with a complaint of headache, probably several episodes have occurred and a pattern has emerged. This pattern is consistent when the headaches are psychogenic in origin.

It is useful to obtain a history of a typical attack and then ascertain the frequency and periodicity of the episodes. Most children are limited in their ability to describe the character and localization of their headaches, and the intensity of pain must be judged more by the child's behavior during an attack than by the description.

Headache due to raised intracranial pressure or to hypertension is rarely constant but may occur daily. It may also occur at night and interfere with sleep. Tension headaches are apt to occur regularly for a while and then be followed by irregular periods of remission. On the other hand, classical migraine is episodic and rarely more frequent than once every two to three weeks.

The headache of migraine has been defined by the World Federation of Neurology's Research Group on Migraine and Headaches as: 'a familial disorder characterized by recurrent attacks of headache, widely variable in intensity, frequency and duration. Attacks are commonly unilateral and are usually associated with anorexia, nausea, and vomiting. In some cases they are preceded by or associated with neurological and mood disturbances. All of the above characteristics are not necessarily present in each attack or in each patient' (quoted by Congdon and Forsythe 1979).

A child who experiences periodic, severe, unilateral headaches accompanied by visual symptoms, nausea and vomiting, followed by sleep, and whose family has a history of a similar problem, certainly has the 'classical' form of migraine. The 'common' form, manifested by diffuse frontal or bitemporal headaches without an aura, is not nearly as clearcut. Many young children cannot define an aura, and in a child it may be very hard to distinguish between common migraine and severe tension headaches. Both may be diffuse, produce nausea and vomiting and be anxiety-related. Complicating symptoms of migraine such as cyclical vomiting, abdominal pain, hemiplegia and ophthalmoplegia should be carefully investigated. If these symptoms are present, the diagnosis of migraine must be made by exclusion after appropriate studies.

The presence of an aura, pallor, malaise and headache followed by somnolence can also suggest a diagnosis of epilepsy. The relationship between epilepsy and migraine is not at all clear. EEG changes reported in migraine have included posterior slow-waves, focal spikes and paroxysmal discharges, but the significance of these abnormal findings in some (but not all) children with migraine is controversial (Brown 1977).

Characteristically, the headache caused by raised intracranial pressure is most severe on rising in the morning and wears off during the day; this is also true of headache associated with school phobia. Tension headaches not due to school phobia are usually more prominent in the evenings, as are headaches associated with eye strain, excessive reading and television-viewing.

The duration of episodes of headache is important. Transient headache lasting a few moments is often an attention-seeking symptom, whereas organic headaches last for hours. Migraine and tension headaches may last from several hours to several days.

The child should be questioned in order to identify possible precipitating factors. Tension and migraine headaches may be precipitated by emotional stress or by motion. Intense exercise and some foods may also bring on a migraine attack. Hunger as a precipitating factor suggests hypoglycemia.

Exacerbating and alleviating factors should also be identified: in adults the headache caused by raised intracranial pressure, and to a lesser extent sinusitis, is made worse by bending, coughing and sneezing. This feature is rarely present in childhood. Both light and movement exacerbate the migraine headache, which is relieved by lying down in a darkened room. Simple analgesics serve to relieve most headaches, and so their efficiency is little guide to the etiology of childhood headaches.

The presence or absence of associated symptoms and signs furnish valuable clues. Vomiting in association with headache should raise the suspicion of increased intracranial pressure, but it may be a feature of psychogenic headache and migraine. If the vomiting is not accompanied by nausea, raised intracranial pressure is a possible cause of the headache.

The classical pattern of migraine is incomplete in many children, and the

135

headache is not always hemicranial in distribution.

The family history should always be investigated when headache is a main complaint. The history commonly reveals that a near-relative suffers from headache, and occasionally it will be found that a relative has had severe intracranial disease which has made the family unduly concerned about the possible significance of headache. It is also important to conduct careful questioning about symptoms which indicate possible visual problems.

Children who complain of headache are often seen because a serious organic condition is feared. The physician should begin by trying to exclude such causes as increased intracranial pressure, brain tumor, cerebral trauma, vascular phenomena, hypoglycemia and hypertension. Sinusitis and allergy can be sought by examination and questioning. If the evidence suggests a visual problem, it may be necessary for the child to have an expert ophthalmological examination, including tests for astigmatism. The possibility of a brain abscess should be considered if the child has congenital heart-disease (especially if over three years of age and cyanotic) and if a child has chronic ear infections. Headache is a late manifestation of brain tumor or abscess, and usually symptoms of intracranial disease are already evident by the time headache occurs.

The examination

Examination of a child complaining of a headache should include careful examination of the eye grounds. The examiner should not be misled by the very marked degree of papilloedema present in pseudotumor cerebri, in which the relative mildness of the headache is out of proportion to the severe degree of papilloedema. It is a simple matter to exclude hypertension as a cause: while it may be assumed that examination of the eye grounds is carefully done, it is surprising how often the measurement of blood pressure is omitted and the diagnosis of hypertension delayed until blurring of vision or hypertensive encephalopathy occurs.

Frequently a child will complain of a significant headache at the time of the examination. The symptoms as described by the child are not in keeping with the child's normal neurological findings and affect. Conversely, a severe debilitating headache may disappear just before or during the examination. It is easy to regard such headaches as 'tension related', 'functional' or caused by psychosomatic symptoms, but adequate explanation is lacking. Vasoconstriction of selected vessels is the most common physiological explanation, but the mechanism is unknown.

Excessive physical investigations may be harmful and lead to further problems, even if the reassurance based on negative investigations appears to be accepted. However, until organic disease can be safely ruled out, the comparative rarity of organic headache should lead neither to negligence over the physical examination nor to lack of follow-up.

THE CHILD WHO MAY BE 'AUTISTIC'

'Affect' refers to the child's emotional relationship with his environment and the way he reacts by demonstration of spontaneous feelings to the people around him.

The distinction between a child with a disorder of affect, such as autism, and one with mental retardation is extremely difficult unless there is unequivocal evidence of earlier normality. The concept of autism is still emerging from simple clinical recognition. There is no specific treatment, multiple types of non-specific therapy have had relatively little success, and the etiology is uncertain.

Autistic or 'ego-defective' behavior also may be an associated finding in mental retardation, speech and language delay, aphasia, hearing loss, seizure disorders (such as infantile myoclonic seizures) and postencephalitic or traumatic syndromes.

The causes of autistic behavior are unknown. There may be a conduction or processing defect in the brain stem or thalamus, or more than one kind of insult to the brain stem at a critical time may be responsible. As the child grows older, the 'process' seems to burn out, but it leaves residual effects. If an organic cause such as a virus or immunological defects is ever shown to be the cause (or most common cause, if more than one insult is blamed), it may be that mentally retarded children are most vulnerable. That would help to account for the difficulty in separating mentally retarded from autistic children.

Autism used to be considered to be related in some way with the family environment and the mother-child relationship, because some of the early reported cases occurred in professional, educated, achieving families. This view is no longer held, although, as with polio and leukemia, epidemiological factors may be involved.

The child who is considered to be autistic relates poorly to other people, avoids eye-contact, and plays with objects rather than people. There may be ritualistic stereotyped movements, such as rocking. He forms interpersonal relationships poorly or not at all, has poor judgment, poor attention-span and is distractible. He 'marches to a different drummer', in that he does not seem to be influenced by the world about him, yet minute changes in routine can bring about violent reaction. Often he is hyperactive, in constant motion, and needs very little sleep. Care may be complicated by a reversal of sleeping patterns. There may be evidence of mental retardation, yet 'islands' of normal or above-normal activity may be striking. An unequivocally mentally retarded child may show a great deal of autistic behavior. Language may be absent or, if present, it may be echolalic, stylized or sing-song. Some autistic children who are mute can learn to communicate with sign language. Behavior can be testing, provocative and difficult to tolerate.

All the features described as being characteristic of the autistic child can be observed in other children, even so-called 'normal' children in certain circumstances. Failure of the child to 'relate' is a highly subjective judgement on the part of the person making it.

The opinion of the examiner, then, is based on skill and intuition. Are the features severe enough, prominent enough and consistent enough to justify the diagnosis of autism?

Although the characteristics seem clear when listed, the natural history of the condition is such that the diagnosis may be revised during future examinations.

CHAPTER 8

Examination of Infants and Young Children (Including Developmental Screening for the Child Over Three Years)

A special approach is needed when examining infants and young children, because the examiner must get as much information as possible in the shortest possible time. The comfort of the infant or child during the examination has a strong bearing on its success.

Answers elicited from the family during the history-taking process are especially valuable in giving a picture of the degree of parental responsibility, reliability and involvement. Details of prenatal and perinatal events obviously are also extremely important in the evaluation of infants.

The evaluation of infants has stimulated the production of a vast amount of literature on neurological maturation and developmental assessment. In his book describing the neurological development of a carefully chosen series of low-risk infants, Touwen (1976) has included an excellent review of the various philosophies and examination techniques used to assess infant development. His own work reinforces the hypothesis that there is wide variation in the rate at which neurological maturation occurs among normal infants. Drillien and Drummond (1977) point out in their discussion of the 'dystonic syndrome' that even high-risk babies who have abnormal signs may improve with time. Even if abnormal signs are present, the future type of clinical pattern may not be predictable. This, in fact, is true at all ages. An isolated physical finding has little predictive value and must be viewed within the larger context of other abnormal signs and factors. Responsible predictions are based on careful observations made over a period of time.

The approach given in the following pages is resolutely pragmatic. Directions are given for special examination techniques which have proved useful. The ages discussed (four weeks, 12 weeks, 24 weeks, 12 months and 24 months) are not developmentally sacred; they are merely identifiable stages. Obviously the procedure must be modified if a severe handicap exists, and an abnormal finding must be carefully investigated, regardless of how long it takes.

The period of observation and inspection preceding the formal examination is especially valuable in the assessment of an infant or toddler. A great deal of valid information can be gained simply by watching how the child moves, communicates, plays and responds to his parents.

A developmental assessment is an important part of the examination of infants, but it is purely a point of reference and should not be used to make a diagnosis of neurological impairment. A developmental examination may be simply an informal appraisal based on clinical experience, or it may be a detailed and formal evaluation performed by a developmental specialist.

The Denver Developmental Screening Test* is a simple, standardized test for detecting developmental delays in infancy and during the preschool years. It is easy to administer, simple to score, and can be used during a general assessment to give something more definitive than a clinical impression. The baby is tested in personal-social, fine motor adaptive, gross motor and language skills. Details of the Denver Developmental Screening Test are given in Appendix B.

Significance of infantile reflexes and automatisms

Early infantile automatisms and postures assumed in suspension often furnish early diagnostic information about delayed development of motor function in a child under 18 months of age. These signs may be much more helpful than conventional neurological signs based on alterations of muscle tone, reflexes and so on. However, they are not in any way specific for cerebral palsy in the sense of a relatively fixed brain-lesion, as opposed to a progressive disease. All of these signs are best interpreted in conjunction with other findings and with the known history. Infantile responses and automatisms may be qualitatively abnormal or asymmetrical, and evidence of abnormality may be furnished by their failure to appear at the normal age, or by their persistence after the age at which they ought to have disappeared. The normal range of variation is considerable and has been studied in detail in a group of normal infants reported elsewhere (Paine *et al.* 1964): Table XVIII shows the percentages of these infants who had lost or acquired certain signs at each month of the first year (Paine 1960).

The Babinski sign (see also p. 89)

The Babinski sign is considered the most characteristic sign of disturbed function in the pyramidal tract (see Fig. 34, p. 88). However, the variability of normal responses in infancy makes its interpretation difficult. Expected responses can include withdrawal, plantar flexion or dorsiflexion of the great toe, and fanning of the small toes. This last response is called the foot-sole response in order to distinguish it from the true sign of Babinski, a consistent isolated dorsiflexion of the big toe caused by supranuclear lesions. The vague and confusing term 'negative Babinski response' should be abandoned and the response to lateral plantar stimulation should be described (Touwen 1976).

The Moro reflex

This reflex is an important special response, in that it is always demonstrable with normal newborn infants, apart from the smaller premature ones. The positive normal reaction is as follows: the baby suddenly extends the upper extremities, then draws them together in front, with the limbs extended in an 'embrace' reaction, the fingers usually being spread (Fig. 42). The femora are also flexed on the pelvis in the full reaction seen in newborns. As the response begins to diminish with age, the clasping phase may be lost first, and only extension is seen.

Retention of the Moro reflex is encountered occasionally among children with

*See p. 4 for supplier's address.

139

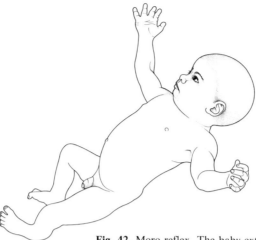

Fig. 42. Moro reflex. The baby extends the upper extremities, then draws them together over the chest. Usually the fingers are spread when the arms are in the 'embrace' position.

TABLE XVIII

Percentages of normal babies showing various infantile reflexes with increasing age

| | Signs that disappear with age | | | Signs that appear with age | | | | |
	Moro	Tonic neck reflex	Crossed adduction to knee jerk	Neck-righting reflex	Support-ing reaction	Landau	Para-chute	Hand grasp
Degree of sign tabulated:	Extension even without flexor phase	Imposable even for 30'' or inconstant	Strong or slight	Imposable but transient	Fair or good	Head above horizontal and back arched	Complete	Thumb to forefinger alone
Age (mths)								
1	93	67	?†	13	50	0	0	0
2	89	90	?†	23	43	0	0	0
3	70	50	41	25	52	0	0	0
4	59	34	41	26	40	0	0	0
5	22	31	41	38	61	29	0	0
6	0	11	21	40	66	42	3	0
7	0	0	12	43	74	42	29	16
8	0	0	15	54	81	44	40	53
9	0	0	6	67	96	97	76	63
10	0	0	3	100	100	100	79	84
11	0	0	3	100	100	100	90	95
12	0	0	2	100	100	100	100	100

From Paine and Oppé (1966).
†Divergence of experience and opinion between different examiners.

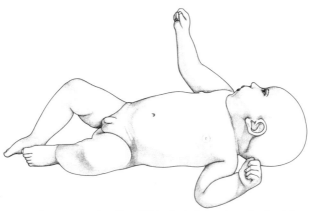

Fig. 43. Tonic neck reflex. With the baby supine, the head is rotated to either side: a positive response is extension of the arm and leg on the side to which the face is turned, with flexion of the limbs on the opposite side.

motor disabilities resulting from cerebral palsy, but this finding is relatively infrequent. The Moro rarely re-emerges following decerebrating catastrophes, whereas the tonic neck reflex commonly does. As indicated in Table XVIII, the Moro is never encountered in fullterm infants after six months of age. Flexion of the hips is the last trace to disappear, and if the test is reinforced by gentle pressure with the examiner's hand against the child's knees, often it is possible to feel an attempt at elevation of the femora until a much later age, although movement of the upper extremities is rarely seen.

The Moro reflex may be confused with the startle response, which is normally present throughout infancy and childhood. The startle response consists of mass myoclonic movement, which may occur during sleep, following a sudden noise or during some event which produces sudden anxiety or fright. It is sometimes accompanied by micturition, defecation or a cry. It is believed (though it has never been proved) that the startle response represents a cortical release phenomenon that becomes less easily elicited as the individual matures, but can be seen when the infant is frightened, or while tired, toxic, sleeping, ill or hungry.

The tonic neck reflex

The asymmetrical tonic neck reflex (Fig. 43) is an important infantile automatism because of its abnormal persistence in cerebral palsy and its reappearance following decerebrating catastrophes or in association with degenerative disease.

Demonstration of an asymmetrical tonic neck reflex is rarely possible in the neonatal period: it is common assumed and may be imposable between two and four months. The imposability of the posture should have disappeared by seven months at the latest. Sometimes the characteristic posture of the limbs develops immediately when the examiner turns the child's head to one side; in other instances there may be a delay of 20 to 30 seconds. The time taken to assume the posture is not critical, or at

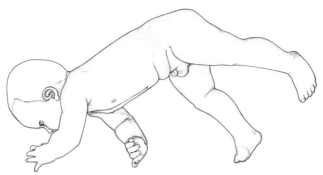

Fig. 44. Neck-righting reflex. With the infant in the supine position, the examiner turns the head to one side. The infant will rotate the shoulders in the same direction, then the trunk and finally the pelvis.

least its diagnostic significance has not been worked out. The degree of obligateness and the length of persistence of the pattern are more important. A normal baby of three or four months may remain in the tonic neck pattern for several minutes if particularly quiet and inactive, but far more often will struggle out of it within half a minute or so. A completely obligate tonic neck pattern, from which the child cannot escape by struggling, is abnormal at any age.

Turning the head to one side may continue to have some effect on the distribution of tone in the limbs until a much later age. This may be demonstrable in the modification of tendon reflexes, ankle clonus, etc., although few detailed studies have been made. Even at an age which some degree is normal, modest degrees of tonic neck reflex should be regarded as abnormal if the reaction is consistently asymmetrical, in the sense of being more spectacular when the head is turned toward the left than toward the right, or vice versa. Whatever degree of tonic neck reflex is present, it is usually more striking when the child is lying supine, but occasionally it will be more impressive when the child is in the sitting position, or even standing supported. Strong degrees of imposable tonic neck reflex almost always are incompatible with balance in independent standing and with independent walking. They tend to disappear as the child learns to walk alone.

A strongly imposable tonic neck reflex after the age of six months or a completely obligate one at any age may be taken as evidence of a degree of significant motor handicap, though not necessarily of mental deficiency.

The neck-righting reflex

The righting reflex follows the tonic neck reflex as the latter disappears with age (Fig. 44). A phenomenon closely resembling a true neck-righting reflex may be demonstrated in the normal newborn infant by the examiner's ability to turn the body toward one side by turning the head. However, in the newborn this is a smooth, immediate and almost simultaneous turning based merely on general hypertonus, and on close observation is clearly different from the two-phase neck-righting reflex seen later in the first year.

142

The neck-righting reflex normally persists to some degree until the child is able to rise directly from the supine position, rather than by rolling over onto the abdomen, getting up first to all fours and then erect. It disappears by degrees, or rather is covered up by degrees by the child's own voluntary activity, and it is best thought of as the mechanism used by small children to rise from the floor in the quadrupedal fashion. It is always abnormal to find an obligate neck-righting reflex, in which the baby can be rolled over and over across the floor like a log despite his most violent struggling. This is encountered chiefly with various types of cerebral palsy.

Abnormally strong tonic neck and neck-righting reflexes are frequently seen with cerebral palsy of various types, at the stage before acquisition of sitting and standing balance. However, it is highly important to remember that the two reflexes are in no way diagnostic of cerebral palsy. Both responses, but especially the tonic neck reflex, may re-emerge following catastrophes such as cardiac arrest or in association with progressive degenerative diseases. If the progressive disease begins early in life, before the tonic neck reflex has quite been lost, it continues uninterruptedly and increases in degree. This may give the false impression of cerebral palsy, and cause the examiner to fail to recognize Tay-Sachs disease if the startle reaction to sound is not particularly exaggerated or if he fails to see the cherry-red spot in the macula.

Placing and supporting reactions

The placing and supporting reactions of the lower extremities sometimes facilitate the evaluation of defects of motor development in infants and very young children. Both are likely to be abnormal in some way if they are affected by any kind of cerebral palsy. The likely principal abnormalities are absence of the normal response, its general disorganization or its exaggeration in a stereotyped, unvarying way. Extrapyramidal involvement usually produces general disorganization of these responses, and generally the supporting reaction is more poorly developed than the placing reaction. The reverse is true in spasticity, in which extensor hypertonus during vertical suspension is an asset in supporting but a liability in placing. Placing in that case is likely to be executed in a stereotyped, mechanical fashion, and invariably with both feet at once, regardless of asymmetrical induction by touching only one foot against the underside of the table-top. Supporting the weight by close adduction of the legs or by standing on the toes also suggests spasticity. Cerebral hemiparesis produces an asymmetrical placing reflex and sometimes an asymmetrical supporting posture.

Placing and automatic supporting are both present normally in the neonatal period and an exact age for their disappearance cannot be set because they are gradually superseded by or integrated into voluntary activity. It is probable that something resembling placing can always be obtained if sufficient traction is exerted to produce discomfort, the reaction then becoming a form of withdrawal response. The normal newborn supports weight in a slightly crouching position, with the hips and knees flexed, in contrast to older children and adults who support weight with the knee fully extended and locked. Though the two types of supporting reaction may merge into one another without any hiatus, there is often a period (usually between two

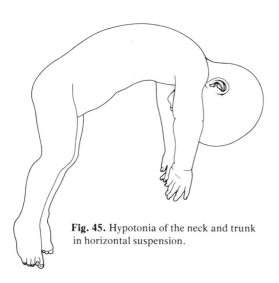

Fig. 45. Hypotonia of the neck and trunk in horizontal suspension.

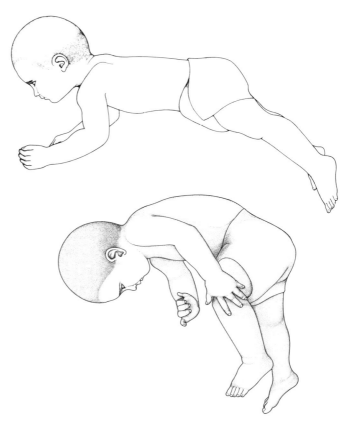

Fig. 46. Landau reaction. The infant is held in ventral suspension and the examiner passively flexes the head, causing extensor tone to be lost.

144

and four months of age) during which the supporting reaction is less effective than it was in the newborn period, in terms of percentage of weight borne. The neonatal form may even disappear, in which case for a month or two before the more mature fashion of support develops, the baby is virtually incapable of supporting any of his weight. This apparent physiological regression in itself does not imply progressive disease.

Stepping and hopping are also gradually integrated into voluntary activity and walking, and are of diagnostic value only if absent, asymmetrical or qualitatively abnormal.

Suspension in space

Adduction, extension or scissoring of the lower extremities while in vertical suspension in space are signs of spasticity (see Fig. 50, p. 152). Abnormal posture in horizontal suspension, without elevation of the head and lower extremities is less specific and merely indicates hypotonia of neck and trunk (Fig. 45). Many spastic babies have hypertonic limbs and a hypotonic trunk, but in the case of future dystonia or choreoathetosis, hypotonus of the trunk is almost universal during infancy once any neonatal rigidity (such as that due to kernicterus or an anoxic insult) has worn off. A normal infant should not collapse limply across the examiner's hand into the shape of an inverted 'U', but there is variation among normal children in the rate at which extension of the neck, spinal column and lower limbs is acquired. The degree of elevation of the lower extremities is less critical; nevertheless, the full Landau reaction should only be defined as being present when there is elevation of the head above the horizontal and upward arching of the spine so that it becomes concave. This degree of spinal extension is not present in all normal infants until about one year of age. When the head is passively flexed, extensor tone is lost (Landau reflex) (Fig. 46). This is also known as the Schaltenbrandt reaction, or as Landau 2 (Touwen 1976). They denote the same condition.

In the case of children who are unable to walk, the attitude they assume during suspension in space should afford valuable information about the nature of the motor deficit. In vertical suspension, the most important clues to look for are those that indicate early spasticity.

The parachute reaction

The parachute reaction (Fig. 47) is a valuable diagnostic sign because its abnormality indicates malfunction of the upper extremities, and may confirm that a supposed cerebral paraparesis (lower extremities only) is actually a tetraparesis (all four extremities), long before a stretch reflex or hyperreflexia can be demonstrated in the arms. The parachute reaction is not present at birth, but should appear around seven months of age (occasionally earlier) and is present in most normal infants at nine months. However, absence in itself should not be considered abnormal before one year of age. An asymmetrical parachute reaction (Fig. 48) implies greater deficit of function on the more abnormal side; a unilaterally abnormal reaction may be seen with hemiparesis, brachial palsy, or with injuries or other painful lesions of one upper extremity or clavicle. The parachute reaction has no specific age of normal disappearance but is much less automatic and less consistently demonstrable after

145

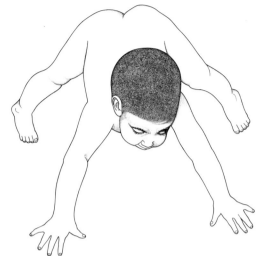

Fig. 47. Normal parachute reaction: horizontally suspended by the waist, face down, the child is lowered toward a flat surface. The arms extend in front, slightly abducted at the shoulders, and the fingers spread as if to break a fall.

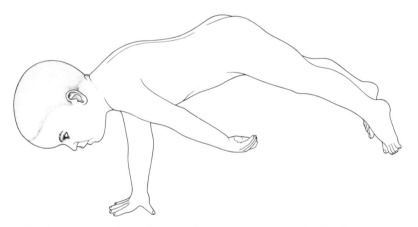

Fig. 48. Asymmetrical parachute reaction: a positive response is elicited only on one side of the body. The response is abnormal when the child's head is unable to stay suspended, the arms do not extend and are reluctant to bear weight or to make plantar contact with a flat surface.

about two years of age. It is more a vestibular reaction than an ocular one, and blindness or bandaging of the eyes makes surprisingly little difference in the reaction of extension of the upper limbs and even in the spreading of fingers. However, there is no increase in finger-spreading when the table-top is near but cannot be seen. The parachute reaction, comprising not only the extension of the limbs as a whole but also the spreading and slight hyperextension of the fingers, tests both proximal and distal function, and since there may be discrepancies between the two, it should always be compared with the child's ability to grasp small objects. Suppression or distortion of the parachute reaction occurs with both spasticity and extrapyramidal dyskinesia. This type of response, combined with a fisted hand, would suggest future spasticity.

146

Future athetosis is suggested by the combination of a poor or absent parachute response, or one which is more abnormal distally than proximally, with delay in acquisition of thumb-to-forefinger grasp for small objects (normally nine to 12 months).

Significance of ophthalmological findings in infancy

Since there are many instances of cranial abnormalities occurring in association with eye defects, the presence of an anomaly in one should make the physician suspect the occurrence of a developmental disorder in the other.

Eye contact

The infant's earliest communication is by eye contact, which develops as the mother and baby interact. The child's ability to recognize a face can be demonstrated by testing within the first 24 hours. This ability of a normal newborn to prefer, and respond to, an object the size of a human face is apparent clinically during the first seven days. How soon depends upon the amount of sedation the infant has received (via the placenta) and the interaction between adult and infant. Many developmentally disabled infants probably are additionally handicapped by diminished ability to make interpersonal contact.

Recognition of form

Recognition of form and a preference for certain objects are present shortly after birth, and highly developed by one month of age. This facility can be recognized by watching the normal one-month-old follow a light in a darkened room.

Findings on funduscopic examination

The optic fundus of a normal one-month-old infant may prove difficult to examine. The pupils are likely to be small and the lids often close in response to stimulation. Even gentle restraint of the infant's lids can make matters worse, and the examiner's ability to distract the baby briefly or to catch the infant's brief gaze may be sorely tested.

The macula of a one-month-infant appears to be less well defined than at three or six months, and therefore is generally considered less mature. Visual acuity at this age is thought to be 20/40 (6/12), though this may be based more on currently used techniques than on true fictional ability. The discs tend to be paler than in older infants. Glial remnants around the disc sometimes give the appearance of early papilloedema. Because of a relative lack of pigment, the retina appears more vascular: this is particularly true of fair-skinned infants. Incomplete pigmentation can be easily confused with the chorioretinitis of maternal infection due to rubella or cytomegalic infection. There is often evidence of previous hemorrhages, particularly at the outer margin of the retina. These occur in at least 50 per cent of infants who have some kind of difficulty in the neonatal period, but the incidence is also high among babies who have had 'normal' deliveries. Detecting the age of hemorrhage usually is not possible on the basis of a single examination.

Very small, white discs are abnormal. They are seen in infants with microcephaly, hydranencephaly and other significant CNS anomalies. Asymmetry (*i.e.* the presence of a small white disc on one side only) is rare and for a variety of reasons suggests aplasia of the optic nerve on the affected side. Absence or asymmetry of the 'light' or 'red' reflex of the maculae is unusual and often is the first evidence of a significant CNS disorder. In some instances the reflected light of the direct ophthalmoscope appears to be diffuse, rather than the crisp, clean point of light against a red background of the normal 'red' or 'light' reflex. The diffuse appearance may be caused by immaturity or local edema, or it can be early evidence of a disorder. Referral for definitive examination by someone skilled in the use of an indirect ophthalmoscope may be necessary to determine whether there is pathology. Often obvious abnormalities of macular formation are missed in the early weeks of life, not because they are not present but because lack of vision, unless marked, is not a common complaint by the parents. Where there is a high degree of suspicion (for example, a history of Tay-Sachs disease in a sibling) macular disease, if present, is readily apparent.

The cornea

The cornea normally measures 8-11mm in the fullterm newborn at one month of age. Asymmetry of the size of the cornea is most often associated with unilateral microphthalmia. Macrocornea may occur in mucopolysaccharide disorders and in the Low syndrome. Although the pupils are likely to be small in early infancy and to dilate poorly (even with mydriatics) because of immature autonomic function, pinpoint pupils without evidence of drug ingestion occur as an isolated finding (congenital mydriosis).

Nystagmus in infancy

Congenital nystagmus is rarely noted before one month of age because most infants do not fix their eyes on one point for a long enough time. The movement is equal to either side of the midline and usually is decreased if either eye is covered. Ocular albinism, which may be familial, is one cause. In some instances nystagmus is due to an error of accommodation. It is unusual for there to be associated abnormalities. Compensatory or associated head nodding (spasmus nutans) is rare before six months. The natural history of the most common form of congenital nystagmus is that it is scarcely detected at one week, apparent by one month and obvious by six months, disappearing gradually during adolescence (see Chapter 4).

Strabismus in infancy

In infants, as in older children, strabismus may be due to an error of accommodation, overaction of muscle groups, failure of a tendon to be inserted properly or failure of central control. The mechanisms by which the CNS compensates for small differences in muscle balance between the two eyes are poorly understood and highly speculative.

Ptosis in infancy

Ptosis is the most common early sign of myasthenia gravis, when it is usually bilateral, but often asymmetrical and occasionally unilateral. Although congenital myasthenia gravis should have cleared by one month, there have been case reports of mixed congenital and acquired forms. Congenital ptosis (a benign condition) may be impossible to distinguish from the ptosis of myasthenia gravis, although clinically in the latter one would expect greater variability with fatigue. A 'Tensilon' test (see Chapter 11) may be necessary. Congenital hyperthyroidism may produce bilateral lid-lag, which, because the lids are puffy, may resemble true ptosis. This lid-lag is always bilateral.

THE FOUR-WEEK-OLD INFANT

A normal one-month-old infant is a delightful individual. Personality is well established and the baby will look at a face intently, remain quiet when spoken to, and might smile in response to a smiling adult. A mother in the first few weeks after birth is probably tired and may be a little depressed, even in the best of circumstances. She may also be anxious about her baby. The examiner must be sensitive to her fatigue and her stress. If a combination of observation and examination suggest the existence of an abnormality, the suspicion should be tested last, not first.

Directions

Watch how the infant and mother react to each other. How is the baby handled and cuddled? Does the mother seem to enjoy the baby? Does the baby regard his mother's face? Does the baby express pleasant anticipation of breast- or bottle-feeding? Note whether the cry is normal (hungry, tired or fretful) or abnormal (shrill, incessant, high-pitched, irritable or weak). Look for facial asymmetry when the baby is crying, and at rest. Check the anterior fontanelle. It should be slightly depressed if the infant is quiet but not sucking and should pulsate visibly, synchronously with the pulse rate. Palpate the head gently, feeling for any bone defects, tenderness, swelling, flattening or prominence of the vessels.

Have the mother undress the baby, noting her skill and interaction with him as she does so. Weigh the baby, and place him supine on the examination table. Make sure the baby is kept warm by covering him, if necessary, with one of his own blankets. At some point during the examination measure the head circumference several times with a steel tape and record the greatest value. Measure the recumbent crown-heel length, and the chest circumference at the nipple line. Note the general appearance of the infant, and look for obvious congenital malformations and skin rashes or lesions. Note the position the baby assumes while supine. See if the movements of the arms and legs are symmetrical, if the limbs move freely and are appropriately energetic. Spontaneous 'bicycling' of the legs (*i.e.* moving the legs as if riding a bicycle) is abnormal at any age. The infant should be able to raise all extremities against gravity without apparent fatigue and the amount of activity on the two sides of the body and of the upper and lower extremities should be roughly equal in an observation period of two to three minutes.

If the baby urinates observe the quality and, if a male, the trajectory and power of the stream. A good stream excludes abnormalities of the lower genito-urinary tract.

Test for a social smile by establishing eye contact and coming face to face 30-45cm (12-18in) apart. A positive response at this age is unusual without touching, but is normally observed after six weeks. Test for the rooting response by placing an index finger on the infant's cheek, about 4cm (1½in) from the corner of the lip. A positive response consists of moving the lips and turning the head so that the mouth is closer to the stimulus. The response usually is present on both sides, but its strength depends on the length of time since the baby was last fed.

Look closely at the infant's hands and fingers, looking for equal use of the fingers on each hand. Touch the palms of each hand with your index finger and expect a symmetrical grasp response. Test for a release and note whether the thumb moves freely outward. A strong finger grasp can also be elicited by touching a knitting needle or pencil against the fingers.

Note the position of the light reflex on the pupils by holding a small flashlight or the light of an ophthalmoscope about 60cm (24in) away from the baby's nose. The light should be symmetrical but slightly toward the nasal side of the center of the pupil. Disregard skin folds at this stage. If the pupils are not in the midline or if the light reflex becomes asymmetrical with forced or spontaneous movement, the finding is unusual and requires further study (see Chapter 4). Exotropia or exophoria (outward turning of the pupil of either eye when the other pupil is in the mid-position) is abnormal at any age. Note the size of the pupils. A large pupil suggests that the iris may be imperfectly formed. Partial or complete aniridia can be overlooked unless a conscious effort is made by the examiner to note its presence. Look for nystagmus (rare before one month of age) and for any abnormalitiy of the sclerae and the corneae. Next test for pupillary response, first by noting the size of the pupils and their symmetry, then, with the pupils in the mid-position test bilateral response by bringing the light towards the nose. The normal response is symmetrical. Test each pupil for direct and consensual response by bringing the light forward from a position a few inches away from each ear to the lateral margin of the pupil.

Test for hearing by ringing a bell 30cm (12in) from the head on either side and watching for lateral movement of the eyes. Response is usually definite, but it may be diminished if there is other noise, or by the infant's mood or fatigue. Stilling of the baby may also be considered a positive response.

Test deep tendon reflexes and try to elicit ankle clonus, gently using one finger. Test for the Babinski response by semi-extending the infant's knee with one hand and stroking the lateral margin of the plantar surface from the heel to the toe, crossing over the distal ends of the metatarsals to the base of the great toe, with your thumbnail, a knitting needle, key or similar edge*. The usual response under one year of age is an inconsistent, variable extension of the big toe. Sustained extension is abnormal if asymmetrical, accompanied by other signs or consistently elicitable. (See Fig. 34, p. 88.)

Gently hold the infant's mouth open by pressing the chin down with the thumb of

---

*Some examiners prefer to stroke the lateral surface from toe to heel to avoid the plantar grasp reflex.

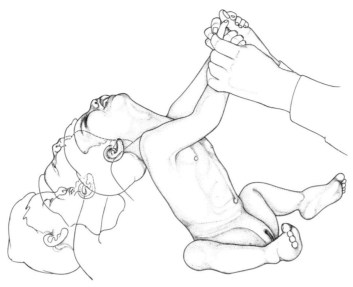

Fig. 49. Head lag on pulling to sit.

one hand and place a small tongue depressor against the upper gum. Observe the tongue movements carefully. If a light has been properly placed, fasciculations will appear as worm-like movements along the surface of the tongue. Note the presence or absence of adder-like movements of the tongue: if present, they suggest immature behavior and probably significant developmental delay. A large tongue may be associated with macrosomia (*e.g.* Beckwith syndrome, glycogen storage disease or hypothyroidism). Atrophy or asymmetry of the tongue is unusual at this age. Where appropriate, taste can be tested by the application of a salt solution and glucose solution to the surface by a cotton applicator.

Elicit the Moro response by slowly lifting the infant a few inches from the table, placing your right hand under the shoulders and the left under the head, then dropping your hand a few inches so that the neck is extended. Be sure the baby's head is in the midline. The usual response at this age consists of extension of the arms and spreading of the fingers, as if in an attempt to embrace something, and flexion of the legs (see Fig. 42, p. 140). There is usually a surprised look on the baby's face and he often cries out. The response may also be elicited by a sudden loud noise or by vibrating the examining table. An asymmetrical Moro response can be a sign of brachial palsy.

Attempt to demonstrate the tonic neck reflex by rotating the head first to one side, then to the other. The arm should extend and the leg flex on the side toward which the infant's face is turned (see Fig. 43, p. 141). Gently pull the infant 15-20cm (6-8in) from the supine position by holding the wrists. Look for head-lag (Fig. 49) and note the infant's ability to overcome the effect of gravity. Lower the infant into the supine position again within five to 10 seconds. Place the baby prone on the examination table. Check the spine carefully for dermal sinuses and other congenital

151

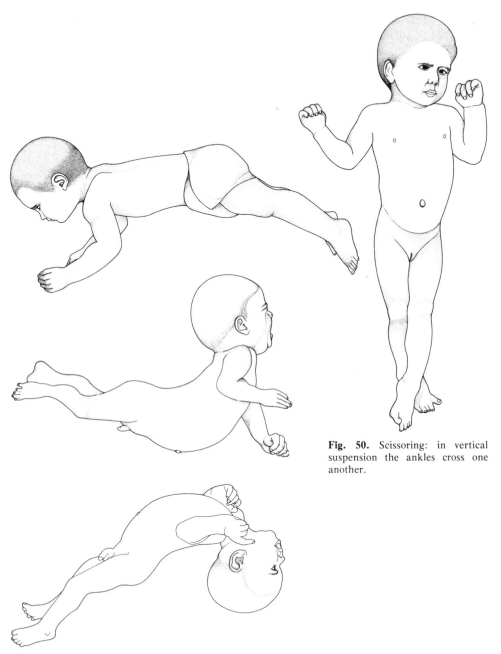

Fig. 50. Scissoring: in vertical suspension the ankles cross one another.

Fig. 51. Horizontal suspension. *(Top)* Normal: the spine is extended, the head and lower extremities are raised. *(Centre)* Hypertonic: there is excessive reflex contraction of muscles, most evident in the ability to maintain this posture. *(Bottom)* Hypotonic: lack of reflex contraction results in 'floppy' or 'rag-dolls' posture.

152

malformations. The baby can be expected to raise his head and chin off the examination table and look to either side. The pelvis will be up off the surface, but the knees should not be tucked under the abdomen. With the baby supine again, test for dislocation of the hip by flexing the knees to a right angle and gently rotate both knees simultaneously, externally and internally.

Grasp the infant so that your right and left thumbs are resting on his left and right clavicles, your palms are under the axillae, and fingers are around his back and pull him into the sitting position. Support his neck and back to make this transition comfortable. Observe for momentary head control. Bring the infant to a standing position and observe neck and back control. Lift him to a tall standing position and then 10-15cm (4-6in) from the surface of the table. Observe any tendency for the legs to scissor or for the arms to flex (Fig. 50). The expected response of the normal infant is to move the legs and arms spontaneously. If briefly suspended over the table by the examiner, then brought down gently so that the toes touch a firm surface and the head is slightly forward, a few stepping movements are usually observed. This response, which is strongly present at birth but often has disappeared by six to eight weeks, seems to be influenced by practice. Next, firmly support the infant under the anterior chest with one hand and lift him from the table. The normal response is for the legs to be raised briefly and for the head to go up. Assess muscle tone in horizontal suspension (Fig. 51). Although there is considerable variation, arching of the back and head usually is associated with other evidence of hypertonicity. The 'rag doll' or inverted 'U' position is evidence of significant hypotonia.

Placing responses, performed by touching the dorsum of the foot against the edge of the table, are virtually always present and easily elicited at this stage (Fig. 52). The response is for the infant to raise the foot and place it on the table-top. Grasp the infant from the rear so that the fingers (but not the thumb) pass through the infant's axillae, with the left hand under the infant's left and the right under the infant's right. The speed of the response is influenced by the temperature of the surface, the vigor of the infant and any distractions. The response is symmetrical.

If meningeal irritation is suspected, check for it by lifting the infant's head with your left hand and the shoulders with your right. When the infant is 10-15cm (4-6in) from the table, gradually lower and raise the head. The normal response in the conscious infant is for this passive flexion and extension to meet with little resistance. The abnormal response is increased resistance, especially against gravity. This increased resistance can be felt by the examiner and may be associated with other evidence of irritability, such as crying and flexion or extension of the extremities. In a one-month-old infant, evidence of meningeal irritation is rarely an isolated phenomenon. Other evidence of meningeal irritation is gained from the awareness and appearance of the child, an increase in fontanelle pressure, abnormal eye-movements, irritability, and, often, an inability to find a position of comfort.

Pick the baby up and talk to him briefly, assessing his alertness. With the baby in a comfortable position, either on his back or with the mother, look quickly at each fundus through a bright ophthalmoscope from a distance of about 1m (3ft); bring the ophthalmoscope closer to the right pupil if you are using your right eye. You should

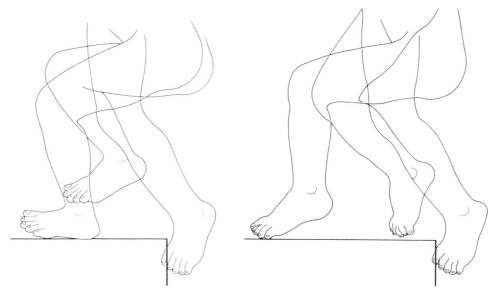

Fig. 52. Placing response. *(Left)* Normal. The child is suspended vertically and the examiner brings the dorsum of the foot up against the edge of the table. The child will plantarflex the ankle and flex the knee and hip, thereby raising the leg and placing the foot squarely on the table-top. *(Right)* Abnormal. The child does not plantarflex the ankle or flex the knee and hip. The foot does not make firm contact with the table-top.

be able to see enough of the lens, maculae, vessels and disc to convince you either that all is well or that more study is required. Next, rotate the baby at arm's length and check whether the eyes move from side to side (see Chapter 4). Finally, transilluminate the head according to the directions given in Chapter 4.

THE 12-WEEK-OLD INFANT

The personality which was emerging at one month should be clearly defined by three months. The mother should know whether she has an alert busybody or a placid gurgler. The three-month-old baby should certainly be settled, *i.e.* reasonably predictable in its sleeping and feeding, and thriving and progressing as expected. Close interaction between mother and baby should be apparent and a social smile should be readily produced when the baby sees a smiling face. The baby should be experimenting with vocal sounds which can be identified as expressions of pleasure, distress or hunger. The baby should respond when spoken to.

Directions

Note the baby's general appearance and look carefully for asymmetries, which may be more apparent at three months. Inspect the eyes, face and head while the mother holds the baby sitting upright on her knee. Check to see if any torticollis is developing and note the degree of head control. Have the mother undress the baby. Weigh him and place him on his back on the examination table, noting his position and movements. Try to get the baby to smile. Measure the chest circumference and crown-heel length, and compare with previous measurements if available. Hold a dangling tape-measure or suspended object in the midline 45cm (18in) above the baby and watch visual pursuit to each side from the midline and from one side across the midline to the other side. Visual pursuit across the midline is rarely done smoothly, so that the infant seems to lose sight of the object then regains it as it passes the midline. Examine the eyes, sclerae, pupils, eye movements and responses to light. Inspect and palpate the head carefully, noting the size of the fontanelle. Measure the head circumference and look for asymmetry or flattening. The fontanelle may be widely patent or virtually closed at three months. With either extreme, associated findings (head circumference, shape, general development) should be reviewed. Ring a bell about 45cm (18in) from and level with the baby's ear and note whether he turns toward the sound.

Hand the baby a rattle. At this age he will not normally reach out for an object. Note the strength of the grasp. Examine the fingers and hands. The hands should be freely open and persistent fisting is abnormal. Feel the muscles, flex and extend the arms and legs. If not voluntary, resistance to passive movement could indicate spasticity. Note the position of the feet: feet kept in extension could also be a sign of spasticity.

Test the deep tendon reflexes. An asymmetrical response or exaggerated knee-jerks would be suspicious at three months. Test for ankle clonus. Test the Babinski response. A reproducible extensor response combined with exaggerated knee-jerks would be a cause for concern. Test the tonic neck reflex, which should be greatly diminished or absent at this age. An obligatory tonic neck reflex is abnormal at any age. Attempt to elicit a Moro response: a full response should not be present, but some babies will still make some arm movements. Examine the tongue, mouth and pharynx. Test for dislocation of the hips, looking especially for an asymmetrical response or limitation of abduction, which could indicate increased muscle tone.

Pull the baby to a sitting position. Note the response of the upper arms and shoulders, and head and back control. The movement should be against gravity and there should be some spontaneous back, neck, and head control, with only a slight head-lag.

Bring to a standing position. The baby should tend to sag at the hips and knees. The weight should be evenly distributed and there should be no extensor thrust. Hold the baby in horizontal suspension, taking care to maintain the head above the plane of the rest of the body. Maintenance of an inverted 'U' position, with hands and feet hanging loosely down, can indicate muscle weakness or hypotonia. Slowly bring the baby down toward the examination table over a period of five to 10 seconds. One would expect to see the neck extend and the arms reach out symmetrically (*i.e.* the arms 'defend' against impact). This response is the first evidence of the emerging 'parachute reaction' (see Fig. 47, p. 146). An asymmetrical response would be abnormal.

Place the baby prone on the examination table. The head should be well up, the

155

weight borne on the forearms, and the chest held off the examining table.

Test for vestibular function (see Chapter 4). Ask his mother to dress him. Be sure a funduscopic examination has been done, and transilluminate the head if this has not been recorded (see Chapter 4).

THE 24-WEEK-OLD INFANT

An average six-month-old baby is an alert, active individual with a definite personality. Most are happy sitting in a baby-chair or lap, mouthing objects, banging a cup for pleasure or attention, and they have very definite likes and dislikes. They attempt to reach for desired objects and, if successful, transfer them from hand to hand. They coo, chuckle and babble and are not yet shy, although they may discriminate strangers from their parents. The history of a normal six-month-old baby should document satisfactory growth and development. Allowances may have to be made for prematurity, hospital admissions and socio-economic disadvantage (to the extent of one month for each month of unusual circumstances). Observation of the acquisition of expected skills over a period of time remains the best method of judging progress if more than one opportunity of examining the baby is available.

The questions asked on the Denver Developmental Screening Test (Frankenberg and Dodds 1967, Frankenberg *et al.* 1971; see Appendix B) are traditional and may be used as part of a baseline against which progress (or lack of it) can be judged three, six or 12 months later. The formal administration and scoring of the Denver test is simple, and it can be used in a standard manner. However, too much time spent on the test may erode the short attention-span of a six-month-old baby.

It is wise first to establish a firm three-month baseline on the Denver scale and to work from that point of reference. The key questions are 'rolls over', 'grasps a rattle', 'laughs', 'squeals', and 'smiles spontaneously'. If the examiner's 'quick glance' or the parents' answers suggest that there are ambiguities, these should be defined and resolved before going further.

Directions

Have the baby sit comfortably in his mother's lap. Listen to his spontaneous vocalizations and observe his facial expressions, alertness and his reponses to his parents' voices; listen for consonantal sounds such as 'Baba' or 'Dada'; if none are heard, ask the parents if the baby makes these sounds at home. Look at his general appearance, head, face and eyes, as described earlier. Dangle a colored ball or tape-measure and observe visual pursuit from one side to the other. Offer a cube or small toy. Note the grasp (it should be palmar) and watch to see if the cube is transferred to the other hand. Look for hand preference (abnormal at this age) and asymmetry in reach and hand use.

Test the baby's hearing while he sits on his mother's lap, if possible with the other parent sitting facing him to distract his attention. Stand behind the mother and gently ring a bell to the side of the baby's head on a level with his ear and 45cm (18in) away. Make sure that the object used to test hearing is out of the baby's line of vision.

156

Repeat on the opposite side, and with a variety of sounds—cup and spoon, high-pitched rattle, tissue paper, and soft-spoken voice ('ss' and 'oo' sounds). The baby demonstrates functional hearing by turning his head to localize the sound. At this age he is able to localize sound in the horizontal plane level with his ear but not at 45° above or below.

Test the baby's distant vision by standing 3m (9ft) away, watching to see if he fixates on a face at this distance and if he will follow a small toy. Use graded white balls on a dark background (either mounted on a stick or rolling across a black cloth) at 3m to observe both fixation and tracking (see Chapter 4).

Stand in front of the mother and baby and hold out your arms. A friendly six-month-old baby may readily hold out his arms in response, indicating a desire to be picked up. Undress and weigh the baby. Place him supine on the examination table, making sure he is comfortable. Examine the sclerae, pupils and eye movements as described previously, using a cover test if necessary (Chapter 4). If the baby is quiet, a funduscopic examination may be done at this point. Examine the mouth and tongue. Measure the crown-heel length of each leg from the anterior iliac crest to the medial malleolus. Measure the head and chest circumferences.

Inspect and palpate the head and neck. Carefully note the size and pulsation of the fontanelle. Look for any unusual head shape such as craniosynostosis, frontal bossing or evidence of enlargement of the posterior fossa, which would suggest the Dandy-Walker syndrome. Look for asymmetrical flattening, which could be caused by congenital torticollis or by the infant constantly lying in the same position in the crib. See if the baby can raise his head spontaneously from the supine position.

Watch the range and symmetry of spontaneous movements of the baby's arms and legs. Often a six-month-old baby is happy to play with his feet. Check the hips for dislocation or spasticity. Passively flex and extend the arms and legs to evaluate joint mobility and muscle tone. Test the deep tendon reflexes and the plantar response. See if the Moro reflex has disappeared, as would be expected. Look for the emergence of the neck-righting reflex by turning the head to one side and noting whether the shoulders, trunk and pelvis follow (see Fig. 44, p. 142).

Turn the baby over to a prone position. When prone he should extend his arms fully and lift himself up to look about by putting weight on his hands. A lively six-month-old may take advantage of this opportunity to demonstrate his skill at rolling from prone to supine.

Pull the baby up to a sitting position. Note any resistance, head-lag, or tendency to fall back. All are signs which require explanation. The baby should sit with minimal support. Marked flexion of the knees while sitting *might* mean spasticity of the hamstrings, and the deep tendon reflexes should then be checked again for hyperactivity. Estimate near vision by seeing if he will fixate on a raisin or small object placed in front of him.

Pull the baby up to a standing position. He should bear his weight on both legs equally, with some flexion at the hips. A strong preference for one leg or the other must be accounted for. If a preference is shown, look carefully for weakness or paresis of the arm on the same side. Test for the beginning of the parachute reaction by grasping the baby around the waist and gently lowering him face down toward the examination table. The arms should extend and attempt to come toward the midline to protect the nose. Any asymmetry of the 'defending' arms is significant. Hold the baby securely in a horizontal position. The head should be extended well above the plane of the shoulders and the legs should also be extended. Test for the Landau reflex by passively flexing the head: the legs should also flex (see Fig. 46, p. 144). Test vestibular function (see Chapter 4).

Partially dress the baby while talking to him, then return him to his mother. If it has not been done previously, do a funduscopic examination at this stage and transilluminate the head if there is no previous record of this procedure.

THE 12-MONTH-OLD BABY

A 12-month-old baby is likely to be reasonably tractable and usually can be won over by quiet, friendly flattery. The attention-span is short, but there is not yet the perversity which characterizes the two-year-old. A 12-month-old baby who is on schedule has learnt to crawl well, pull to stand, and to cruise along pieces of furniture. He may walk if one hand is held, and perhaps take a few steps unassisted. A minority of babies are 'bottom shufflers'; they usually do not crawl, and walk late, but get around quite fast on their bottoms in a sitting position. A 12-month-old baby should also be able to feed himself up to a point, though he will not be very competent with a spoon. He may have one recognizable word beside 'Mama' or 'Dada' which is appropriately used. He can wave 'Bye-bye' and clap hands in imitation. He may be very shy of strangers and cling tightly to his mother when approached.

The general history should focus on emerging skills in motor development and communication, as well as checking on general health and evidence of satisfactory growth. Bear in mind that lack of stimulation and lack of opportunity can be important factors in apparently delayed development.

Directions

Watch and listen while you take the history. Observe how the yearling explores a new environment, how he moves around, uses his hands, and how the parents control him. Note the presence or absence of toys, bottles or blankets brought along for comfort, distraction and stimulation.

Ask the mother to sit the baby on her lap. Offer a toy and note hand use, reaching skills and grasp. Put a small object or raisin in front of him and watch for prompt visual recognition and a neat pincer movement of the thumb and fingers when picking it up. The response should be symmetrical, and a pincer grasp in one hand but not the other should be investigated.

Check the baby's hearing, as at six months, with a variety of high- and low-pitched sounds. Move behind the baby when he is momentarily distracted and test his hearing by quietly crackling paper, shaking a high-pitched rattle and gently ringing a bell below and above each ear, but outside his visual field at a distance of approximately 1m (3ft). The baby should turn toward the sound, and should be able to localize sounds at 45° above and below the plane of the ear.

Take off the shoes and give one to the baby to hold. Observe finger, arm and hand movements as the shoe is transferred from one hand to the other. Make an informal quick assessment of the mobility of the joints and muscle tone. Look at the shoes for clues to motor skills. The unmarked shoes of a baby who has never crawled or stood up are as clear an external 'footprint' as those of the baby who has worn out the top of the toe but not marked the sole. The counterparts of these 'footprints' are the bilaterally worn but symmetrical inner toe of shoes of the child who has spastic diplegia or the lack of wear on the heel of the child who has a hemiplegia.

Ask the mother to undress the baby. Observe whether the undressing process gives a clue to a motor defect or movement disorder. Re-check the muscle tone of the arms and legs and mobility of the joints, and check deep tendon reflexes and plantar responses. Take the baby, weigh him and have him sit on the examination table. Measure the chest. Gently turn the baby into the supine position. Examine the eyes and do a funduscopic examination at this time if the baby is quiet, or this may be done later on the mother's lap. Examine the head, neck, mouth and pharynx. Test for the neck-righting response (see examination at 24 weeks).

Pull the baby up to a standing position. Note how he bears his weight. Hold him horizontally and try to demonstrate the parachute response by bringing his nose toward the examining table. The arms should extend and sweep forward smoothly to protect the face and nose. Measure the head. Partially dress the baby and talk to him; put him on the floor facing his mother and see how he negotiates the terrain.

THE 24-MONTH-OLD TODDLER

A child just past his second birthday has changed from a malleable toddler to a runabout with a strong sense of independence, so he may be very difficult to evaluate. An older child can be diverted by verbal cues, pictures, running the water faucet, washing and drying hands, and other subtle (and not so subtle) forms of bribery. A two-year-old may not be won over by these measures and may assert his right to be in control by sitting determinedly on his mother's lap and refusing to co-operate. A display of temper during the examination causes a confrontation, wastes time, and undermines the confidence of the parents in the validity of the examination. Tantrums can occur at any age, but are most likely to occur with two-year-olds or with children who are generally at that level of development. None of us likes being manipulated, particularly in our own territory of the examination room: an answer may be to move the territory to the child's home. Observations made in the home are valuable at any age, particularly if the child is developmentally disabled, but the amount of time required may seem disproportionate to the information gained. However, there are situations in which observations made at home can actually save the physician's time. If a two-year-old has a tantrum or begins to cry in the examination room, it is probably the wrong time to attempt a neurological examination and at the same time become involved with resolving child-rearing practices. The latter indeed may be the principal problem. The best way to handle a child who is in control of his parents and the examining situation is to watch him and try to assess how he has managed to manipulate his world.

159

In some cases it may never be possible to do a detailed inspection and orderly neurological tests at this age, but an accurate evaluation should be possible, even though the method of examination is unorthodox. Information gained from quick informal observation is vital, and the most should be made of this opportunity to assess the child before actually touching him. An unusual appearance, growth failure, abnormal motor development and deficiency in communication may be observed. Motor skills, co-ordination, language skills, vision, hearing and social awareness sometimes can be evaluated informally while the child is moving around the room. The level of development needs to be defined as clearly as possible before formal examination begins. Time is precious, so if the child's attention-span obviously is short, the pertinent part of the history must be secured quickly.

A normal two-year-old helps with simple household tasks, can kick a ball, throw a ball overhand, build a tower of four to 10 cubes, walk up steps, turn a door-knob, combine two words and scribble with a crayon. Although the parents indicate that the child does indeed combine words, he may not choose to demonstrate his language skills beyond the word 'No'. It is important to enquire both during and after the examination whether the observed behavior and skills (dressing, undressing, talking) are typical of those seen at home.

Directions

As the two-year-old comes into the examination room, observe the interaction between parent and child. Parents usually give the child every opportunity to do well. Try to interest the child in a toy or object and watch to see if the response is appropriate for his age. Give the child ample opportunity to become familiar with the examining situation before touching him. Most children will allow an examiner to touch them after a 'gift' has been offered and received. Often a truck, bell or tape-measure is accepted briefly by the child and quickly returned. If so, use a more attractive toy or make the gift more attractive by moving the wheel of the truck, ringing the bell, or showing how the tape-measure disappears back into the holder. Initially the parents may serve usefully as a go-between in the exchange of toys, but the examiner should aim to establish rapport with the child and gain his co-operation without involving the parents.

If the exchange of gifts has been successful, you can be reasonably sure that you, too, have been accepted, at least until something happens to provoke the child's anxiety. Give the child some colored 2.5cm (1in) wooden cubes, and show him how to build a tower. Then ask him to do likewise, watching his arm and hand movements. Give him plain paper and a pencil and see if he will draw. Most two-year-olds will produce a linear scribble. One way to ensure that the child is ready to be examined is to play peek-a-boo. Hold your hands in front of your face. Watch through your fingers to see if your attempt has been successful. By moving your face or hands, by using your voice and by moving your body to various positions, it should be possible to test for social response, attention-span, interest, visual pursuit, gross evidence of strabismus and response to auditory as well visual cues. If the child is interested in the light from an ophthalmoscope and is willing to 'blow the light out' (which can be done successfully with the co-operation of the examiner), this facilitates testing for

160

symmetry of facial movement and visual pursuit, and should enable the examiner to glance briefly at the fundi. This portion of the examination can be done at any convenient place in the examining room, and the child may be standing, playing at a table or sitting with either parent.

Removal of clothing is the next step. The child should be seated wherever he is likely to be happy. You can probably obtain most of the information needed to judge motor skills by partially undressing the child, but a co-operative youngster may be willing to demonstrate his skills in removing shoes and socks. Look for skill and symmetry in the use of hands and fingers. Inspect the shoes for wear, then hand the shoes to the child and look at the legs for evidence of abnormalities such as tight heel-cords, foot deformities or asymmetrical development. Test the deep tendon reflexes and the plantar responses.

Try to engage the child in fetching, carrying, throwing and kicking. Pick the child up and try to elicit a symmetrical parachute response by handing him, nose-down, to a parent. Estimate muscle strength and tone by watching how well he climbs, runs and moves around.

DEVELOPMENTAL SCREENING FOR THE CHILD OVER THREE

The basic neurological examination should include an appraisal of the child's developmental abilities to see if they are consistent with expectations developed from the history, the presenting problem and indirect observation. If a discrepancy is found between intellectual development and motor development, the physician can then emphasize the parts of the neurological examination which will help identify the cause of the discrepancy. The tests used by the physician should be simple, short and reliable for screening purposes. They should not be a substitute for definitive psychological studies. Equivocal or abnormal results obviously indicate the need for formal testing. The tests discussed below simply document the physician's clinical appraisal. If recent valid psychological or developmental assessments are part of the child's record and are available, the screening tests could be omitted.

The tests can be done at any convenient point in the examination. There is an advantage in administering them before beginning the formal neurological examination: a child will often settle into the actual physical examination with less anxiety after 'success' has been obtained with pictures, pencil and paper. The examiner must be careful not to devote a disproportionate amount of time to these tests. Parents and children have a way of postponing the formal neurological examination, the former by prolonging discussion of developmental accomplishments, the latter by drawing picture after picture.

It is useful to consider the observed developmental functions under the traditional headings of gross motor, fine motor, vision and perception, hearing and language, and social skills. (Examination of gross and fine motor skills is discussed in Chapter 9).

There are many tests which are appropriate for screening purposes, and indeed they often yield information about the child's functioning in more than one sphere.

The examiner should become expert in three or four but may need to use only one or two, and the choice will depend on the age of the child. For the younger child the Denver Developmental Screening Test is appropriate, and is discussed in the section on examination of infants (p. 139). For the child of three years or over it is useful to start by looking at pictures, as initially this does not require too much co-operation from the child. Unless they are very shy, most children of three to four will name pictures of simple objects when asked, and an older child can be asked to tell you what is happening in a more complex picture.

A useful formal test of receptive language skills is the Peabody Picture Vocabulary Test, which is quick to use for screening purposes. It requires no expressive language skills by the child, and can be used from 2½ years of age up to adulthood.

Peabody Picture Vocabulary Test*

Directions

Have the child sit comfortably in a position to look at the Peabody Test Book. Ask the child to choose from a group of four pictures on a page which one best represents the word you read aloud. Start with a page and test a word which should be within the child's expected capacity. Continue until the 'ceiling' is established (when a child has missed six out of eight consecutive test words). Subtract the total number of words missed from the score. Using tables, the raw score can be compared with expected scores for age and equivalent IQ.

Discussion

The Peabody Picture Vocabulary Test is a very satisfactory test for screening purposes, and only takes about 10 minutes to administer. The results correlate well with IQ, and give a good indication of the child's receptive language skills.

Slosson Oral Reading Test*

Directions

With children of six years or over, reading ability can be tested by using the Slosson Oral Reading Test. Ask the child to read from a list of words below his expected grade-level and continue until he can no longer read any of the words correctly. An error is counted for each word mispronounced or omitted and for each word which takes more than five seconds to pronounce (unless there is a speech impediment). The raw score comprises the total number of words pronounced correctly. The reading level is obtained by dividing the raw score in half and then dividing this figure by 10. For example, a raw score of 96 gives a reading level of 4.8.

Discussion

This test of reading ability gives an indication of the child's reading achievement, which can be compared with the result of the Peabody Test and with the child's current school-placement. Inconsistent findings (*e.g.* a normal Peabody test score

*See p. 4 for suppliers' addresses.

162

TABLE XIX
Criteria for scoring 'Draw-a-Person'

1. Head present
2. Legs present
3. Arms present
4. Trunk present
5. Length of trunk greater than breadth
6. Shoulder indicated
7. Both arms and legs attached to trunk
8. Legs attached to trunk and arms to trunk at correct point
9. Neck present
10. Outline of neck continuous with that of head or trunk or both
11. Eyes present
12. Nose present
13. Mouth present
14. Both nose and mouth in two dimensions; two lips shown
15. Nostrils indicated
16. Hair shown
17. Hair on more than circumference of head, non-transparent, better than scribble
18. Clothing present
19. Two articles of clothing, non-transparent
20. Entire drawing, with sleeves and trousers shown, free from transparency
21. Four or more articles of clothing definitely indicated
22. Costume complete without incongruities
23. Fingers shown
24. Correct number of fingers
25. Fingers in two dimensions, length greater than breadth, angle subtended not greater than 180°
26. Opposition of thumbs shown
27. Hand shown, as distinct from fingers or arms
28. Arm-joint shown: either elbow, shoulder or both

In determining the mental age of a child, the basal age is three. For each group of four criteria met by the drawing, the child is credited with one additional year.

Modified from Bakwin and Bakwin (1972).

and a low reading level) indicate a need for a careful study of why the child is not learning (see Chapter 9).

Drawing co-ordination

Drawing and copying skills should be examined next, as these will give some indication of developmental level, visual-motor integration and co-ordination. In addition, something will be learnt about the child's personality, self-image and ability to follow directions. Two useful tests are described here.

Draw-a-person
Directions

Make sure the child is sitting comfortably at a table. Give him a sheet of white paper and a pencil and ask him to draw a person. Watch silently, but in an interested fashion, noting the child's grasp of the pencil and his use of the 'dynamic tripod'—the thumb, index finger and middle finger functioning together for fine co-ordinated movements (Rosenbloom and Horton 1971). After the child has finished, ask whether the picture represents someone special—for example a parent or sibling.

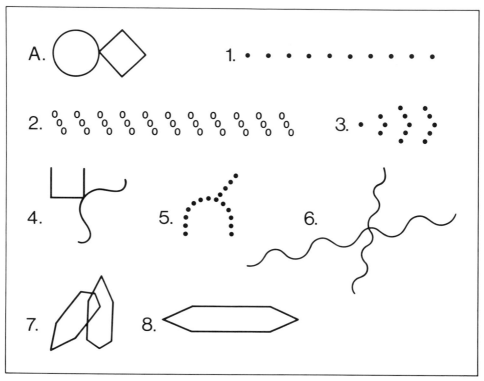

Fig. 53. Bender Gestalt test for assessing visual-motor function. Each design is presented individually for the child to copy.

Discussion

There are some pitfalls in this test: an inexperienced examiner may read too much into the drawings, and they may be difficult to interpret if the child has a physical handicap. Bakwin and Bakwin (1972) have devised a scoring system, modified from the original of Goodenough (1926). A credit of one year is added to a basal age of three years for every four features added. Thus a four-year-old would be expected to draw the head, legs, arms and trunk. A five-year-old would be expected to show that the length of the trunk exceeds the breadth, would indicate a shoulder and would show both arms and legs attached to the trunk, with the legs at the correct point (Table XIX).

Slosson Drawing Co-ordination Test
Directions

Copying figures is a rough guide to developmental level, visual-motor integration and co-ordination. A three-year-old is expected to copy a circle and a vertical line, a 3½- to four-year-old a cross, a 4½-year-old a square, a five-year-old an 'x', a 5½-year-old a triangle and a six-year-old a diamond. The Slosson Drawing Co-ordination Test (Slosson 1967) is a very simple, easily administered test which gives a quantitative measurement of the child's figure-copying skills.

164

TABLE XX

Check-list for assessment by observation of developmental level of preschool children*

Age (yrs)	Historical (or observed) items	Items to be tested
2	Runs well Walks up and down stairs—one step at a time Opens doors Climbs on furniture Puts three words together Handles spoon well Helps to undress Listens to stories with pictures	Builds tower of six cubes Circular scribbling Copies horizontal stroke with pencil Folds paper once
2½	Jumps Knows full name Refers to self by pronoun 'I' Helps put things away	Builds tower of eight cubes Copies horizontal and vertical strokes (not a cross)
3	Goes upstairs, alternating feet Rides tricycle Stands momentarily on one foot Knows age and sex Plays simple games Helps in dressing Washes hands	Builds tower of nine cubes Imitates construction of bridge with three cubes Imitates a cross and circle

4	Hops on one foot
	Throws ball overhand
	Climbs well
	Uses scissors to cut out pictures
	Counts four pennies accurately
	Tells a story
	Plays with several children
	Goes to toilet alone
		Copies bridges from a model
		Imitates construction of a gate with
		  five cubes
		Copies a cross and circle
		Draws a man with two to four parts—
		  other than head
		Names longer of two lines

5	Skips Names four colours Counts ten pennies correctly Dresses and undresses Asks questions about meaning of words	Copies a square and triangle Names four colours Names heavier of two weights

From Paine and Oppé (1966).

Ask the child to copy each of a set of figures on the form three times in the designated boxes, using a crayon (if very young) or pencil. The number of drawings is determined by the child's age, and rulers, compass and erasers are not allowed.

Discussion

The drawings are scored 'plus' if the child's figure matches the example, and 'minus' if distortions are apparent. The child should be able to copy all the figures expected for his age-level, without distortion. Details for scoring are given in the test manual.

Bender Gestalt Test

Directions

The Bender Gestalt Test is a further test of visual-motor function. It is useful for studying the effects of loss of abilities, organic brain defects, aphasias and mental retardation by documenting the child's response to a constellation of visual stimuli.

Have the child sit comfortably, with a pencil and an adequate supply of plain white paper. More than one sheet may be necessary for children who are confused, disturbed or retarded. Present the designs individually (Fig. 53) and ask the child to copy each one. The test is scored by looking for distortions of shape, rotation, substitution of circles for dots, perseverations, integration of parts, angles in curves and incorrect angles. Details of the scoring and administration of the test can be found in *The Bender Gestalt Test for Young Children* (Koppitz 1964).

Discussion

The Bender Gestalt Test has been found to give remarkably consistent results for children who have similar clinical patterns. Because the responses are predictable, easily scored and consistent between examiners, the test has been accepted as a dependably objective measure. The test helps define the child's probable maturation in visual-motor perception and intellectual ability and the severity of neurological and emotional problems.

A list of developmental levels between two and five years is given in Table XX.

CHAPTER 9

Higher Cortical Function

Introduction

Most of the interesting and characteristically human activities depend on the activity of the cerebral cortex. Intellectual ability, personality, memory, attention and morality are all examples of such functions. It is clear that if the brain becomes damaged such functions can be disturbed, but it is not easy to assess the rôle of the brain in disturbances of these functions, or their failure to develop in a child. Surprisingly extensive degrees of brain damage can leave the intelligence relatively intact: on the other hand, higher cortical functions are influenced by a variety of factors, including genetic factors, the social and physical environment, an individual's general state of health, nutrition, oxygen supply and cerebral vascular structures. How much and in what circumstances higher cortical function can be influenced by the conscious effort of the individual, and can be superimposed upon the primitive responses, are matters of speculation.

Professionals such as psychologists can assess these functions. The psychologist has a whole battery of tests for assessing intelligence, but it is important to realize that the tests only assess function and one cannot deduce from them very much about brain pathology. Thus, while discrepant measures between different parts of an intelligence test are common among brain-damaged invididuals, such discrepancies on their own cannot be taken as evidence of brain damage.

An important and related issue concerns the extent to which developmental delay can be regarded as evidence of neurological dysfunction. There is rather a poor correlation between many of the so-called developmental tests (such as the Bayley or the Griffiths) and later intelligence tests, and the professional should be aware of the range of normal development. The developmentally delayed child who subsequently proves to be mentally retarded may have had no classical neurological signs but with sophisticated examination techniques may be shown to have brain damage.

There is now reliable evidence that behavior disorder is more common among children with brain damage, but again, disturbed behavior on its own usually cannot be taken as evidence of brain damage. For example, while some overactive children do have brain damage, many children labelled as 'overactive' have no evidence whatsoever of brain damage. Similarly, other behavior disturbances seen in brain-damaged children occur equally frequently among normal children. While the more gross stereotypies (*e.g.* spinning movements) are not commonly seen except among mentally retarded and neurologically damaged children, most disturbed behavior is elicited by the same triggers in the normal child as in the brain-damaged child. Thus family discord disturbs children, and the brain-damaged child is more vulnerable to such events than his normal peers.

While the physician himself will want to undertake some simple assessment of the child's intellectual ability and personality, in many instances he will feel the need to enlist the help of a psychologist. Child psychologists usually will have taken a first degree in psychology and then gone on to supervised postgraduate work with children. They have a whole range of standardized instruments to help them assess the child, and also have some understanding of the ways in which children learn both intellectual and social skills. Child psychologists are able to advise parents and teachers on how to help children with difficulties. However, it is not within the scope of this book to discuss the various techniques and tests used by psychologists. Rather, in this chapter we shall consider the pediatrician's rôle in assessing the child.

Among the common situations presenting to the pediatrician are language delay or disorder, learning problems and behavior problems which are thought to have an organic basis, and it is the rôle of the pediatrician in relation to children with these problems that will be considered.

Psychological tests are standardized on normal individuals, and not on children with motor, mental or sensory handicaps. Social problems and language difficulties can also influence the results. The help of a skilled psychologist is needed to interpret a particular test for a particular child. An individual test, appropriately administered according to the child's age, circumstances and social background, has predicitve value. Variability arises from the lack of standardization for handicapped children rather than from the tests themselves. For groups of children the test-retest reliability is about 98 per cent, whereas for an individual child the figure is about 90 per cent.

Psychological tests are best used as a point of reference—to define the present problem and to find out what can be done to make the future as favorable as possible. The tests should identify a child's strengths and weaknesses, skills and possible strategies for learning, and projective tests should assess personality, imagination and resourcefulness.

A skilled psychologist will select the most appropriate test for the purpose of the evaluation, so the physician must specify what information is wanted. After the results of the test have been educed, the psychologist will define how they were achieved and how reliable they are (Meadows *et al.* 1981).

LANGUAGE PROBLEMS
General comments
A neurological examination is a necessary part of the evaluation of a child who has a speech and language problem. This may be a child who is not talking at all at the age by which some speech would be expected, whose language is inappropriate in content in relation to his age, or who has had some speech and has lost it temporarily or permanently. The concern about language may be the primary cause for referral, or the discrepancy may be noted as an incidental finding in the course of the examination. While speech and language are intimately related, they should be distinguished. Language refers to the symbols with which we think and which we use for expression, whereas speech is one medium by which language is expressed: there are others, such as the written word. A speech problem (*e.g.* a stutter) may exist without a language problem.

Language is dependent on a receptive unit, which consists of the ear and auditory

TABLE XXI
Development of speech and language

Age (mths) at which behavior should be established	Receptive language behavior	Expressive language behavior
3	Random activity arrested by sound; appears to listen to speaker; may smile at speaker; looks in direction of speaker	Random vocalization; primarily vowel sounds; vocal signs of pleasure; social smile, cooing and gurgling; smile in response to speech
6	Responds differentially to angry vs pleasant voice; responds to own name; recognizes words like 'bye-bye', 'Mama', 'Daddy'	Responds vocally to social stimuli; begins to mimic sounds; protests vocally; squeals with delight
9	Responds with gestures to words such as 'up', 'come', 'bye-bye'; stops activity when own name is called; stops activity in response to 'No'	Begins to use word-like sounds, some jargon; imitates sound sequences; imitates intonation pattern of speech
12	Accurately imitates pitch variations; responds to simple questions ('where is the dog?') by looking or pointing; responds with gestures to a variety of verbal requests	First words appear; jargon well-established; announces awareness of familiar object by name
15	Recognizes names of various parts of body	True words heard embedded in jargon or with gestures
18	Identifies pictures of familiar objects when they are named	Uses words more than gestures to express desires
21	Follows two consecutive, related directions ('pick up your hat and put it on the chair')	Begins combining words ('Daddy car', 'Mama up')
24	Understands more complex sentences ('after we get in the car we'll go to the store')	Refers to self by name

Courtesy of Dr. Carol Towne.

pathway, a processing unit—the brain—and the expressive unit. This expressive unit organises the neuromotor control of the larynx, oropharynx, mouth, tongue, teeth and lips. Satisfactory language depends on normal functioning of the entire apparatus, so the physician must assess each component and try to find out where the defect may be. Exact definition of the problem may require the aid of other specialists, and both the physician and the family must know what to expect from any specialist who may be involved. Sometimes several consultations and a period of observation are necessary before a definitive diagnosis can be reached. Stages in the development of language and speech are shown in Table XXI.

Infants begin to communicate almost from birth. At first communication is receptive only, and demonstrable by response to voices and sounds. At about three weeks of age the earliest attempts at expressive behaviour are made, and a pattern of spontaneous random vocalization begins which eventually will develop into babbling and cooing. By six months the baby is laughing and squealing, and may begin to imitate sounds of speech. Response to specific words and commands by gestures, activity and 'games' begins before the baby actually says his first word, sometime around 10 months. Sheridan (1974) gives the following guidelines for the normal number and variety of spontaneously produced words at different ages:

15 months — two to six words

18 months — two to 20 words; understands commands and points out named objects

21 months — primitive sentences or phrases of two or three words

24 months — 50 words or more; asks questions in terms of what? where? who?

30 months — uses pronouns and prepositions and can repeat short, simple nursery rhymes

36 months — 250 words; forms plurals; asks questions why? how?

48 months — tells stories and can describe experiences; asks meaning of words, particularly abstract ones.

In spite of the predictability of language development, there is enormous variation in the actual timetable. Health, heredity, nutrition, environment and verbal stimulation can all affect the development of speech in a normal child. Twins are notoriously slow talkers, preferring to use their own particular type of Lilliputian communication with each other, and it is a truth universally acknowledged, if not statistically proven, that little girls talk earlier and more volubly than little boys.

The wide variations that occur in normal language development may make it difficult for the examiner to decide when a language delay is abnormal. A serious language disorder needs intervention at the earliest possible moment, yet a great deal of harm can be done by needlessly upsetting the family and child if the 'delay' is an extreme variation of normal. In general, the ability to speak in short sentences by two years of age is almost always followed by normal or higher than normal intelligence, but the converse is not true. Investigation of some children who fail to speak at 2½ years may lead to no definite diagnosis, and the child will speak approximately normally between six months and a year later. However, investigation at this age may reveal indications of processing problems found in older learning-disabled children. Failure to speak meaningful sentences by three years should always be considered abnormal.

Causes of language delay

Mental retardation

The most common cause of language delay is mental retardation, so the evaluation must include a thorough developmental assessment. A careful developmental history will show that delay has occurred in all areas, except possibly in gross motor development. If apparent retardation is compounded by a hearing impairment, serious emotional disturbance or aphasia, it may be very difficult to define the extent of the language disorder.

A child who has delayed speech because of retardation will react normally to sound and will listen to sounds around him, although his attention-span may be short. Spontaneous babbling may begin as expected at six to eight months, or be delayed. If mental impairment is not too severe, words may be late but will emerge eventually. Intonation may be normal or it may have a 'sing-song' quality. The child may be echolalic. The vocabulary can be in keeping with that expected of the child's mental age, or it can be inconsistent, so that clearly enunciated unusual words are used inappropriately, as in the rapid, perfunctory and ritualistic 'cocktail-party' chatter sometimes heard from hydrocephalic children.

Impaired hearing

Although hearing loss is a much less common cause of delayed speech than is mental retardation, it must be sought and specifically excluded. Symptoms of a communication disorder antedate expressive language, and even mild degrees of hearing loss can interfere with the development of speech and language.

Types of hearing loss can be classified as conductive, sensorineural, mixed and central. In childhood, eustachian-tube dysfunction secondary to otitis media is the most likely cause of a conductive hearing loss. Sensorineural hearing loss is caused by damage to the inner ear and the associated nerve fibers, and interferes with both auditory sensitivity and discrimination of sound. Proper function of the sensorineural system is essential for speech and language formation: the more severe the deficiency, the greater the problem in the acquisition of speech and language skills. The mixed type of hearing loss occurs when a conductive disorder is superimposed on a sensorineural hearing loss. Deficiencies in either the conductive or the sensorineural systems, or both, constitute a peripheral hearing impairment. A central auditory problem occurs when the brain cannot process the signals sent in by an intact peripheral hearing system.

If peripheral deafness has an early onset it is unusual for the child to present with this complaint, and unfortunately the diagnosis is often delayed until there is evidence of retarded speech development or other signs of backwardness. It is important, therefore, to test the hearing of all infants whose history suggests any of the known antecedents of deafness or who show signs of malformations associated with the possibility of deafness. Deafness must be *specifically excluded* in any child who:

(*a*) has a family history of congenital deafness;

(*b*) shows signs of a genetic condition associated with deafness—Waardenburg syndrome (white forelock, heterochromia of iris, deafness); Pendred syndrome (goitre and deafness); first arch syndrome; Klippel-Feil syndrome; syndromes with retinitis pigmentosa (Usher, Laurence-Moon-Biedl, Refsum, Cockayne);

(*c*) shows evidence of having mucopolysaccharidosis, neurofibromatosis or heredo-familial degeneration of the nervous system;

(*d*) whose mother developed rubella, toxoplasmosis, syphilis or cytomegalic inclusion disease during pregnancy;

(*e*) was premature and/or suffered anoxia and injury at birth;

(*f*) has a history of neonatal jaundice;

(*g*) received ototoxic drugs;

(*h*) has cerebral palsy;

(*i*) has recovered from an infection of the central nervous system;

(*j*) has recovered from mumps;

(*k*) has a history of frequent ear infections;

(*l*) *whose parents suspect deafness.*

171

Deafness often is suspected earlier by parents than by attending physicians, especially if the baby has an older sibling, and any question of hearing loss raised by a parent must be rigorously investigated. The deaf infant's extraordinary awareness of visual cues and his response to vibration may delay recognition of a serious hearing deficit. Deaf babies babble at the usual time, but the babbling ceases at about seven to eight months of age. What vocalization remains lacks the inflection of normal speech, and the baby laughs and cries infrequently and in a monotone.

Hearing can be tested clinically only by observing the child's response to a sound stimulus. The stimulus used and the methods of observing the response vary according to the age, intelligence and anticipated degree of hearing loss. Absence of response is held to imply loss of hearing, but this interpretation is not always correct because response to sound is dependent on several factors, such as attention, as well as on the reception of sensory information. Minor or even moderately severe hearing loss is difficult to detect in ordinary clinical practice because of background noise, so the services of an audiologist should be sought whenever there is suspicion of deafness.

Central auditory processing difficulty

A central auditory problem may be suspected if the child obviously responds to sound but lacks the ability to communicate verbally in a manner appropriate for age and development. Central auditory dysfunction (sometimes known as developmental aphasia) may present as delayed speech, immature use of vocabulary and syntax, inability to process rapid speech, or difficulty with selective attention. In severe cases no speech develops at all. In the mildest situations the child will have apparently normal language skills but may experience a great deal of difficulty with schoolwork. The diagnosis of central auditory dysfunction is a strong possibility when there is a language delay, intact peripheral hearing and ability to communicate by non-verbal methods. Diagnosis is made by an experienced speech and language pathologist.

New computerized neurophysiological techniques to study reception and processing of sound have begun to be used clinically in a few centers. This neurometric study analyses the reception and processing of sound by recording the electrophysiological response to multiple, short auditory stimuli. Brain-stem responses to these auditory stimuli (those that can be recorded 1 millisecond to 9 milliseconds after the stimulus) can be distinguished from 'noise' by digital filtering (Fridman *et al.* 1982). The impulse is received in predictable fashion by the cochlea, auditory nerve and pons during the early part of the tracing, and then by the temporal, parietal, occipital and central areas 50 to 500 milliseconds later. A characteristic wave from an electrode placed in the midline on the scalp will show that the signal was received by the midbrain. If the waves do not occur in the expected, predicted pattern this is evidence of a defect in the ability to process auditory information. If peripheral hearing is intact, neurometric testing can be a useful adjunct in the study of central auditory dysfunction (see Chapter 11).

Orofacial abnormalities

Far less common causes of delayed onset of speech are structural orofacial abnormalities, such as cleft palate, which are often associated with a conductive hearing loss. Although such abnormalities as cleft palate, micrognathia, severe malocclusion and tongue-thrust may contribute to delayed development of speech, dysarthria, which may be severe, is the more likely cause. It is extremely rare for a short frenum to cause difficulty with speech, in spite of ample folklore to the contrary, but severe 'tongue tie' may lead to some difficulty in articulation.

Social deprivation

Social deprivation does not usually lead to delayed development of speech in a child who has no other problems, but the content of the language may be quite immature because of the lack of verbal stimulation and the constant inhibition of normal language development.

Multiple languages

A normal child may experience a little delay in mastering expected language skills if two languages are spoken at home; however this is usually corrected by school age, by which time most children exposed to two languages since birth are bilingual. However, if a child has any type of problem which could influence the acquisition of language skills, trying to learn a second language while struggling with the first could lead to difficulties with both.

Dysarthria

Structural dysarthria is based on visible anatomical defects such as cleft lip or palate, missing or widely separated incisors (a common cause of lisp), disproportionate size of the palate, the tongue, or the pharynx, and, very rarely, tongue-tie. Milder degrees of malformations may be compensated for by an intelligent child who hears correct spoken language and whose other essentials for speech are normal. However, when relatively mild anatomical variation is associated with a neurogenic, psychogenic or environmental problem, the two together may cause a greater degree of dysarthria than either would on its own.

Neurogenic dysarthria can originate in the lower motor neuron, as in palatal paralysis due to old poliomyelitis, diphtheria, Guillain-Barré syndrome or injury to the palatal nerves at tonsillectomy. Nuclear agenesis (Moebius syndrome) can also result in dysarthria if bulbar nuclei other than the facial are involved.

Congenital suprabulbar paresis can result in a dysarthria very similar to that of athetotic cerebral palsy, but without any affectation of musculature elsewhere in the body.

Cessation of speech

A child may cease speaking for a variety of reasons. Petit mal status—a convulsive episode characterized by an EEG pattern of continuous spike and wave discharge—may occur without evidence of a previous seizure, although the history usually reveals a change in behavior. Psychomotor seizures, documented on the EEG by spike complexes in the temporal area, may also cause mutism. A severe bilateral acquired hearing loss, such as that following mumps or treatment with an ototoxic drug, may also cause cessation of speech. However, drug-related deafness is usually accompanied by vertigo. A child with a degenerative disease of the central nervous system in which clinical onset is in childhood rather than infancy will lose speech as part of the general deterioration inherent in the disease. Acquired aphasia from injury or intracranial pathology can also cause mutism, but in that case usually there are other abnormal central nervous system signs. Sometimes mutism is a manifestation of hysteria, the symptom commonly following a traumatic incident in the child's recent past.

The term 'elective mutism' is used in psychiatric literature to describe a child who is capable of speaking in a fluent and articulate way in some situations but is unable to do so in others. The children described have been intelligent and have had no organic disease. The condition may appear, for example, at the time of the first separation from the family. Most psychiatrists agree that the first step is to eliminate the situation in which the mutism occurs.

Elective mutism is diagnosed by exclusion. Some children who at first seem to have elective mutism go on to develop the signs of other conditions in which mutism is not 'elective' but is a symptom. For example, sudden cessation of speech is a common finding in a child who later develops autistic traits.

There are times when the exact cause of cessation of speech will never be known. For example, a bright seven-year-old girl had a mild febrile illness after which she stopped talking for five years. Multiple diagnostic tests yielded no definite results. She started to talk again while attending a residential school for the retarded, at which time her intelligence quotient was 50-60. Encephalitis was suspected but never proven.

The evaluation

The evaluation of a child with language delay should begin with a careful exploration of present communication skills as observed by the family. When an infant is being examined it is important to ask how the baby responds to people and to sounds around him. Does he turn toward the sound of unseen voices? Does he awaken if a dog barks or the telephone rings nearby? Does he enjoy music? Does he ever wake from sleep if his mother enters his room and moves around it? Does he imitate speech? How does his language development compare with that of his siblings? If the child is older than his sibs, how does he communicate with them?

A careful history should be taken of the child's language and speech development, and of general mental and physical development. The medical portion of the history should search for clues to known causes of deafness and retardation, including complications of pregnancy, perinatal problems, infections and the administration of ototoxic drugs. Careful listening to the family's narrative for evidence of emotional problems is important, and of course a meticulous family history must be taken in order to exclude genetic causes. The physician should try to obtain a clear idea of the verbal climate of the home in terms of the extent of verbal stimulation, and for the child in particular.

The examination

While the history is being taken and before the formal examination, careful observation can be made of the baby's responses to people and sounds and to his spontaneous vocalization. A deaf infant's dependence on visual cues gives him an extraordinarily alert expression. With older children, this period of indirect observation is also an extremely valuable time in which to get an idea of spontaneous speech. What the child says casually to himself, to his mother or to the physician during the early part of the visit is likely to be the truest sample of his speech. Often much can be learned by judicious listening while taking the medical history and during the initial discussions with the mother, while the child is not aware that his vocalizations are being appraised.

The child may be completely mute, may make sounds only but have no spoken words, may speak little or a normal amount, or may chatter constantly. All these points are worth noting, although the implications of the quantity of spontaneous speech on the part of the child often shed more light on the psychiatric aspects of his situation than on the neurological ones. The physician's office or clinic is an unfamiliar place, and it is probable that a majority of children react by speaking less, or occasionally more, than they normally do at home or in familiar surroundings. Nevertheless, this information should be taken into account for whatever it may be worth.

Testing material for younger children

In order to elicit speech (and language) from the young child the examiner needs to have materials available with which the child will be familiar. In order to select appropriate material the examiner must know something of his patients' social and cultural background. A child from the country will distinguish cows from sheep much earlier than an urban child. A London two-year-old will identify a red double-decker bus; a Philadelphia two-year-old will not. A two-year-old who has not had books around him will fail to use picture material appropriately, but most will be able to. Providing he has used picture material, books with clear simple pictures of well-known objects are useful. The human body (eyes, nose, mouth, tummy) and clothes the child wears are also common to many cultures. In most developed countries a furnished doll's house is useful. If picture material fails to elicit speech, other good objects are household and particularly kitchen material: cups and plates, spoons and forks. Transport is another almost universal interest of children; cars, buses, horses, trains and airplanes are early-used words by most children.

In normal conversation with both adults and children 'what' is a great conversation stopper. Of course a co-operative child will enjoy naming objects, but a shy child will be inhibited. If you stand over a child pointing at an object and wait while he doesn't answer, you may decide your patient is mute. Kneel down behind the child and start discussing the material; ask him a question quite casually and answer it yourself if he doesn't immediately respond. Look for receptive language (has the doll got a nose?) before trying to elicit expressive language.

Comprehension of speech

An idea of the child's comprehension of speech can be gained by his response to commands and his ability to point to the correct one of a group of common objects or pictures when the examiner names it. Complex two- or three-step directions should be given to children of school age, including such things as 'Put the penny on top of the block', or 'Give me the penny when I touch the block with my finger, but not before'. Many children who appear to have pure disabilities of expression will prove to have more subtle defects of comprehension when tested by these methods.

Finally, if there is any suspicion of hearing loss the child should be given a series of tests, both while he has the opportunity of watching the examiner's facial expression and lip movements, and again while the examiner is behind him and unseen.

The Peabody Picture Vocabulary Test (see Chapter 8) is a simple, reliable means of estimating the child's receptive language ability and comprehension.

Perception of sound
Defective hearing must be unequivocally excluded or proven in the evaluation of any child with language delay, and the physician must decide on the basis of his examination whether additional specialized tests are needed.

With aphasic or autistic children, best results are obtained by using relatively faint sounds which are unusual enough to be interesting, and by presenting each sound only a few times before going on to another one. Rattles, squeaking toys, clicking 'crickets', devices to imitate bird or animal sounds, or even rustling the fingertips are usually effective if hearing is normal, but a louder sound or one presented often may be ignored. This method may document a certain level of hearing, even though an audiologist has stated that the child is deaf. Autistic children often react inconsistently to a sound, or only after a delay of several seconds. Of course this is not to say that turning the head or eyes or pointing to the source of a sound is any evidence that spoken language is normally perceived at a cerebral level, and it is equally possible for a person with normal hearing to have impaired ability to localize sounds. Testing with whispered voice is another conventional approach, but it is important to note any distortion in repetition of what has been whispered. Distortion may reflect diminished auditory acuity, or, alternatively, difficulty in prompt and accurate production or reproduction of a particular sound.

Both in testing by whispered voice and in conversation it is important to note whether the child answers appropriately or whether he repeats the directions verbatim. Echolalia is perhaps most easily recognized from the response to questions. Children who are highly distractible or hyperactive or who have short spans of attention, and also some aphasic children, are most satisfactorily tested if the eyes are covered. Many such children become so interested in visual stimuli that they ignore auditory stimuli.

Testing language skills of very young or unco-operative or developmentally disabled children can be difficult and time-consuming. Mary Sheridan's STYCAR Hearing and Language Tests (1976b, c) require only time and simple equipment to administer, and they can yield valuable information if administered exactly according to directions by an examiner with patience, experience and skill.

TABLE XXII
Audiological tests

Test	Description	Principal uses
Pure-tone threshold	Measures faintest tone subject can hear. Frequencies from 250 to 8000Hz presented through ear-phones measure air conduction. Bone conduction measured by vibrator placed in mastoid area	Indicates whether hearing loss is conductive, sensorineural, or both
Speech reception threshold	Measures faintest intensity at which listener correctly repeats 50 per cent of sporadic words	Checks on validity of pure tone threshold. Sets proper level for speech discrimination test
Speech discrimination	Evaluates listener's ability to discriminate speech by presenting standard word-lists	Loss of ability to discriminate words is characteristic of sensorineural lesions
Loudness recruitment	Measures whether listener shows 'recruitment', an abnormal increase in perception of loudness	Loudness recruitment indicates possible cochlear dysfunction. Recruitment tests would be positive if hearing loss caused by ototoxic drugs, noise injury and Menière disease
Central auditory	Staggered, sporadic word-lists, filtered speech, competing messages; binaural integration test presented to listener through earphones to detect possible central auditory processing difficulties	Diagnostic value in detection of central auditory processing dysfunction as a cause of a child's language disorder
Impedance audiometry and tympanometry	Measures middle-ear function electro-acoustically. Variations in air pressure are created in external canal and response from a probe sealed into canal is depicted on graph. Measures acoustic reflex threshold	Studies integrity and mobility of tympanic membrane and ossicles. Monitors bilateral contraction of stapedius muscle in response to unilateral sound. Excellent screening tool for middle-ear pathology in children
Evoked response audiometry	Records electrical responses in brain to auditory stimuli. Use of computers for detailed analysis can extricate auditory activity from background electro-encephalographic activity	Record indicates how signal is being processed, first in cochlea, auditory nerve and brainstem and later in cerebral cortex. May help in the diagnosis of central auditory processing difficulty
Electro-cochleography	Records electrical activity within cochlea and cochlear nerve by use of electrodes placed within ear canal or in middle ear	Most sensitive indicator of functional status of peripheral auditory system

Pure tone audiometry

Co-operative and intelligent children over the age of three or four years can be tested with pure tone audiometry. Their perception of pure tones of different frequencies may be tested either by asking them to press the button when they hear a sound, in the conventional type of examination, or by some kind of 'play' testing. If several loudspeakers are placed in different parts of the room, the child may be observed to turn his face toward the one from which the sound comes, but this test of localization involves other abilities in addition to simple hearing.

One frequently finds that there is difficulty in obtaining a reproducible record or that serial tests over a period of nine months or a year are highly inconsistent. Such a situation suggests some central defect in transmission of auditory input, or one of the developmental aphasisas, and should not be considered to imply lack of skill on the part of the examiner. If consistent curves are obtained, severe hearing loss (more than 50 decibels), especially if the loss is greater for higher frequencies than for low, is characteristic of nerve deafness or of a deficit more centrally located but at present difficult to define. Hearing loss of the conductive type involves less severe diminution of auditory acuity and shows bone conduction to be better than air conduction. This is the reverse of the situation in the normal individual or in cases of nerve deafness.

Impedance audiometry

Also known as tympanometry, this is a technique developed to evaluate the mobility of the eardrum, the condition of the ossicles and eustachian-tube function by recording the movement of the eardrum throughout a range of pressures in a closed cavity. The test takes only a few minutes to perform and the child's co-operation, beyond sitting reasonably still and quiet, is not required. However, most audiologists feel that impedance audiometry, though technically simple to do, should be combined with other diagnostic audiological studies (Table XXII).

Physical examination

Physical stigmata of certain syndromes associated with hearing loss or mental retardation, or both, may be apparent. Obviously a careful examination of the ears, oropharynx and tongue is needed.

Multiple handicaps

Language delay with or without hearing loss or retardation may be one of several handicaps present in a developmentally disabled child, and the physician must delineate all handicaps present so that remediation for the language delay can be integrated into the over-all rehabilitation plan.

Communication has the highest priority in the habilitation of the handicapped child, and communication specialists have the responsibility to recommend the means of communication best suited to that individual, be it speech improved by elocution, sign language, electronic aids or total communication.

Additional studies

Further steps in the evaluation of a child with language delay depend, of course, on the working diagnosis. If the apparent reason for the delay is a hearing loss, the physician must make every effort to ascertain its etiology by searching for congenital and acquired causes by history and confirmatory laboratory studies.

BEHAVIOR PROBLEMS

Behavioral assessment

Behavior disturbances are more common in the neurologically damaged child than they are among ordinary children and the physician should always review the child's behavior. It is obviously beyond the scope of this book to discuss the full assessment of children's behavior, but some general guidelines can be given.

It is not usual for a child of average ability to display disturbed behavior in the clinician's office (but see overactivity below). In general, therefore, the decision to refer a child to a psychiatric colleague will be based on the history obtained from the parents and, if possible, from teachers or other caretakers. Often the correlation between parents' and teachers' views of the child is not high, and while this merely may reflect different views of the same behavior, it can also reflect the fact that much behavior is 'situation bound'. The child may be almost impossible to live with at home and yet be causing no trouble at school.

Certain screening questionnaires concerned with children's behavior have been validated and may be found useful, although they are probably of more use in screening populations of children or in gathering epidemiological data than in assessing an individual child. Richman and Graham (1971) have described and used a behavior scale for three-year-olds, and also useful for older children are the Rutter Scales (1970) for both teachers and parents and the Conners (1969) scales for teachers.

Given the shortage of child psychiatrists (and the expense of referral), the physician should base his decision to refer on two factors. The first is the seriousness of the behavior problem—how far is it disrupting the child's development or learning, and how far is it disrupting the child's social environment. The second is whether the behavior is a temporary phenomenon or likely to persist. To take the second issue first, sometimes an obvious trigger may be identifiable as causing the disturbed behavior. Thus a preschool child may be disturbed by being admitted to hospital; subsequently he may be clinging, have temper tantrums, night-waking, and generally prove difficult to manage. Given an ordinary family background, such behavior should subside over about three to six months. Similarly, while the death of a loved grandmother (providing mourning is handled appropriately) or changing school may cause disturbed behavior for several months, they do not presage longer-term disturbances. On the issue of the 'seriousness' of the behavior problem, often the decision is more difficult. For example, a parent may say 'He's driving me mad', but often it is difficult to know how much weight to give to such a remark. In taking a history it is useful to get an account of the pattern of a child's behavior over a whole 24 hours. It may prove that 'after-school' is a period of friction in the family but that the rest of the day is relatively peaceful. Similarly, get the pattern for the week—how are things at weekends? If the family can cope with each other most of the time the situation isn't too bad; in fact one might say it is normal. If the problem is considered to be serious, then referral to a child psychiatrist is appropriate. However, some problems perhaps are more appropriately managed by the pediatrician, and next we shall consider one of the most common 'behavioral' referrals—the overactive child.

179

The child who is 'hyperactive'

In the United States (far more than elsewhere) the complaint of hyperactivity is a common cause of referral to a physician. Sometimes parents seek help because of increasing frustration with their child's behavior: they may feel that their problems will disappear if a definite cause can be found and appropriate therapy given. Sometimes the referral is initiated because a teacher or school psychologist feels that an organic problem must be present to explain the symptoms, and recommends a neurological examination 'because there must be something wrong with him'.

The term 'hyperactivity' is at best a vague description of excess gross motor activity, and there is no agreement about its exact meaning. The term is used loosely by physicians, psychologists, educators and administrators, and by writers for the popular press. Unfortunately, the term 'hyperactive child' is a pejorative label which immediately identifies a child as being a trouble-maker and difficult to manage in the classroom. Too often the expectation is realized because the child senses what behavior is anticipated. The matter is further complicated by the fact that hyperactivity, short attention-span and distractibility are often (but not invariably) found in the syndrome known as 'minimal cerebral dysfunction', and that a child with a specific learning disability may be restless in the classroom simply out of frustration, or may be hyperactive because his learning disability is part of the larger problem of minimal cerebral dysfunction.

A pragmatic method of evaluating the symptoms of hyperactivity in a particular child is to consider various degrees of activity as a spectrum of behavior ranging from the normal activity of childhood to the constant, uncontrolled activity of an autistic child. Many children go through a period of intense activity which begins at the runabout stage near the second birthday, intensifies through the next two years, and then gradually decreases by the time of school entry at five. They seem to delight in experiencing their new motor skills to the fullest degree. Some will settle down quite quickly in the normal course of development. Others with a highly active personality are overactive well beyond the age at which it is acceptable. These children may be a source of concern to their parents and teachers. Their activity is considered inappropriate for their home or school surroundings and differs markedly from the behavior of their siblings at the same age. These children seem to go into 'overdrive' and become exuberantly noisy when stimulated, for example, by social activities and holiday excitement. Yet these same children will sit quietly for long periods of time if they are doing something they like. A child who can watch a favorite television program quietly, play with a cherished toy and enjoy an outing may be considered normal, even though he becomes 'hyperactive' if bored, restless, overstimulated or tired. The active child is likely to turn into a busy, energetic adolescent who may overextend himself with educational and social activities. Many successful adults who thrive on doing prodigious amounts of excellent work in a short time under pressure were 'overactive' children. The question, then, is what constitutes normal behavior? Any acceptable standard obviously is influenced by family, school, environmental and cultural norms.

If the hyperactivity is accompanied by behavior which is detrimental to the child and to people around him, some kind of intervention may be needed. A child with

180

poor judgement, poor impulse-control, short attention-span and excessive activity, especially at school, disturbs, distracts and upsets those around him. This type of hyperactivity may be caused by boredom, frustration, emotional problems or psychiatric disorders, or by minimal cerebral dysfunction, with or without a specific learning disability. The behavior problem may be strikingly absent outside the schoolroom, at the weekend or during vacations. A random, purposeless type of hyperactivity may be associated with mental retardation.

In the United States, a child who is in constant motion, whatever the surroundings or situation, who has a short attention-span, poor impulse-control, mood swings, distractibility, normal intelligence and no evidence of abnormal neurological findings is considered to have the hyperkinetic syndrome. Although the condition is cited as being present in 4 to 10 per cent of all American school-age children, it is rarely identified in the United Kingdom and some investigators question whether it exists at all, since most of the symptoms can be attributed to various conduct disorders (Bax 1972, 1978; Sandberg *et al.* 1978). There is no question that children on both sides of the Atlantic show the same symptoms: the cause of the difference in incidence appears to lie in diagnostic usage and definition.

Organic brain-damage resulting from anoxia, head injury, meningitis or encephalitis can lead to the syndrome of 'organic drivenness', first described by Kahn and Cohen in 1934. A child who manifests organic drivenness in its extreme form is in constant motion and cannot be left alone. He has no judgement and no sense of danger. He will quickly turn the physician's office into a shambles, pulling open drawers, overturning wastebaskets and throwing whatever can be grabbed. The care of such a child is extremely difficult and frustrating. Constant vigilance is required, and the child often needs far less sleep than the rest of the family. Frustrations may accumulate to breaking-point for the parents and the physician must keep in mind the possibility of child abuse when dealing with the family of an organically driven child.

Although organic drivenness may be considered clinically as the extreme form of the continuum of hyperactivity, evidence from neurometric analysis suggests that there may be a specific type of brain damage associated with the syndrome. Over 90 per cent of children who are found to have increased delta activity (5Hz) and poor coherence in the frontal areas have clinical correlates of constant hyperactivity and short attention-span. Many children with these neurometric findings have a history suggestive of an organic cause for their hyperactivity (John 1977). Of course this evidence does not imply that 90 per cent of all hyperactive children will exhibit this finding. The sample is biased, in that children with the most severe form of hyperactivity are most likely to be referred to a medical center, and the clinical findings were linked to a specific neurometric abnormality, rather than vice versa. The broad implications of neurometric studies of hyperactive children must be based on the results of carefully designed research on a large sample. Nevertheless, neurometric analysis is a promising tool, in that it produces objective results rather than clinical impressions.

An autistic child may be continually hyperactive, day and night, the activity being totally unrelated to people or surroundings. This type of hyperactivity may be the same as in organic drivenness. Many autistic children and many severely retarded children have a peculiar type of repetitive, ritualistic, stereotyped movement (stereotypies) superimposed on excessive motion. These include rocking, head-banging, twisting the hair or fingers, twirling, flapping the hands, or drizzling sand through the fingers. Sometimes it is very difficult to tell whether a very hyperactive child with bizarre movements is psychotic, brain-damaged or retarded. In these cases the etiology is not nearly as important as helping the family to cope with an almost impossible situation.

The evaluation

Because of its manifestations and effects on the family, hyperactivity is a symptom for which help is sought frequently. It should be emphasized, however, that the opposite type of behavior should be of equal concern, especially as a child who becomes withdrawn, mute or depressed may not be brought to the physician because the family or teacher is satisfied with his conduct: 'He causes no trouble at all'.

Evaluation of the symptoms of hyperactivity demands skill, flexibility and patience on the part of the physician. The child may not be co-operative and the parents can be defensive about the child's behavior, apprehensive about anticipated criticism of his upbringing, uneasy about a possible organic cause and ready to unleash a torrent of frustration. The parents should be able to sense from the very beginning of the interview that the physician is not going to be judgmental about the child's behavior. He should find something good to say about the child at the outset, to reinforce positive behavior and encourage co-operation. He must establish rapport with both child and family, instill confidence, do the best examination possible and remain in control. It is not an easy task.

Hyperactivity may be a simple behavior problem or a symptom of an emotional disorder, or it may be associated with a definite organic condition such as mental retardation, cerebral palsy, a seizure disorder or a degenerative disease. Whatever the cause, the physician must get an idea of the dimension of the problem and its effect on the child's home and school environments. A plan of management should be developed after the symptom is put into perspective.

During the interview, indirect observation should be proceeding. The physician should ask whether the observed behavior is that which concerns the parents, and whether it is typical. For example, a child whose parents are surprised by the excessive degree of his activity in the physician's office might simply be reacting to unhappy past experiences with physicians or to new surroundings. The family should be given a chance to recite the child's accomplishments and strengths and to state what the child does best in order to give a clue about the family's attitude toward the child. It is far easier to manage a child who is cherished in spite of provocative and difficult behavior than one whose hyperactivity is a sign of family disorganization and who is the 'whipping boy' (sometimes literally) for the frustrations of the rest of the family. If he hears his mother say to all and sundry, 'He is a monster, I just can't control him', indeed he will exhibit monstrous behavior with impunity. It is important to find out how the family tries to control the child and who in the family seems to do it best. Conversely, it may become apparent that the child controls the family in that his actions determine where they go and what they do. In that case he has no incentive to change.

Discussion of the symptom of hyperactivity should include the times it occurs and the circumstances, to see if it is triggered by a particular situation or environment. Was the child always hyperactive or was the activity precipitated by a particular event such as school entry, promotion into a particular grade, the birth of a sibling, a change in the family or a move to a new home? Although the evaluation is focused on hyperactivity as the presenting complaint, there may be associated traits which have a bearing on the management of the problem, such as recklessness and inability to perceive danger. Careful note should be made of any behavior which suggests regression or a seizure disorder.

The duration of the hyperactive behavior is important. Is it episodic or constant? Is it a problem because it occurs in the 'wrong' place—the supermarket or schooi—or is the child in perpetual motion, whatever the surroundings? One weary mother's lament, 'It isn't what he does that's bad; it's just that he does so much of it', illustrates the latter situation. If the child is retarded, allowance must be made for the intellectual deficit, since a backward child can be expected to exhibit a certain amount of activity which would be considered immature in a normal child of the same age.

The history must include careful questioning about organic illnesses which could produce hyperactivity, a good developmental history, a systematic description of the child's school progress and present school setting, a detailed family history, and tactful enquiries into the home environment. Any clues in the history which indicate an associated neurological condition should be pursued. A few rare degenerative disorders (Wilson's disease, for example) may begin with what appears to be behavioral hyperactivity.

The examination

The physical examination of a hyperactive child who is tired, tense and apprehensive presents a formidable challenge, but the physician must do the best neurological evaluation possible in the circumstances. He will need to engage the child's interest by being flexible. Since hyperactivity frequently is associated with the minimal cerebral dysfunction syndrome, the part of the examination which tests fine motor co-ordination and balance might be done first. School progress is often a problem, and it might be best to do some developmental screening tests early while the attention-span is still good.

Intervention

If the intervention is necessary, certain tools are available to improve or mitigate the situation. A young hyperactive child who is about to enter school is at risk of learning difficulties, which may compound the hyperactivity. The physician may need to assist the family by smoothing the path and making sure the school setting is the best one available. An older child whose activity seem to be school-related may need careful educational assessment. The physician can be of service in prodding the school to do the assessment and in providing any pertinent records.

Behavior modification is used sometimes to enable the family and teacher to concentrate on one particular aspect of the child's behavior (such as head-banging) which is upsetting. A family having to cope with an extremely hyperactive, organically driven child may benefit from counseling, family therapy, and such indirect measures as respite care.

Treatment of a hyperactive child with drugs is a more specific tool. The primary purpose of drug therapy is to control the behavior which is upsetting others. A secondary purpose is to give 'control' of the situation back to the parent, who then can influence the child's behavior dramatically by giving enough diazepam, chlorpromazine or thioridazine to reduce the symptoms. Individual tolerance to a particular drug and the placebo effect make it difficult to measure a drug's efficiency. Although administration of tranquilizers is empirical treatment for the symptom rather than the cause, their judicious use may reduce the level of activity enough to take some pressure off the family and allow an opportunity to institute changes in the environment which will be of lasting benefit.

Diet therapy, which gives the family control by using specific food as a weapon, may be effective, not for its content but as a symbol of authority and as an easy explanation of failure (an unauthorized cookie eaten yesterday explains today's bad behavior). Parents are happier with a specific reason, and they can take the blame or assign it, according to their own needs.

It is impossible to judge the efficacy of the gluten-free diet, the low-sugar diet or the allergy-free additive-free diet because the number of variables is large and true believers usually are unwilling to participate in a controlled experiment. Moreover, as yet there is no objective way of gathering a consistent sample on which to test a well-designed research project. Anecdotes of success are convincing for almost all diets and are difficult to prove or disprove.

Hyperactivity is a symptom, not a disease, and there is no single specific therapy. All the physician can do is evaluate the symptom, assess the impact of hyperactivity, and meet the needs of the child and his family by recommending the best combination of remedial measures.

THE CHILD WHO HAS A LEARNING DISORDER

A child can be said to have a learning disorder when his difficulty in mastering expected educational material is out of proportion to his presumed mental ability. Such difficulty is often the reason for referral to an array of specialists, each of whom will evaluate the child from the point of view of his own discipline. Such specialized study may result in a well-designed, specific program or it can give rise to conflicting opinions, muddled priorities and no clear plan of action. The physician is the one professional who can evaluate the child as a whole. The learning disorder can be assessed in relation to the child's general well-being and development, and remediation can be worked out against a background of the home, the school and the community.

The physician must determine the validity of expectations for the particular child. If a learning disorder does indeed exist, the physician should then determine whether it is of endogenous origin, involving a central nervous system dysfunction, or whether it is caused by social, environmental or educational conditions. Usually both aspects are involved. For example, physically handicapped children of normal intelligence may do poorly in school because the educational system simply is not sufficiently flexible to provide a proper program.

The terminology of learning disorders is complex and controversial, and usually reflects the interests of those who make up the classifications. It differs from author to author and from year to year. The physician's task is to recognize conditions underlying the learning disorder which can be corrected or ameliorated, such as seizures, emotional disorders and visual or auditory handicaps; to identify basic conditions of which learning disorders are an intrinsic part, such as mental retardation; and if no overt neurological condition is present, to describe neurological findings accurately enough to enable educational specialists to classify the specific learning disability and develop appropriate remediation.

Causes of learning disorders

One common cause of an alleged learning disorder in the early years of the child's schooling is simply unrealistic expectations. A child of average ability whose parents and siblings have already achieved academic success may appear to be dull because he doesn't measure up to the high standards set by the family. Failure to measure up will generate feelings of inadequacy, and he will not attempt educational tasks because he fears he will fail.

Immaturity is another common cause of alleged learning disorder. Many children, especially boys, are not yet ready to cope with formal learning at the time at which they are expected to enter school. In addition to intellectual immaturity, neurological immaturity may be manifested by an inappropriate degree of activity, short attention-span and distractibility, all of which traits are quite normal in a younger child. The neurological immaturity may be compounded by the frustration of being unable to meet the academic demands. The late developer requires patience and fortitude rather than a battery of tests.

Mild mental retardation is a common endogenous cause of a learning disorder. For example, the problem may remain undetected until a formal learning situation exposes deficiencies in cognitive thinking. Sometimes the stress and exigencies of entering school can trigger symptoms of a serious emotional problem or an adjustment reaction, and the learning disorder may be the earliest manifestation of a larger problem. Tumors of the nervous system and degenerative diseases can also cause personality changes and changes in the child's learning pattern: deterioration of school performance then becomes a signal of the development of an organic neurological condition. Obviously difficulties with vision or hearing can affect a child's school performance.

Minimal cerebral dysfunction

The exact meaning of the term 'minimal cerebral dysfunction' is controversial: the definition is in the eyes of the beholder. The educator equates it with school under-achievement, while the psychologist emphasizes behavioral aspects and the physician considers it evidence of immaturity of the central nervous system. The clinical hallmarks of a child with minimal cerebral dysfunction are short attention-span, distractibility, poor impulse-control, mood swings, clumsiness, difficulty with fine motor co-ordination, visual-perceptual problems and right-left confusion. The child with minimal cerebral dysfunction is sometimes overactive but not invariably so, and he may also have a specific learning disability. Mentally retarded children can also exhibit traits of minimal cerebral dysfunction. Any attempt to exclude mental retardation from a definition of minimal cerebral dysfunction is based on administrative rather than neurological reasons. Although minimal cerebral dysfunction, like mental retardation, is associated with prematurity, circumstances which could lead to anoxia at birth, delayed development and adverse socio-economic factors, there is no simple cause and effect relationship. No specific cause has yet been identified by the standard investigative techniques available.

A child with minimal cerebral dysfunction may have a problem in achieving satisfactorily in school simply because the traits exhibited do not accord with acceptable classroom behavior. If there is also a specific learning disability (that is, a defect in central processing) the problem becomes much more complex. Some children have specific learning disabilities which handicap them severely, but they show no evidence of minimal cerebral dysfunction.

Learning disabilities
The exact definition of a learning disability, like that of minimal cerebral dysfunction, is the subject of considerable debate (Rapin 1982). Definitions in the literature range from the simple to the unwieldly: 'A child with learning disabilities is one with significant intradevelopmental discrepancies in central motor, central perceptual or central cognitive processes which lead to failure in behavioral reactions in language, reading, writing, spelling and/or content subjects' (Kas 1966, quoted in Chalfant and Scheffelin 1969). Specific learning disabilities include ' . . . those children who have a disorder in one or more of the basic psychological processes involved in understanding or in using language, spoken or written, which disorder may manifest itself in imperfect ability to listen, think, speak, read, write, spell or do mathematical calculations. Such disorders include such conditions as perceptual handicaps, brain injury, minimal brain dysfunction, dyslexia and developmental aphasia. Such terms do not include children who have learning problems which are primarily the result of visual or emotional disturbance, or of environmental, cultural or economic disadvantage'.*

It is beyond the scope of this book to go into the psychological and educational details of the various forms of central processing deficiencies. The physician should try to determine whether there is a central processing disorder such as dyslexia or developmental aphasia, and then seek help from a specialist.

If the child must be tagged with a specific type of learning disability, the

*The Education for All Handicapped Children Act of 1975. Pub. L. No. 94-142, 89 Stat. 773. Codified at 20 U.S.C. 1401-1453 (1976), and Suppl. I (1977).

physician must be sure that the label does not oversimplify a broad problem and that the program prescribed is appropriate and necessary. Glib acceptance of a label such as 'dyslexia' can involve the child in a uniform remedial program designed for all children who happen to bear that label. However, it might not be the right program for that particular child. Many children can learn to compensate for a learning disability and do well in school and in life, even though test results are compatible with failure. These children may benefit from nothing more than remedial work, possibly a change of school, and an enlightened family attitude. Another child will need an individually planned educational program. The physician who knows the child and the family is in a unique position to evaluate the importance of a particular remedial effort in the child's over-all habilitation.

Clearly there are neurophysiological components which are poorly understood. For example 'neurometrics', the analysis of neurophysiological data by computer technology, is a new experimental technique which attempts to measure the ability of the brain to process information (see pp. 222-225). It is a promising tool in the search for a demonstrable organic basis for specific learning disabilities (John 1977). As yet it is available in only a few places. Theoretically, children with specific learning disabilities should show some lack of symmetry and alterations of electrical activity in areas of the brain assumed to be vital for particular functions, such as the occipital area for vision, the central area for movement, the frontal areas for marked behavioral difficulties and the temporal areas for auditory and language function. In practice, however, some children with such findings do well in school.

The evaluation

A detailed history obviously is a vital part of the neurological evaluation of a child with a learning disorder. A chronology of school experiences, including nursery school, can show at what level difficulties began. The child may never have adjusted well; the problem may have begun in a specific grade when the curriculum was beyond the child's ability; or the child may have had a serious illness or changed school or teachers. It is important to gather information about the child's friends in and out of school and about behavior problems in school, at home, or in the community. Most children are willing to talk about their school-work and can be encouraged to discuss or demonstrate it. The physical and social ambience of the school being attended can be brought out by adroit questions about class size, quality of teaching, discipline, physical resources, physical barriers and the time it takes to travel to and from school.

Aspects of the medical history which may have a bearing on learning disorders are those concerning the child's birth, serious illness and accidents, upper respiratory infections and bouts of otitis media. Clues to the presence of a seizure disorder or visual or auditory handicaps should be pursued. A developmental and school history can reveal whether the child is on schedule or shows some evidence of immaturity or developmental delay. The educational accomplishments of the parents and siblings will give an insight into the academic expectations for the child. Occasionally specific learning disabilities are familial, so it is important to know if any siblings or relatives ever had the particular educational difficulties shown by the child.

The examination

The all-important period of indirect observation while the history is being taken might reveal hints of immaturity or of traits found in minimal cerebral dysfunction if the child squirms, wriggles, fidgets, interrupts and flits from one object of interest to another. However, a visit to the doctor can bring out the worst in all of us, and no firm conclusion should be made on the basis of a brief period of observation in adverse surroundings. While the physician is busy with the history he can listen to the child's spontaneous speech for content and articulation.

It is wise to begin the actual examination with tests that have a bearing on school performance, since that subject is uppermost in the parents' minds and the scope of the remainder of the examination depends on the findings. Administration of the Peabody Picture Vocabulary Test (see Chapter 8) is a good beginning, giving a rough idea of the child's intellectual potential and receptive language skills. Age-appropriate tasks involving reading and writing can be carried out next. The Slosson standardized word lists (see Chapter 8) are also useful. The examiner should listen for accuracy, fluency, reversals, omission of sounds and blending of sounds. A nine-year-old child can be asked to write and print his name, telephone number and birthday and to draw a person. A child over five years of age should be able to copy a circle, a square and a triangle. Older children can be asked to copy more complicated shapes, such as those in the Slosson Drawing Co-ordination Test or the Bender Gestalt Test (see Chapter 8).

'SOFT' NEUROLOGICAL SIGNS

The term 'soft neurological signs' is used differently by different people. Often it is used to refer to signs which are either difficult to elicit or difficult to interpret. Some so-called soft neurological signs disappear with age, and their persistence beyond a certain age may be significant.

They may occur, though not invariably, in a child with minimal cerebral dysfunction, with or without a learning disability. Touwen (1979) has developed a quantitative examination technique (and reporting format) which standardizes the examination of a child who might have minor neurological dysfunction. The validity of his procedure depends on strict adherence to protocol. A separate examination is required if his method of testing is to be included in the evaluation. A few simple but useful tests are described here.

Directions

Give the child both a large and a small stove-bolt (see Fig. 1, p. 3). Ask him to thread the large nut on to the large bolt right up to the head of the bolt. Get him to repeat this with the smaller stove-bolt. Observe the quality of eye-hand co-ordination and any difficulty in setting the nut on the thread.

Ask the child to put the tip of his index finger very neatly to his nose three times with each hand. If he is over six years of age, ask him to repeat the test with each hand with his eyes closed. Hold out your index finger: ask the child to put the tip of his index finger on the tip of your index finger three times. Repeat with the other hand. If the child is over six, ask him to repeat this with his eyes closed. Note the accuracy of placement and look for tremor and involuntary 'overflow' associated with movements of the hand not being used, and with the face.

Have the child close his eyes tightly, put out his tongue and extend his arms forward with fingers spread apart. Look for vertical or horizontal deviation of the hands, asymmetrical posture and fine involuntary movement of the tongue, arms and hands. Ask the child to pronate and supinate each hand rapidly on his lap, first one at a time and then in unison.

Discussion

The stove-bolt test is a highly subjective test of eye-hand and fine motor co-ordination for children over three years of age. It is also an excellent way of getting children to co-operate, since they usually find it enjoyable. A child with poor co-ordination will have considerable difficulty in threading the nut onto the bolt and screwing it toward the head, and often will drop it. Many four- and five-year-old children can manage it and few children over the age of six have any difficulty. The dominant hand is used to thread the nut: the other hand holds the bolt.

Proper placement of the finger on the nose with the eyes open indicates satisfactory eye-hand co-ordination and visual tracking. Performance of the tests with the eyes closed is a means of assessing proprioceptive and cerebellar function. A slight tremor and overflow movements are often seen in very young children and in those with immature neurological development. Rarely, benign essential tremor may be a cause. Tremor and inability to place the finger properly, with constant deviation to one side, could also be a sign of cerebellar dysfunction, but it is likely that there would be a history and neurological signs indicative of a cerebellar lesion.

The arms-outstretched position can reveal tremor and small involuntary movements, which are normal in young children but indicative of developmental delay beyond the age of five years. Abnormal involuntary movements of a greater degree usually are of primary (cerebral palsy) or secondary origin (*e.g.* drug intoxication). Deviations from the horizontal or vertical positions are considered unusual in children over six years of age: the most common cause is hypotonia. Asymmetrical deviation can be caused by unilateral motor deficit, or muscle or joint disease.

Most six-year-old children can perform pronation and supination tests. Difficulties may be an indication of immaturity of the nervous system, resulting in poor co-ordination. The movements usually are more rapid and accurate with the dominant hand. A considerable tendency to mirror-movement is normal among pre-school children and may persist into adult life, especially when the child is learning or practising unfamiliar patterns of movement. However, strong mirror-movements which cannot be suppressed by attention or effort are abnormal. A common cause in childhood is hemiparesis, in which mirror-movements are seen in the affected extremity when the opposite (normal) one is moved. This overflow may be in either direction but is usually more spectacular in the paretic limb when the normal limb is moved than vice versa.

189

Laterality

It is also useful to check the child's laterality. Eye preference, hand preference and foot preference should be looked for.

To check eye preference, ask the child to pick up a short cardboard tube or a paper towel with a hole in it and to look at you through the hole. Record which eye is used. Crumple the paper and play 'catch' with it, noting hand preference (if any) and skill in throwing and catching. Place the crumpled ball on the floor and ask him to kick it. Repeat at least twice. Then ask him to put it into the waste basket. Note the preferred hand used for drawing and writing.

Test further for ability to lateralize by asking him to imitate your gestures, 'Do as I do', then giving him directions to carry out: 'Put your right hand on your left ear'.

The tests for eye, hand and foot use merely establish the child's preference. According to Touwen (1979), 'handedness' is established at age six and 'footedness' at about age eight; however, one would expect to see a strong preference for one hand between the ages of three and 4½ years. Strong or exclusive use of one hand or foot by a younger child should alert the examiner to the possible existence of a motor defect.

The question of the importance of dominance and right-left orientation has been the subject of many studies. Bergès and Lézine (1965) have published normative data on the ages at which normal children can be expected to distinguish right from left, both on themselves and on the examiner. As would be expected, there is considerable variation. A normal child of six is doing well to differentiate his own right and left consistently and may not be able to do so for other persons for another one to three years. Anxiety and immaturity can also interfere with successful completion of the tests.

Conclusions

Visual and auditory acuity must be scrupulously checked by careful screening, and all equivocal results must be followed up by definitive study. Color vision should be tested. Defective color recognition is not a learning disorder, but inability to recognize color could handicap a child in a classroom if color coding is used extensively as a teaching tool.

The basic neurological examination should seek to exclude chronic illness and to define any handicap, especially those which have a bearing on the child's ability to learn. Tasks of fine motor co-ordintion, balance and laterality are often abnormal in a child with a learning disorder, but abnormality is not a *sine qua non* of minimal cerebral dysfunction or a specific learning disability. These tests must be interpreted in relation to the whole clinical picture. Inability to stand on one leg for 10 seconds is not a significant finding in a bright, healthy 10-year-old who has no other abnormal findings. The same sign in a healthy 10-year-old who is failing in school, cannot hop without falling, has poor handwriting and a short attention-span, corroborates the existence of minimal cerebral dysfunction accompanied by a learning disability.

Planning

The result of the neurological examination should enable the physician to identify whether the learning disorder is the result of central nervous system dysfunction, or whether it is caused by environmental or social factors. Sooner or later, perhaps after referral to a psychologist, a speech pathologist and an educational specialist, an education program might be devised and the child might be placed in a particular school. The school the child attends should be one in which he is successful, even though that success may not be measured by being in the proper grade or by the expectation of finishing the standard course of studies in the allotted time.

The proper school for the child is one in which he feels good about himself and has confidence in his abilities. Many special techniques have been developed to increase concentration, improve co-ordination, control behavior and overcome a host of learning disabilities. These educational innovations help a child to make up lost ground, strengthen his weakness, and feel more competent about his schoolwork. If he feels competent and secure, rather than isolated and ridiculed, has a sense of success and is functioning well in a program geared to his abilities, he will appear to function more like a person of the same mental age and the learning disorder will appear to diminish.

CHAPTER 10

Implementation

The foregoing pages have described a selective neurological examination and an approach to the evaluation of some common clinical problems. The assessment has involved an examination of previous records, a detailed analysis of the child's medical and developmental history, a clinical impression gained from as thorough a neurological examination as possible in the circumstances, special laboratory studies, and consultation with other professionals. The end result of the evaluation should be a working diagnosis, recommendations for direct treatment if appropriate and for medical management of the child's current needs, and a discussion of the problems which the child and family may face in the future.

The parents should be encouraged to accept and understand the child's condition and to participate in his care to the best of their ability. They will need guidance in getting the child to accept his handicap and to feel comfortable about himself to the greatest possible extent. If the prognosis is poor, every effort must be made to ensure that proper emotional support is given.

Achievement of the maximum degree of independence possible is the primary goal for the handicapped child. Obviously, the degree of independence will be defined by the limitations of the child's handicap, and planning must be realistic, but positive. Priorities must be set to develop those skills which that particular child will need most. Communication skills, mobility, activities of daily living and gait must all be given appropriate emphasis in the child's habilitation plan.

The family may also need help with social problems. A handicapped child can have a devastating effect on family relationships, finances and way of life. Inevitable problems will arise in school placement. Questions of vocational training, sexuality, and eventual independent living in the community will arise. The question of guardianship may need to be faced.

The physician who has made the initial neurological evaluation may not be the one who follows the child, but he is responsible for setting the wheels in motion. The best neurological evaluation in the world would be a complete waste of time if the physician's responsibility ended at the door of the examination room. The implementation process must be initiated in the manner most likely to ensure that recommendations and the habilitation plan are followed.

A common cause of unsatisfactory implementation is poor communicaton. The physician may not have been able to describe the problem and the recommendations in a useful manner. Sometimes the family is anxious and hostile, and may choose not to hear what is said. The physician may be perceived as the messenger of ancient times, who was beheaded for bringing bad tidings. Poor communication back to the referring source also may diminish the effect of the recommendations. The recommendations might not have been sent in a usable form—or they might not have been transmitted at all. A local treatment facility charged with the responsibility for carrying out specific therapy may be unable to do so effectively because the physician

192

did not specify exactly what was needed or what the priorities were.

Another obstacle to successful implementation is diffusion and overlap of responsibility. In the United States the care of a handicapped child may be shared by a general practitioner, a pediatrician, one or more medical and surgical specialists, a speech and language pathologist, an audiologist, a clinical psychologist, a social worker from the medical center, an educator, an educational psychologist, a school nurse, an educational administrator, a public-health nurse, and a case-worker from a community agency. No one person is in charge to see that the over-all plan is followed and the priorities are kept in order. The family becomes confused by the plethora of specialists, and by conflicting opinions. The opportunity for long-term follow-up is lost and the child is medically abandoned.

The co-operation of the family is essential to the success of the habilitation plan. Co-operation is based on trust, confidence and understanding, and a positive commitment on the part of the family may take time to evolve. A social worker can provide essential counseling and support and facilitate communication between the physician and the family, and between the family and community resources, including school, local treatment facilities and agencies. The social worker may also play an important rôle as an advocate for the child and family, to ensure that mandated services are provided effectively.

One person must be in charge to keep the child's over-all needs in the proper perspective, to make sure that specific recommendations are being followed, and to give the family a focus for continuing discussion. The physician who provides the care usually is in the best position to assume this responsibility, but in some cases the social worker, the speech and language pathologist or the psychologist may be more suitable. The person in charge should be the one to whom the family relates best and who has the opportunity to form a long-term therapeutic relationship.

Plans for a handicapped child invariably involve the use of community resources. The family will have confidence in the physician's recommendations if they are obviously based on familiarity with services for the handicapped in the community, and with details of government health-care systems which could benefit the child. The physician who provides care within the community can give enlightened support and advice if he has first-hand contant with the resources available in his community. He should know the staff and level of competence of local treatment facilities, the services offered by private agencies for the handicapped, and details of parents' groups organized to help with a particular disability. He should also have first-hand on-site experience of local preschool and school programs so as to be familiar with physical barriers, the staffing pattern, the curriculum offered and the quality of medical and health support given.

A 'successful' neurological evaluation is one in which the correct diagnosis, reached efficiently with minimal stress to child and family, is accompanied by practical recommendations, complete co-operation of the family, and satisfactory implementation. Circumstances usually preclude the achievement of this ideal, and the end result may have to be the best compromise possible. The work of a compassionate, experienced physician includes obtaining the trust and co-operation of the child and the family and making sure that recommendations are carried out.

CHAPTER 11

Special Investigations

Additional information may help to clarify the clinical history and examination, but each of the possible sources has certain limitations. Invasive procedures should be kept to a minimum, although some of these techniques (*e.g.* biopsy) have improved markedly.

This chapter and appendices on pages 227 to 235 discuss some of these methods, which may require additional equipment or facilities. Test kits will be needed for the Denver Developmental Screening Test. A detailed and systematic record is necessary for the genetic history. Chromosome analysis requires special laboratory facilities, with highly trained technical assistance. For computerized axial tomography, expensive equipment and a specially trained radiologist with an interest in pediatrics will be needed. Electroencephalographic facilities must recognize the special treatment needed by young children if useful traces are to be obtained. For evoked potentials, acquisition of neutrophysiological data entails the use of computer technology, with its attendant problems. For gas liquid chromatography, as with other laboratory procedures, reliable equipment and the integrity of all those involved are essential. Radioisotope studies also require special facilties, and should be done only for specific indications. Nuclear magnetic resonance and positron emission tomography are discussed briefly because it seems likely that these procedures will become more widely available.

Most laboratory tests measure associated phenomena which affect homeostasis generally, but not a single event at the cellular level. Although many are not invasive, or only minimally so, their lack of specificity limits their usefulness. If it were possible to do so, identification of anatomical, electrical or chemical events at the synapse would be preferable, so that disorders of neurosecretion, neurotransmission and neurochemistry could be identified more precisely. There is increasing evidence that neurosecretory function and the appearance of certain cells during electron-microscopy can be closely correlated. Therefore the gaps that have existed between neuroanatomy, neurophysiology and neurochemistry are becoming smaller.

Other valuable techniques are becoming available: fluorescin-microscopy, for example, can be used to identify neurotransmitters. After a histological section has been exposed to formaldehyde, pathways have been demonstrated from the medulla to the spinal cord, from the substantia nigra to the striatum and from the tegmentum to the hypothalamus, amygdala and hippocampus. Norepinephrine and dopamine secretory cells give green fluorescence and 5-hydroxytryptamine (serotonin) give pale yellow fluorescence. These neurotransmitters almost certainly play important rôles in tardive dyskinesia, Huntington's chorea, Parkinson's disease and other disorders.

COMPUTERIZED AXIAL TOMOGRAPHY

Description

Computerized axial tomography (CT) combines radiology and computer science to provide a non-invasive method of identifying structures within the cranial vault or the entire body. The amount of radiation required for a head is no more than that used for radiological examination of the skull.

Principal uses

This test is indicated when a non-invasive procedure is needed to determine the anatomical integrity of the brain. It is particularly useful if space-occupying lesions (*e.g.* tumor or abscess), sequelae of trauma (*e.g.* hematoma) or anatomical changes are suspected. Enhancement by comparing similar cross-section views before and after the administration of a contrast material increases the amount of information that can be obtained.

Method

The head or body of the subject is placed in a position so that a beam of x-rays can be exposed and recorded from various angles, according to a predetermined program.

The area within the skull is considered to be divided into small cubes and each can be given an 'address'. The density of x-rays within each cube can be obtained and rated between 1 and 1000. A density map of a layer of cubes, taken across a cross-sectional plane, can be constructed by computer and printed out. A second examination can be performed after intravenous administration of contrast material (this test is similar to an intravenous pyelogram). The densities of the tissues and further identification of vascular structures can be compared with the previous study by subtraction techniques, done by computer analysis, as well as by interpreting the print-outs themselves.

Results

The degree of resolution of the reconstructed 'layers' depends on the size of the cubes and the limits of the equipment in determining how much the densities of central nervous system tissues vary from fluid. It is possible to determine alterations in ventricular size, displacement caused by blood or tumor, the location of calcified areas, and the relationship of the central nervous system to bony landmarks.

An example is a 10-year-old boy with Dandy-Walker syndrome and an absent corpus callosum (Fig. 54). He was reported to have had a gradually increasing head-circumference, which measured 60cm at the time of examination. There was no evidence of mental, motor or growth retardation. Visual acuity was 20/60, 20/60 and visual fields were constricted, in addition to papilloedema.

Limitations

Because of the great cost of purchasing and installing the equipment, computerized axial tomography usually is carried out only in medical centers, so its

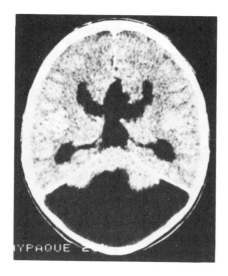

Fig. 54. CT scan of 10-year-old boy with Dandy-Walker syndrome. Note 'bat wings', a characteristic of absent corpus callosum. [By courtesy of Drs. Eric Faeber and Catherine Foley, Departments of Radiology and Pediatrics, Temple University School of Medicine at St. Christopher's Hospital for Children, Philadelphia.]

availability is limited. The method is of questionable value from the cost:benefit point of view in identifying abnormalities for which no specific therapy is available. Only about 10 per cent of children with seizure disorders, significant motor or mental delay or a history of a significant postnatal cerebral insult will have abnormalities which are detectable by CT. There are no clear indications for using the method for children who have apparently non-progressive but chronic disorders: it depends on local availability rather than generally accepted criteria.

Further reading

Hounsfield, G. N. (1973) 'Computerized transverse axial scanning (tomography). I: Description of system.' *British Journal of Radiology.* **46,** 1016-1022.
Ambrose, J. (1973) 'Computerized transverse axial scanning (tomography). II: Clinical application.' *British Journal of Radiology.* **46,** 1023-1047.
Perry, B. J., Bridges, C. (1973) 'Computerized transverse axial scanning (tomography). III: Radiation dose considerations.' *British Journal of Radiology.* **46,** 1048-1062.

RADIOISOTOPE IMAGING AND NUCLEAR MAGNETIC RESONANCE IMAGING

(This section has been contibuted by H. Theodore Harcke, M.D., Director, Division of Nuclear Medicine, Alfred I. duPont Institute, Wilmington, Delaware.)

Radionuclide imaging studies usually are performed to obtain physiological information. They complement computed tomography (CT) and ultrasound, which provide superior anatomical details of brain matter and the ventricular system but may not reveal functional changes. In some instances a radionuclide study may be requested as an alternative if CT is not available.

Imaging is dependent upon the injection of a radioisotope whose distribution in the body can be detected. A variety of tracers are used (Table XXIII), often serving as the label for a non-radioactive carrier compound. The non-radioactive carrier is

TABLE XXIII
Isotope studies*

Isotope	Suggested dose	Form	Use
In^{111}	0.5mCi†	DTPA**	CSF pathways
Tc-99m	20.0mCi	DTPA	Brain scan
Tc-99m	200μCi/kg	Pertechnitate	Brain scan

*Available from St. Christopher's Hospital for Children, Philadelphia. Only those applicable to CNS are included.
**Pentetate calcium trisodium.
†mCi = millicurie—adjust for weight (adult dose).

selected because of its physiological behavior in the part of the body being investigated. Both tracer development and advances in the imaging equipment have made possible several methods of patient evaluation.

Recently, nuclear magnetic resonance imaging, a totally new approach to medical imaging, has shown considerable promise. It is anticipated that this will become an important clinical tool, since it provides good resolution and requires no exposure to radiation.

Radioisotope imaging
Brain scan

The brain scan begins with the intravenous injection of a radioisotope tracer, followed by three phases of imaging. Technetium 99m pertechnetate (Tc-99m), alone or in compound, is the most commonly used tracer, with aqueous potassium perchlorate being given orally 10 to 30 minutes before the injection. Perchlorate competitively blocks Tc-99m uptake in the choroid plexus, thereby eliminating a potential source of confusion when the images are interpreted. Alternative tracer compounds are Tc-99m-diethylene-triamine pentacetic acid (DTPA) and Tc-99m-glucohelptonate (GH).

Phase 1. The radionuclide angiogram (flow study) evaluates cerebral blood-flow. Beginning at the time of the tracer injection, serial images of the head and neck are obtained every 0.5-1.5 seconds. The arterial, capillary and venous phases of cerebral perfusion can then be assessed. If the images are stored in a digital computer, graphs of activity *vs* time can be generated for selected regions of the brain. The radionuclide angiogram is the key phase when the brain scan is used to assess patients suspected of cerebral vascular disease and vascular malformations (Fig. 55)[1]*.

Phase 2. Blood pool (immediate static) images of the cranial vault in anterior, posterior and lateral projections may be obtained immediately following the angiogram phase. Local areas of increased or decreased tracer activity reflect regional hyper- or hypoperfusion, usually following the pattern seen on the flow study.

Phase 3. Delayed static images are used to assess the integrity of the blood-brain barrier. Multiple views (anterior, posterior, right and left laterals) are obtained two to four hours after injection. If there is a breakdown in the blood-brain barrier the

*For references throughout this section, see 'Further reading' at end of section.

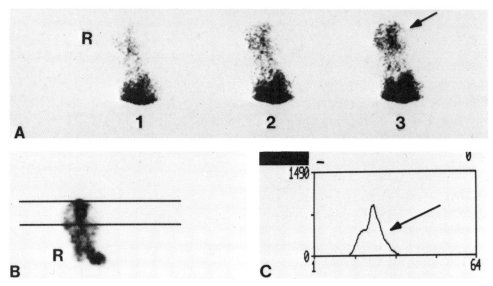

Fig. 55. Radionuclide angiogram of two-year-old boy who had a cerebral vascular accident after surgery for congenital heart-disease. **A.** Serial anterior images at 1.5-second intervals show a perfusion deficit in left hemisphere (arrow). **B.** Computer-generated composite of flow images with **(C)** profile analysis reflect decreased flow (arrow). [A normal profile is symmetrical.]

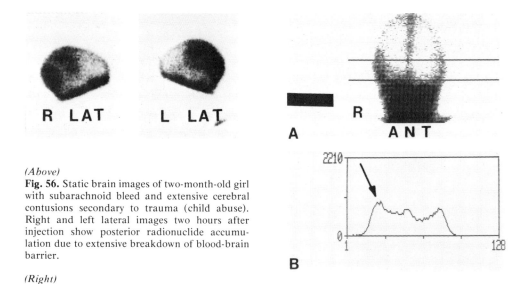

(Above)
Fig. 56. Static brain images of two-month-old girl with subarachnoid bleed and extensive cerebral contusions secondary to trauma (child abuse). Right and left lateral images two hours after injection show posterior radionuclide accumulation due to extensive breakdown of blood-brain barrier.

(Right)
Fig. 57. Static brain image with computer profile: 13-year-old boy with tuberculous meningitis. **A.** Abnormal right temporal activity in anterior image and on **(B)** computer-generated activity profile (arrow). CT scan at the time of this study was interpreted as normal.

198

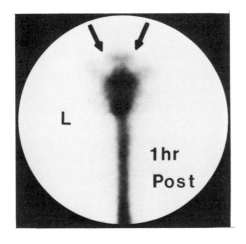

Fig. 58. Radionuclide cisternogram: four-month old boy with extraventricular obstructive hydrocephalus. One hour after Tc-99m-DTPA administration through lumbar puncture, tracer has reached basilar cisterns and there has been retrograde filling of the lateral ventricles (arrows).

radionuclide will leave the vascular compartment and accumulate in the extravascular tissues. This focal collection of activity is seen as an abnormal density on the images (Fig. 56). Most intracerebral pathology results in a breakdown of the blood-brain barrier. Trauma, abscesses, tumors and infarcts may look similar, but often can be specifically identified because of the patient's history or the patterns on scan images (Fig. 57)[2,3].

Cisternography

The cisternogram is used to assess the cerebrospinal fluid (CSF) spaces and the dynamics of CSF movement. Indium-111-DTPA is the radiopharmaceutical of choice when imaging is required more than 24 hours post-administration. For children, there is usually no need to image after 24 hours and Tc-99m DTPA, which has a shorter half-life than In-111, can be used. Tracer administration is usually by means of lumbar puncture, but it may be placed into the CSF by other accepted routes (*e.g.* cisternal puncture, indwelling intraventricular catheter). After tracer injection, serial images of the spine and cranium are obtained to document dispersion in the CSF. Following lumbar injection, the tracer normally moves to the basilar cisterns within one hour, does not enter the ventricular system, and moves over the convexities of the brain within 24 hours. There is considerable resorption by this time. Communicating hydrocephalus is diagnosed when the tracer enters the ventricular system and/or is delayed in passing over the convexities (Fig. 58)[3].

Nuclear tomography

Advances in imaging equipment and digital computers permit tomographic planar images to be obtained after radionuclide injection. This development produces an image similar to that obtained by radiographic computed tomography and shows radionuclide distribution in the reconstructed section. However, at present resolution is in the order of 1 to 2cm, much less than on CT. Tomography possesses an advantage over conventional brain-scan images, in that it removes the influence of scalp activity and therefore increases the contrast between a lesion and the adjacent tissue.

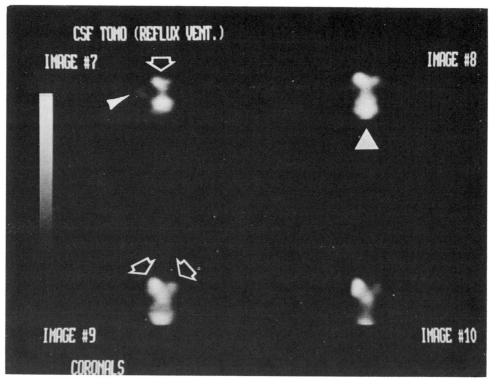

Fig. 59. Single photon emission tomography (SPECT) imaging. Serial coronal sections of the brain from anterior to posterior were obtained as part of the cisternogram of a child with extraventricular obstructive hydrocephalus. A clearer delineation of reflux into the lateral ventricles (open arrows) is possible. Compare these images with Figure 58. Other structures demonstrated are the Sylvian fissure (image 7, closed arrows) and basal cisterns (image 8, closed triangle). [Images by courtesy of Dr. David L. Gilday, The Hospital for Sick Children, Toronto.]

Development of new radiopharmaceuticals that are distributed on a metabolic rather than a pathophysiological basis has spurred development of two types of tomographic equipment. The first is single-photon-emission computed tomography (SPECT), generally performed by rotating the nuclear camera detector head(s) around the patient in a series of steps after tracer injection. This method produces a set of images which can be reconstructed into tomographic sections by digital computer (Fig. 59)[4]. The second-type is positron-emission tomography (PET), a more sophisticated tomographic unit currently being developed and tested. PET units use a special group of radioisotope tracers that emit positrons. These interact with nearby electrons to produce gamma rays, which are then sensed by an array of detectors surrounding the patient. The images produced are computer-reconstructed tomographic sections. By linking the positron emitters to common metabolites (such as glucose), functional mapping of the brain has been made possible. The association of patterns of metabolic activity with disease states has already produced exciting information. During an epileptic seizure, for example, focal increased glucose has

200

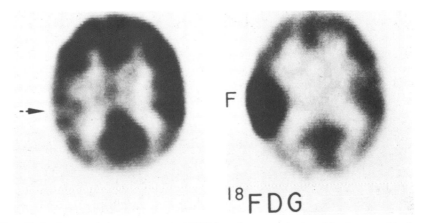

Fig. 60. Positron emission tomography (PET) imaging. Inter-ictal and ictal scans of brain of five-year-old boy with right focal motor seizures. Distribution of fluorine-18 labeled 2-deoxy-2-fluoro-D-glucose is compared. Hypometabolism (decreased activity) is seen in left temporo-parietal cortex (arrow) on inter-ictal scan. During seizure activity [right facial twitching and epileptiform EEG spike activity in the left frontotemporal region] there is hypermetabolism (increased activity) in the right temporoparietal cortex (F). [Figure from Alavi *et al.* (1982), by courtesy of Dr. Abass Alavi, with the permission of Dr. David Kuhl, UCLA School of Medicine, Los Angeles, who provided the case.]

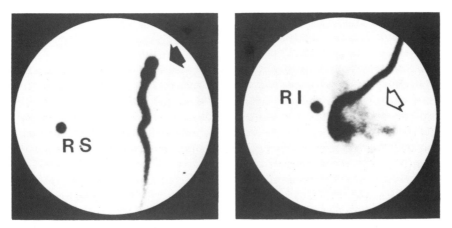

Fig. 61. CSF shunt evaluation: five-year-old girl with ventriculoperitoneal diversionary shunt for non-communicating hydrocephalus. Serial imaging documents patency. Five minutes after injection of shunt reservoir (closed arrow) activity is noted in proximal portion of tubing. (RS is an external marking at right shoulder.) 20 minutes after injection the tracer has passed through the tubing and diffused within the peritoneal cavity (open arrow). (RI is an external marker at right iliac crest.)

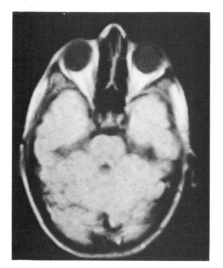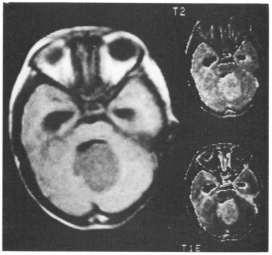

Fig. 62. Normal and abnormal NMR brain images. *(Left)* Normal section of brain of 13-year-old girl. Image obtained with 3.5 K Gauss magnet, using spin-echo pulse sequence. *(Right)* Brain section of 6½-year-old with posterior fossa tumor. The spin-echo image demonstrates low-intensity mass in posterior fossa, with displacement of fourth ventricle and enlargement of temporal horns. Calculated T_2 and T_1 images reveal the long T_2 and T_1 of the mass, which was a medulloblastoma. [Images by courtesy of Dr. Catherine Mills, Radiologic Imaging Laboratory, University of California, San Francisco.]

been documented by PET imaging (Fig. 60). Its application in the diagnosis of other forms of brain pathology which show no anatomical changes is also anticipated[5,6].

Other imaging studies

CSF leak test. This test is actually a variation of cisternography, in which the tracer is placed into the CSF and allowed to circulate. The nostrils and/or ear canals are packed with cotton-wool after the injection and sequential imaging is performed with the packs in place. If there is a leak the packs will absorb the labelled CSF, and occasionally this is apparent on the images. After several hours the packs are removed and if no leak has been visualized on the images, the packs are measured for radionuclide activity in a scintillation well counter. When there is a CSF leak the pack(s) which absorbed the CSF will show higher levels of tracer activity.

CSF shunt elevation. Most CSF shunts for hydrocephalus have a subcutaneous reservoir or flushing device connecting the intracranial and extracranial portions of the apparatus. A small volume of radionuclide activity (Tc-99m or Tc-99m DTPA) can be placed into the reservoir under sterile conditions and observed by serial imaging. Normally, distal movement through the shunt tube will occur and the tracer will diffuse into the peritoneum, atrium, etc. at the tube's tip (Fig. 61).

Shunt blockage distal to the reservoir will prevent movement.

Nuclear magnetic resonance (NMR) imaging

This is a new technique which is still at a developmental stage and is currently undergoing clinical trials. It differs completely from conventional radiology and nuclear medicine in that no radiation exposure occurs. Physically, the NMR apparatus is not unlike other imaging devices, in that the body is surrounded by a cylinder; however, in NMR this houses the magnet. With the patient in the magnetic field, the section of the body to be imaged is exposed to a series of radio-frequency (RF) pulses. Some atomic nuclei act like tiny magnets and are sensitive to this sequence. Initially they align themselves with the magnetic field. The RF pulse sequence provides energy which serves to deflect the nuclei from their alignment. In returning to the aligned state, part of the absorbed energy is released as a detectable RF signal. This behavior in the magnetic field is measured and processed by digital computer to create an image by sampling many small volumes of tissue at known locations in a plane.

To date, hydrogen, which is present most abundantly as water in the body, has been shown to differ in its NMR characteristics in various body structures. This permits organs to be differentiated on the computer-reconstructed tomographic sectional images, analogus to CT. Images produced may reflect the distribution of nuclei (*e.g.* proton density images) or the relative time increments required for the return of nuclei to the relaxed or aligned state after pulsing (*e.g.* T_1 and T_2 relaxation times). Studies under way suggest that NMR imaging will be useful in studying the brain in a variety of pathological demyelinating diseases and tumors (Fig. 62)[7-9].

Further reading

1. Savage, J. P., Gilday, D. L., Ash, J. M. (1977) 'Cerebrovascular disease in childhood.' *Radiology,* **123,** 385-391.
2. Kim, E. E., DeLand, F. H., Montebello, J. (1979) 'Sensitivity of radionuclide brain scan and computer tomography in the early detection of viral meningoencephalitis.' *Radiology,* **132,** 425-429.
3. Gilday, D. L. (1976) 'Pediatric neuronuclear medicine.' *In:* Harwood-Nash, D. C., Fitz, C. R. (Eds.) *Neuroradiology in Infants and Children.* St. Louis: C. V. Mosby. pp. 505-608.
4. Ell, P. J., Kahn, O. (1981) 'Emission computerized tomography: clinical applications.' *Seminars in Nuclear Medicine,* **11,** 50-60.
5. Alavi, A., Reivich, M., Jones, S. C., Greenberg, J. H., Wolf, A. P. (1982) 'Functional imaging of the brain with positron emission tomography.' *In:* Freeman, L. M., Weissman, H. S. (Eds.) *Nuclear Medicine Annual.* New York: Raven Press. pp. 319-372.
6. Kuhl, D. E., Engel, J., Phelps, M. E., Selin, M. S. (1980) 'Epileptic patterns of local cerebral metabolism and perfusion in humans determined by emission computed tomogram of ^{18}FDG and ^{13}NH$_3$.' *Annals of Neurology,* **8,** 348-360.
7. Pykett, I. L. (1982) 'NMR imaging in medicine.' *Scientific American,* **246,** 78-88.
8. Oldendorf, W. H. (1982) 'NMR imaging: its potential clinical impact.' *Hospital Practice,* **17,** 114-128.
9. Witkofski, R. L., Karstaedt, N., Partain, C. L. (Eds.) (1982) *NMR Imaging. Proceedings of an International Symposium on Nuclear Magnetic Resonance Imaging.* Winston-Salem, North Carolina: Bowman Gray School of Medicine of Wake Forest University.

CHROMOSOMAL ANALYSIS

Description

Chromosomal analysis is a method of studying genetic material in cells grown in tissue culture. Lymphocytes are most commonly used, but studies for special conditions may require culture of fibroblasts (for mosaicism and biochemical defects), bone-marrow cells (for blood dyscrasia) or amniotic-fluid cells (for prenatal diagnosis). The most common abnormalities reported are alteration in the

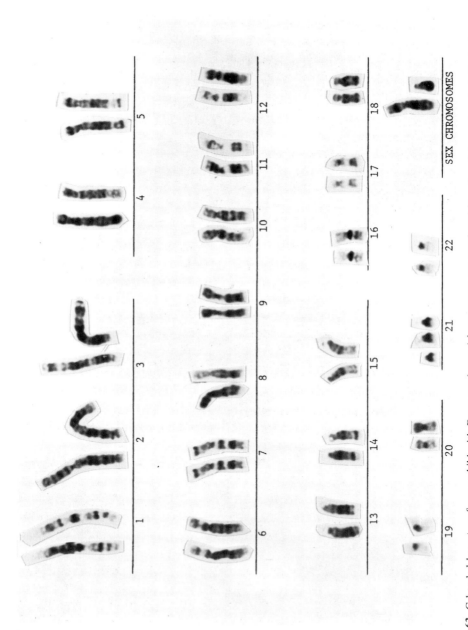

Fig. 63. G-banded karyotype from a child with Down syndrome (chromosomes are numbered in order of decreasing size). Each chromosome is identified by its unique pattern of bands. In G-banding the fixed cells are treated with trypsin, followed by Giemsa staining. Note that there are three chromosomes 21 (trisomy 21).

number of chromosomes, translocations (balanced or non-balanced), deletions and fragile sites.

Principal uses

Chromosomal analysis documents the presence of a condition which has been suggested clinically. It can be used to confirm the obvious (*e.g.* a child with typical trisomy 21; Fig. 63), or it can be a diagnostic tool if evidence of a chromosomal disorder is less certain. This type of analysis contributes to the better understanding of genetic disorders. If accompanied by skilled genetic counseling, which must be an integral part of chromosomal analysis, it may lead to the prevention of congenital defects. Some parents also welcome evidence of a definite cause for their offspring's condition.

Any individual who is mentally retarded and for whom a specific diagnosis is not apparent can be considered a candidate for chromosomal analysis. Children who have congenital anomalies, except those known to be inherited as Mendelian traits, are also candidates.

Banding techniques have increased the usefulness of chromosome analysis, since they can identify small deletions and rearrangements. For example, a small deletion in chromosome 13 occurs in some children who have retinoblastoma of the sporadic type. This deletion has not been found in the autosomal dominant form, and its absence may be suggestive that further cases of retinoblastoma may occur in that particular family.

There is a chromosomal defect when aniridia and Wilms tumor occur together, but in the sporadic cases of aniridia with normal chromosomes there have been no reported instances of Wilms tumor. (Children with aniridia with a chromosomal defect usually also have mental retardation, hypogonadism and Wilms tumor.)

Method

Usually the test is performed by placing the lymphocytes from 5-10cc of blood, or a few drops of whole blood, in appropriate tissue-culture media, stimulating by phytohemagglutinin, arresting the cells in mitosis, harvesting the lymphocytes, swelling the cells with hypotonic fluid and staining as required. Subsequent examination with photomicrography completes the process.

Although various body tissues have been grown in tissue culture, lymphocytes are the most useful. Culture conditions may alter the appearance of chromosomes on banding and may enhance sites of chromosome fragility.

Limitations

The widespread use of chromosomal analysis is limited by its expense and by the need for sophisticated laboratory techniques and skilled interpretation. The laboratory method itself has some weaknesses. Failure to find an abnormality in one tissue may not rule out abormalities in another. (In some instances chromosomes grown from culture of skin cells have shown abnormalities that were not found in the blood, and vice versa.) The resolution of the chromosomes may be poor because the lymphocytes have failed to divide adequately. Small fragments of

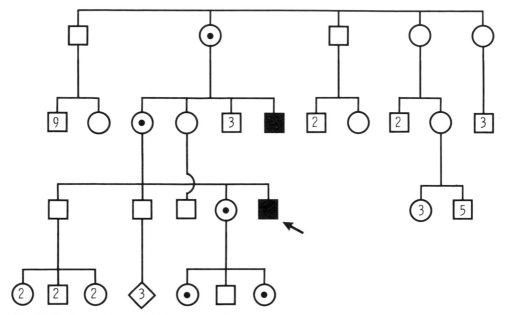

Fig. 64. Pedigree of 'fragile-X' chromosome. [Figs. 63 and 64 courtsey Dr. Hope Punnett, Cytogenetics Laboratory, Department of Pediatrics, Temple University School of Medicine at St. Christopher's Hospital for Children, Philadelphia.]

chromosomes are not always interpretable with today's understanding. Some abnormalities within the chromosomes may not be definitive: for example, a mother who appears to be normal may have similar chromosomal abnormalities to those of her mentally retarded child. It is not clear why the mother should be mentally normal and the child retarded.

An example of a human chromosome marker is the 'fragile-X' syndrome, which can be recognized clinically in males by the association of macro-orchidism and mental retardation. The pedigree of an affected family is shown in Figure 64. The 29-year-old male (arrow) had been placed in an institution early in life. His intelligence had been measured in the 50-60 range. His right testicle first reported to be '?large' at 13 years of age, now measures 8 × 6 × 3cm. His height is 131cm (67in); head circumference is 57cm (22½in). Otherwise his physical features and results of examination were unremarkable. Three female relatives have been found to have the same marker X chromosome. A photomicrograph shows a typical 'fragile X' chromosome (Fig. 65).

Comment

It is unclear whether information from chromosome studies of other mammals and other species can be applied to human genetics. It is known that 'trisomy' with clinical signs suggesting Down syndrome occurs in the chimpanzee and orang-utan. In addition, the fruit fly *(Drosophila melanogaster)* has mutants (3D3-3D4) which have poor learning ability, as judged by performance tests. These 'dunce' mutants have an alteration in cyclic AMP phosphodiesterase activity.

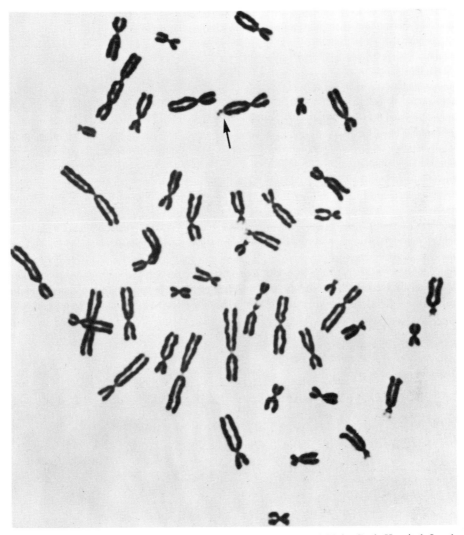

Fig. 65. 'Fragile-X' chromosome (arrow). [Courtesy Paediatric Research Unit, Guy's Hospital, London.]

Further reading

Adinolfi, M., Benson, P., Gianelli, F., Seller, M. (Eds.) (1982) *Paediatric Research: a Genetic Approach.*
    Clinics in Development Medicine No. 83. London. SIMP with Heinemann Medical; Philadelphia:
    Lippincott.
de Grouchy, J., Turleau, C. (1977) *Clinical Atlas of Human Chromosomes.* New York: Wiley.
Yunis, J. J. (Ed.) (1977) *New Chromosomal Syndromes.* New York: Academic Press.

TABLE XXIV

**CSF protein values during first year
of life**

	CSF protein (mg/dl)*	
	Range	Mean
Birth preterm	65-150	115
Fullterm	20-170	90
One month	20-150	62
Three months	20-100	46
Six months	15- 50	37
Nine months	15- 30	24

*Normal adult < 35 mg/dl.

CEREBROSPINAL FLUID

Cerebrospinal fluid (CSF) is obtained most commonly by lumbar puncture, but may also be obtained by ventricular puncture or, in very experienced hands, cisternal puncture. Contra-indications to lumbar puncture should be noted. These are:

(1) infection in skin or deeper tissues at the site of puncture;
(2) papilloedema, unless due to benign intracranial hypertension or papillitis;
(3) suspicion of posterior fossa mass;
(4) suspicion of supratentorial tumor, or supratentorial subdural hematoma;
(5) bleeding diathesis or anticoagulant therapy;
(6) pre-existing compression of the spinal cord.

The technique for lumbar puncture should be familiar, so it is not described here. Samples of CSF are taken, their appearance noted, and then sent to the laboratory for analysis. If the CSF is bloodstained, a portion should be centrifuged and the supernatant fluid examined for xanthochromia. If present, this confirms a pre-existing hemorrhage. The fluid should also be examined for cells, and the number and character noted. Biochemical analysis usually includes protein, glucose and chlorides. Normal values of CSF protein at ages up to nine months are shown in Table XXIV. Table XXV shows the composition of normal lumbar CSF and serum. Many trace metals have been detected in the CSF, but no specific disease states have been associated with their presence or absence.

Two newer techniques which have become available are the estimation of myelin basic protein and oligoclonal banding of CSF IgG. Although abnormal values have been found in certain conditions, raised values are not diagnostic of specific disorders. However, these techniques may have a future.

In certain circumstances enzyme studies may be helpful. The following enzymes are known to be present in CSF: lactic dehydrogenase and its isoenzymes (increased in both bacterial and viral meningitis); lysozyme (high levels are associated with lymphomas, and the increase usually parallels changes in lactic dehydrogenase); and creatinine phosphokinase (increased after seizures).

TABLE XXV
Composition of normal lumbar CSF and serum*

	CSF	Serum
Osmolarity (mOsm/l)	295	295
Water content (%)	99	93
Sodium (mEq/l)	138	138
Potassium (mEq/1)	2.8	4.5
Calcium (mEq/l)	2.1	4.8
Magnesium (mEq/l)	2.3	1.7
Chloride (mEq/1)	119	102
Bicarbonate (mEq/1)	22	24 (arterial)
CO_2 tension (mmHg)	47	41 (arterial)
pH	7.33	7.41 (arterial)
Oxygen (mmHg)	43	104
Glucose (mg/dl)	60	90
Lactate (mEq/l)	1.6	1.0 (arterial)
Pyruvate (mEq/1)	0.08	0.11 (arterial)
Lactate/pyruvate ratio	26	17.6 (arterial)
Fructose (mg/dl)	4	2
Polyols (μmol/1)	340	148
Myoinositol (mg/dl)	2.6	1.0
Total protein	35mg/dl	7gm/dl
prealbumin (%)	4	trace
albumin (%)	65	60
alpha$_1$ globulin (%)	4	5
alpha$_2$ globulin (%)	8	9
beta globulin (beta$_1$ + tau) (%)	12	12
gamma globulin (%)	7	14
IgG (mg/dl)	1.2	987
IgA (mg/dl)	0.2	175
IgM (mg/dl)	0.06	70
kappa/lambda ratio	1	1
beta trace protein (mg/dl)	2.0	0.5
fibronectin (μg/ml)	3	300
Total free amino acids (umol/dl)	80.9	228
Ammonia (μg/dl)	24	37 (arterial)
Urea (mmol/l)	4.7	5.4
Creatinine (mg/dl)	1.2	1.8
Uric acid (mg/dl)	0.25	5.50
Putrescine (pmol/ml)	184	
Spermidine (pmol/ml)	150	
Total lipids (mg/dl)	1.5	750
free cholesterol (mg/dl)	0.4	180
cholesterol esters (mg/dl)	0.3	126
cAMP (nmol/l)	20	
cGMP (nmol/l)	0.68	
HVA (μg/ml)	60	
5-HIAA (μg/ml)	0.04	
Norepinephrine (pg/ml)	200	350
MHGP (mg/ml)	15	
Acetylcholine (mg/dl)	1.8	
Choline (mM/ml)	2.5	
Prostaglandin PGF$_2$ alpha (pg/ml)	92	
Insulin (mμ/ml)	3.7	36
Gastrin (pmol/l)	3.4	
Cholecystokinin (pmol/l)	14	
Beta endorphin (pmol/l)	145	10
Phosphorus (mg/dl)	1.6	4
Iron (μg/dl)	1.5	15

From Fishman (1980): reproduced by permission
*Average or representative values are given. Many trace metals have been detected in the CSF, but no specific disease states have been associated with their presence or absence.

TABLE XXVI
Therapeutic levels of anticonvulsants

Drug	Therapeutic level*	
	$\mu M/ml$	$\mu g/ml$
Phenobarbital ('Luminal')	65-150	15- 35
Carbamazepine ('Tegretol')	13- 42	3- 10
Primidone ('Mysoline')	14- 46	3- 10
Phenytoin ('Dilantin')	20- 89	5- 10
Ethosuximide ('Zarontin')	180-850	10-120
Valproic acid ('Depakene')	400-700	60-100

Source: Department of Laboratories, St. Christopher's Hospital for Children, Philadelphia.

GAS LIQUID CHROMATOGRAPHY

Description

Gas liquid chromatography (GLC) is a method for obtaining a quantitative measurement of drugs or other chemicals from a tissue sample. Equilibrium of anticonvulsants and other drugs is reached in serum, a stable and easily accessible tissue.

Principal uses

This method is used for the regular monitoring of serum levels of people receiving anticonvulsant medication. Monitoring prevents over-medication, provides an objective means of judging the value of a particular drug for a particular individual, and gives specific evidence of compliance or lack of compliance in taking the drug. Differences in individual tolerance to medication prescribed by arbitrary calculations can be verified and corrected. GLC is particularly helpful if more than one drug is being used.

Method

The effluence of a small amount of serum (0.1cc) is mixed with a gas. Following the passage of this mixture through a specially prepared glass or metal column, which has been packed with an absorptive material, the residue is burned. Alterations in the material during nitrogen (or other) ionization are measured over a fixed time, compared with known samples and reported on a unit basis. (The method lends itself to automation.)

Results

Laboratory standards vary, depending on the method used. Table XXVI gives typical values of therapeutic levels of anticonvulsants.

Limitations

The test is of limited value if medication is taken irregularly or, obviously, if laboratory techniques are suspect.

Variations in method

High-pressure chromatography differs in several important respects. The column is relatively short and the procedure is carried out at room temperature. Following passage through the high-pressure column, changes in the effluent are measured as it passes through an ultraviolet light.

AMINOACIDEMIA (SERUM) AND AMINOACIDURIA (URINE)

Abnormalities of amino acid metabolism can be detected by chromatography of the serum or urine. Significant amounts of amino acid are almost always three or more times the normal levels and give characteristically abnormal patterns. Depending on the method used, nutritional factors, recent ingestion of food in unusual amounts, or the administration of certain drugs may produce 'slightly abnormal' patterns. Generalized aminoaciduria usually is associated with renal abnormalities or with defects in gastro-intestinal absorption.

Disorders associated with metabolic disease should be considered in infants and children who have evidence of mental retardation, seizures, spasticity, progressive neurological deterioration or growth retardation, or whose bodies or urine have a distinctive or pungent odor.

Reported defects of amino acid metabolism include:

phenylalanine	proline, hydroxyproline
tyrosine	glutamic acid
methionine	urea-cycle amino acids
cysteine	histidine
tryptophane	beta amino acids
valine, leucine, isoleucine	lysine
glycine	threonine

CREATININE PHOSPHOKINASE LEVELS

Elevated levels of creatinine phosphokinase (CPK) are found in muscular dystrophy. Serum CPK is consistently high in the sex-linked pseudohypertrophic type, and smaller elevations have been noted in limb-girdle and facioscapulohumeral dystrophy, as well as in myotonic dystrophy (Table XXVII). CPK levels may also be elevated in the acute stages of polymyositis in childhood.

ELECTROMYOGRAPHY

Electromyograms (EMGs) are recorded chiefly to investigate patients with muscular weakness (local or generalized) suspected to be due to a disorder of the lower motor unit. Thus a study of the electrical activity of affected muscles is indicated for children suspected of myopathies, peripheral neuropathies or of diseases

TABLE XXVII
Serum CPK levels in neuromuscular diseases

Disease	Serum CPK level (iu/litre)	Estimated 90% confidence level
Normal	8-60	<60
Muscular dystrophy:		
Affected fetus	>100	>100
Affected newborn	>100	>100
Duchenne type (sex-linked)	>1000	>1000
Female carriers	10-500	>100
Limb girdle	10-500, but may be 1000	>100
Facio-scapulo-humeral	10-200	>60
Dystrophia myotonica	10-200	>60
Congenital myopathies	10-200	Variable
Polymyositis/dermatomyositis	Normal, but may be >1000 in acute phase	Variable
Neurogenic atrophies:	Normal	
Benign Kugelberg-Welander type	10-200	<60 under 6 yrs
Glycogenoses (e.g. McArdle syndrome)	Up to 1000	>100
Malignant hyperpyrexia		
Acute	>1000	>1000
Subclinical	10-200	Variable

of the lower motor neurons in the spinal cord or brain stem. The EMG is abnormal in a non-specific way in cases of spasticity, dystonia, athetosis, and so on, but is not of differential diagnostic value for suprasegmental spinal or cerebral disease with our present state of knowledge. EMGs are also useful to test existent muscle power of individual muscles in such cases as infants with myelomeningoceles, for whom the usual clinical testing of muscle power is limited or technically difficult. The presence or absence of EMG evidence of denervation has some prognostic value in peripheral neuropathies such as Bell's palsy.

Electromyographic units involve the use of concentric needle-electrodes from which the changes in electrical potential associated with activity of the muscles are recorded, amplified and displayed by an electron beam moving across the screen of the cathode-ray oscilloscope. Usually the same amplified input is also fed into a loudspeaker, producing the noise pattern of normal muscle action or the pips of fibrillation, which the experienced examiner can identify by ear just as accurately as he can visually identify the potentials on the screen, but this is not essential unless permanent records are required.

A detailed discussion of EMG abnormality is beyond the scope of this book, but the physician should be familiar with the basic principles.

(1) *Insertion potentials*. Normally a small amount of electrical activity is produced when the needle is inserted. This is increased in hyperirritable muscles, as in polymyositis for example, and is prolonged in cases of myotonia congenita and myotonic dystrophy.

(2) *Movement potentials*. Moving the needle about has a similar effect to its original insertion.

(3) *Activity at rest.* Normal resting muscle is silent. The most characteristic finding in denervation, whether from a peripheral neuropathy or from disease of the anterior-horn cells, is fibrillation, which represents the spontaneous contraction of individual denervated muscle-fibers. Fibrillations are lightning-quick and of small amplitude (50-100 μV). Fasciculations represent the discharge of a motor unit (all the muscle fibers innervated by a single lower motor neuron), and have amplitudes (100-500 μV) comparable to the normal trains of action potentials seen in slight voluntary effort in normal muscle. They can occur from irritation of a nerve root or, in childhood, more frequently from active irritative disease of the anterior horn-cell or bulbar motor-neuron. Fasciculations are of much greater amplitude than fibrillations.

(4) *Slight voluntary activity.* In normal muscle a slight, suitably graded, sustained voluntary contraction results in a train of action potentials occurring more or less regularly. These are similar to fasciculations in amplitude and in their appearance on the oscilloscope screen, except that they occur in a regular series and only on voluntary effort, rather than irregularly at rest. Giant action potentials, as high as 1000 to 3000 μV, may be seen in Werdnig-Hoffmann progressive spinal muscular atrophy; potentials of this magnitude are abnormal and suggest a disease of the anterior horn-cells rather than of peripheral nerves. In muscular dystrophy and other myopathies the action potentials are smaller and are splintered or polyphasic.

(5) *Maximal voluntary contraction.* In normal muscle, maximal contraction results in an 'interference pattern' of continuous activity of rather uniform amplitude. This is less strong, less well-developed and of irregular amplitude in myopathies, whereas in neuropathies it is more uniform but of lower than normal amplitude. Electrical activity ceases promptly on relaxation of normal muscle, but relaxation is delayed in myotonia congenita and myotonic dystrophy: this is easily seen on the oscilloscope screen.

As has been mentioned, electromyography is of limited use in suprasegmental disease, except to differentiate it from disease of the lower motor unit. In spasticity there may be normal-appearing action potentials in a muscle supposedly at rest; attempted activity or passive movement produce increased activity. The stretch reflex is easily displayed in this manner. Very similar increased electrical activity is seen with dystonia, chorea, athetosis and other types of adventitious movements, which differ only in the fluctuation of the interference pattern, in its timing, and in the activation of antagonist as well as agonist muscles in dystonia.

ELECTRONYSTAGMOGRAPHY

The electronystagmogram (ENG) measures the rate and amplitude of eye movements. It is based on the existence of an electrical potential between the cornea and retina. Eye movements interrupt this electrical field, and recording equipment can detect these through electrodes placed near the eyes. Alterations in eye movements, with or without the eyelids closed, can be recorded during changes in rotation of the head, caloric testing or other events.

213

The test gives objective evidence of patterns which have been recognized clinically. For example, the nystagmus associated with patients who experienced vertigo of organic etiology can be distinguished from that of 'dizziness' (the feeling of weakness or faintness), which is subjective. The patterns associated with ocular albinism, congenital nystagmus, search nystagmus and eye diseases can be distinguished from each other and from physiological nystagmus—for example, that associated with end-point gaze (more than 90° to either side). Nystagmus of central origin lasts longer than labyrinthine nystagmus and may be enhanced rather than inhibited by visual fixation. (The use of strong convex—20° diopter—glasses eliminates visual fixation.)

ELECTROENCEPHALOGRAPHY

Description

The electroencephalogram (EEG) is a record of spontaneous electrical activity in the brain during various clinical states. The record can be taken from the scalp while the subject is awake, asleep, hyperventilating, or during spontaneous or induced seizures.

It is generally recognized that there is a resting potential on the surface of a cell which can be altered by chemical change. The resulting action potential spreads to adjacent axons and synapses, so that recordings of the scalp EEG become compound harmonic waves representing various cortical and subcortical events. Responses to controlled auditory, visual and other stimuli have gained acceptance as additional clinical tests.

Principal uses

The EEG has been most useful in the recognition and classification of patients with seizure disorders. It is non-invasive and requires minimal co-operation on the part of the patient. Virtually all metabolic and disease states affect the EEG responses of the central nervous system.

Although the diagnosis of epilepsy is based primarily on clinical findings, an electroencephalogram is useful for confirmation of the diagnosis, for monitoring the response to therapy and for detecting a specific abnormality in the central nervous system. The tracing is unlikely to be normal in a true idiopathic convulsive disorder. A normal tracing accompanied by a history of recurrent seizures should make one sceptical of the history, or should indicate the need to look for a metabolic or vascular cause. Ominous multiple spike-waves of 1-2Hz suggest a serious cerebral insult, such as tuberous sclerosis, and the physician should make every effort to arrive at an exact diagnosis.

Method

Suitable recording equipment is now more sophisticated than the string galvanometer of 100 years ago, but the principle is unchanged. Placement of scalp electrodes by the so-called 10-20 system has gained wide acceptance: this technique allows the electrodes to be placed in the same relative locations from subject to subject, and more importantly, from hemisphere to hemisphere.

Electrode placement on the scalp begins with the identification of three landmarks: the *nasion* (midpoint of the naso-fontal junction); the *inion* (external occipital protruberance at the midline); and two *pre-auricular* points (cartilage of the ear in front of the external auditory canal). Using a tape-measure, measuring calipers and a marking pencil, electrodes can be placed at symmetrical points.

The amount of energy produced in any area is measured in microvolts squared and will vary according to the duration of the test, the thickness of the skull and the child's clinical state (awake, drowsy, sleeping). On a conventional clinical tracing the graph represents a compound harmonic. The dominant rhythm can be estimated by counting the number of waves per second, which is reported in Hertz units (Hz).

During sleep (without the use of an hypnotic) abnormalities may be observed which are not seen in awake recordings. Hyperventilation for two minutes is commonly used to bring out latent abnormalities in the EEG and occasionally may induce a seizure.

Needle electrodes are contra-indicated when doing EEGs on children. Although less time is required to attach them and movement artifacts are reduced, it is impossible to convince a child that multiple needles do not hurt. If the first EEG has been a frightening experience, it becomes very difficult to get satisfactory follow-up tracings.

Results

The data from the EEG recording system are interpreted by visual inspection of the graph (Fig. 66). In the newborn period the EEG tracing looks rather flat. The EEG of a young child usually shows random 3-7Hz waves and some low-voltage fast activity. The basic rhythm becomes more regular as the child matures (Tables XXVIII and XXIX), and by six years of age the pattern is made up mostly of 5-7Hz waves. By 10 years alpha waves (8-12Hz) predominate. During adolescence some slow-wave activity (6-8Hz) is not uncommon and may be interpreted incorrectly if adult standards are used. A normal adult's EEG would be expected to show alpha waves and, less commonly, a beta rhythm with a frequency of 13-50Hz and lower voltage.

Because the recognition of patterns affected by age, state of consciousness and various physiological and pathological states is becoming increasingly sophisticated, detailed analysis of EEGs by computer technology will become more common.

Limitations

The clinical EEG is of limited use in young children who are unco-operative or whose clinical condition makes recording difficult. By its nature, the EEG tracing is a reflection of various processes, so that changes in it may not be of primary clinical interest. For example, the clinician may be interested in detecting evidence of a seizure disorder but the effect of medication may obscure the typical pattern seen in that disorder by producing faster waves than normal.

There is considerable variation among clinicians in interpreting EEG records. This is of particular significance in the interpretation of borderline-normal records,

TABLE XXVIII
Development of EEG*

| | Years | | | | | |
	4	6	8	10	12	14
	%	%	%	%	%	%
Delta (1.5-4.5Hz)	25	23	20	17	15	12
Theta (4.5-7.5Hz)	37	31	26	21	16	13
Alpha (7.5-13.5Hz)	26	33	40	47	54	60
Beta (13.5-20.0Hz)	12	13	14	15	15	15

Courtesy Dr. Michael Bergelson.
*Expressed as relative power in left temporal area.

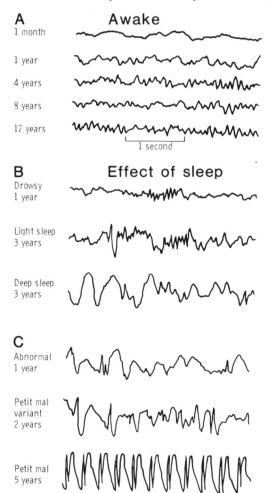

A Awake
1 month
1 year
4 years
8 years
12 years
1 second

B Effect of sleep
Drowsy 1 year
Light sleep 3 years
Deep sleep 3 years

C
Abnormal 1 year
Petit mal variant 2 years
Petit mal 5 years

Fig. 66. Electroencephalograms of infants and children. **A.** tracings from comparable areas of the scalp, illustrating variations with age of electrical activity in the motor cortex. All were obtained during a quiet phase just before sleep. **B.** The effects of sleep: variations among normal children. **C.** Abnormal waves. [From *Nelson Textbook of Pediatrics*, by permission of W. B. Saunders Co., Philadelphia.]

TABLE XXIX

Percentages of types of activity at various ages*

Age (yrs)		Delta	Theta	Alpha	Beta
4	Central	27.0	37.5	28.0	7.5
	Temporal	25.0	36.5	26.0	12.5
	Occipital	21.0	32.0	40.0	7.0
	Frontal	30.0	31.0	17.0	22.0
6	Central	25.0	35.0	31.0	9.0
	Temporal	22.5	31.0	33.0	13.5
	Occipital	18.0	27.0	47.0	8.0
	Frontal	28.0	29.0	20.0	23.0
8	Central	23.0	32.0	34.5	10.5
	Temporal	20.0	26.0	40.0	14.0
	Occipital	16.0	22.0	53.0	9.0
	Frontal	27.0	26.0	23.0	24.0
10	Central	21.0	29.5	37.5	12.0
	Temporal	17.0	21.0	47.0	15.0
	Occipital	13.0	17.5	59.0	10.5
	Frontal	25.0	23.5	26.0	25.5
12	Central	19.0	26.5	40.5	14.0
	Temporal	14.5	16.5	54.0	15.0
	Occipital	11.0	13.5	64.0	11.5
	Frontal	23.5	21.0	19.5	26.0
14	Central	17.0	24.0	43.0	16.0
	Temporal	12.0	13.0	60.0	15.0
	Occipital	9.0	10.0	68.0	13.0
	Frontal	21.0	19.0	33.0	27.0
16	Central	15.0	21.0	46.0	18.0
	Temporal	10.0	10.0	64.5	15.5
	Occipital	7.0	8.0	71.0	14.0
	Frontal	20.0	16.5	36.0	27.5

Courtesy Dr. Michael Bergelson.

*Percentage of microvoltage from each area represented by age and location. This example of frequency analysis is included to show that recording and analysis of EEGs by computerized systems can be applied to children of various ages.

when the inexperienced electroencephalographer, unfamiliar with the normal variations caused by clinical states of sleep or hyperventilation, poor technical quality of the tracing and factors of age, may conclude erroneously that a convulsive disorder exists.

The physician also should remember that many people have considerably abnormal EEGs without ever having had seizures. For example, from time to time patients with spastic cerebral palsies are seen who have very frequent spike-wave discharges in their EEGs, but have never had a convulsive episode. Individuals who are entirely normal may also have EEG abnormalities. Conversely, it must be remembered that the EEG is merely a 20- or 30-minute sample of the electrical activity of the child's brain, and the inter-seizure records of children who have epilepsy may be repeatedly normal. This is particularly true in the case of temporal-lobe seizures and in idiopathic grand mal, but a higher percentage of children with all types of seizures show EEG abnormalities than do adults. Petit mal is the only type of epilepsy in which one almost always can obtain a typical EEG discharge in the resting record, or at least on hyperventilation or photic stimulation.

NERVE-CONDUCTION STUDIES

Nerve-conduction studies should be carried out on all infants and children suspected of having neuromuscular disorders. A superficial nerve such as the median, posterior tibial, ulnar or peroneal can be stimulated and the conduction velocity determined from the evoked motor response. Slow conduction-times are found in various neuropathies. Normal conduction velocity in adults is 50-70m/sec: in new born infants it is much slower, but by the age of three years it has reached adult standards. Most neuropathies are more severe distally, so reduced conduction velocity is readily measured. If the involvement is chiefly proximal, as in Guillain-Barré syndrome, there may be little or no reduction of peripheral conduction speed. Most neuropathies of childhood are mixed in nature, although certain toxins—such as lead—produce a pure motor neuropathy, and a few rare sensory neuropathies exist.

EVOKED POTENTIALS

Description

Information regarding the processing of sensory information is gained from evoked potential measures, also known as evoked responses. These are the averaged electrical activity of the brain in response to the presentation of specific stimulation— *e.g.* a blank light-flash, a visual pattern or a click. The early portion of this evoked potential wave-shape reflects the sensory content of the stimulus, while the later portion reflects the interpretation of the stimulus. Information about the co-ordination of the two halves of the brain with respect to evoked potentials is also very important, and is reported in terms of amplitude and wave-shape asymmetry.

Principal uses

Measurement of evoked potentials establishes the ingregrity of receptor sites and the peripheral nerves which serve them. Evoked responses to visual and auditory stimuli may help in the diagnosis of visual impairment or hearing loss in an infant or child who is otherwise untestable. Possible indications for somatosensory evoked potentials include subacute combined degeneration of the cord, vascular cord lesions and polyradiculoneuropathy.

Method

A dependable source of intermittent stimulation (visual, auditory or tactile) is selected. Recording electrodes are placed in convenient, previously selected positions. In most instances the ratio of the response of the stimulus to the noise in the background pattern is usually such that the individual stimulus alone cannot be identified. By using the external stimulus as time 0 and by cueing the responses through the use of the computer of average transients, the random waves of the background noise become flat. The signal artifact, which is brief (2msec, for example) and the responses which follow it can be identified and stored temporarily on a cathode-ray oscilloscope. Later these can be photographed or transcribed onto an XY plotter.

Because units consisting of more than one cell and nerve are involved in clinical practice, multiple stimuli are needed and the average response is used. The number of stimuli may vary from 50 to 3000, depending on the nature of the procedure.

Visual evoked responses can be recorded from the scalp in the occipital areas up to 600msec after the stimuli. A checker-board pattern, the light and dark areas of which are suddenly reversed, is often helpful because changes are produced without changing the total luminance of the pattern.

Somatosensory responses can be recorded after percutaneous electrical stimulation of large afferent fibers at the fingers, wrists, toes, ankles and knees. This is done by administering a signal by a square-wave generator (0.2msec waves at 5 per second with a current of 5 to 15mA). In order to minimize the differences in the measurement of latency, convenient points of reference are used: for example, Erb's point in the shoulder area may be used for recording impulses in the medial nerve, and a lower area lateral to the spine for stimulation of the peroneal nerve.

Results

The responses for each kind of stimulus (visual, auditory and tactile) are recorded separately. These are compared with those of other 'normal' individuals obtained with identical equipment and in similar circumstances. The responses to various stimuli can be classified, according to their latent periods, as short (less than 30msec), medium (30-75msec) and long (75msec and above). The longer the response the more likely it becomes that other factors, including attention span and fatigue, will alter the pattern.

Cortical responses to visual stimuli usually are symmetrical in the posterior hemispheres of normal subjects. Alterations of visual evoked responses after a pattern shift are to be expected and are often a valuable way of measuring function.

Brain-stem auditory evoked responses (recorded from the mastoid or temporal areas) are relatively unaffected by sleep, coma, or even large amounts of barbiturates. These responses are seen 1 to 8msec after the stimuli. This is a useful investigation when a hearing loss is suspected, but there is difficulty with conventional tests of hearing.

Somatosensory evoked responses measure conduction velocity of the largest-diameter nerve fibers. Adequate testing will demonstrate the integrity of these fibers. Electrical stimulation strong enough to produce activity in small-diameter fibers is too painful for clinical use. Abnormal results of somatosensory evoked potentials have been reported in association with many disorders in adults, but technical difficulties and the lack of consistent normal values have limited the use of this test in infants and children.

Further reading

John, E. R. (1974) 'Assessment of acuity, color vision and shape perception by statistical evaluation of evoked potentials.' *Annals of Ophthalmology,* **6,** 55-66.
Greenberg, R. P., Ducker, T. B. (1982) 'Evoked potentials in the clinical neurosciences.' *Journal of Neurosurgery,* **56,** 1-18.

MUSCLE BIOPSY

Muscle biopsy is used chiefly to investigate presumptive disease of the lower motor unit. This unit comprises the lower motor neuron, the central and dorsal roots, the peripheral nerve, the neuromyal junction and the muscle itself. Muscle biopsy and electrical studies of muscle and nerve are the principal aids to differential diagnosis of the site of disease at this level. All too frequently, muscle biopsy is a disappointing procedure and too often non-diagnostic, but this can be avoided by careful planning and proper technique. It is the responsibility of the physician in charge of the patient to select which muscle is to be biopsied, and it should be a muscle with significant weakness but not one that is so atrophic as to be almost totally replaced by fat, with little histological evidence of its original disease. A muscle rated as 3+ or 4+ on the MRC scale (see p. 73) is usually the best choice. Muscle recently studied by electromyography should not be selected for biopsy. Standards of normal are better developed for some muscles than for others, and the biopsy of quadriceps or gastrocnemius is easier to interpret than one of the glutei or a muscle less frequently sampled.

The biopsy should be performed by a competent and experienced surgeon. A sufficiently large sample of muscle must be taken and the specimen should be fixed and sent to the laboratory without delay. Interpretation must be made by an experienced pathologist or by a pediatrician or neurologist with special knowledge in this field.

Only a limited number of conditions can be differentiated by muscle biopsy. The chief distinction is between a myopathy, disease of the muscle itself and denervation, but in most cases it is not possible to determine whether denervation is the result of disease of the peripheral nerve or of the lower motor neuron itself. Certain types of

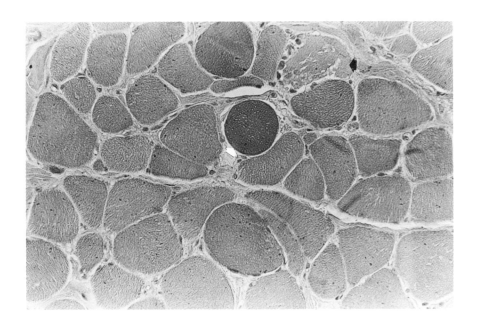

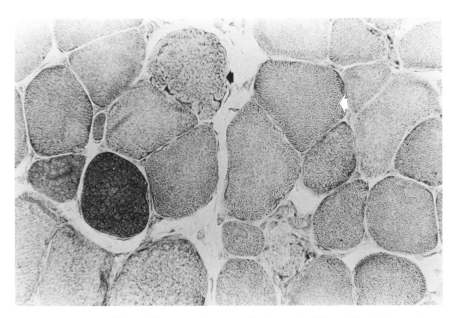

Fig. 67. Seven-year-old boy with progressive muscular dystrophy. *Upper:* Muscle biopsy shows marked variation in fiber size and increased endomysial tissue. Open arrow indicates an 'opaque' fiber and closed arrow a necrotic fiber undergoing phagocytosis. *Lower:* Most fibers have a relatively normal intermyofibrillar network pattern (open arrow) but a few have a disrupted pattern (closed arrow). [Courtesy Dr. Harold Marks, Department of Pediatric Neurology, Alfred I. duPont Institute, Wilmington, Delaware.]

myopathy also can be differentiated with some confidence, such as muscular dystrophy (less reliably between different types of this) from myositis and the various relatively benign congenital myopathies.

An example is C.R., a seven-year-old boy with a two-year history of increasingly frequent tripping and falling, and increasing difficulty in climbing stairs. On neurological examination he was found to have diffuse weakness, more proximal than distal; hyporeflexia; hyperlordosis; and marked calf hypertrophy. The results of enzyme assays were: CPK 21,700 Iu/1, LDH 1540 Iu/1 and SGOT 820 Iu/1. Marked abnormalities associated with myopathy were evident in the EMG. The results of the muscle biopsy were also characteristic of progressive muscular dystrophy (Figs. 67a, b). In this instance the electrocardiogram was normal.

NEUROMETRIC EVALUATION

Detailed analysis of the electroencephalogram and of evoked sensory responses following auditory and visual stimuli can now be done by a neurometric examination, a recently developed technique which uses computer technology to obtain qualitative electrophysiological data which can be analyzed statistically with reference to a normal data-base. At present the technique is still in the process of changing from a research project to a clinical tool which will yield quantitative data in the study of neurophysiology.

Principal uses

Neurometric evaluation may be particularly sensitive to cognitive dysfunction and early signs of neuropathology, and it is said to provide a subtle, objective and quantitative assessment of various aspects of brain function, supplementing conventional neurological and psychometric procedures. It is especially useful in obtaining data from individuals who are difficult to test, such as hyperactive children, since test conditions require minimal co-operation on the part of the subject.

Neurometric evaluation provides a valuable quantitative method of extending the study of children with convulsive disorders. It may provide evidence for a specific organic cause of seizures in a particular area of the brain. A possible clinical application is in the study of learning disabilities: it may help to determine whether a child's inability to learn is caused by faulty processing, or is related to emotional problems or difficulties in the environment.

Method

The full international 10-20 EEG system (19 electrodes) is recorded simultaneously (bipolar derivations are constructed by computer). While the channel is made, the computer automatically monitors every channel for eyeblink and movement artifacts. After resting measurements have been recorded, standardized visual and auditory stimuli are presented. The information is stored on a computer disc, which is then sent to an appropriate facility for computer analysis. That analysis provides the following quantitative measurements:

222

(1) spectral analysis of the spontaneous EEG, evaluated in relation to normative data describing the expected composition of the EEG spectrum as a function of age in normally developing individuals;

(2) symmetry of wave-shape and amplitude of the EEG between bilaterally symmetrical scalp locations;

(3) amplitude and variability of brain responses evoked by visual and auditory stimuli;

(4) symmetry of amplitude and wave-shape of the evoked responses;

(5) wave-shape (morphology) of evoked responses in comparison with wave-shapes observed in normally functioning individuals;

(6) changes in evoked response morphology with changes in stimulus characteristics, reflecting sensory acuity and perceptual reactivity.

The information in Figures 68-70 can also be shown topographically as a z-score, so that a comparison of an individual with others of similar age can be represented visually as being normal or 1, 2 or more than 3 standard deviations from the norm for that age. it is also possible to represent an 'expected pattern' for a particular age or disorder. It is possible to make a variety of representations of the data after they have been recorded in a form suitable for analysis by computer programming.

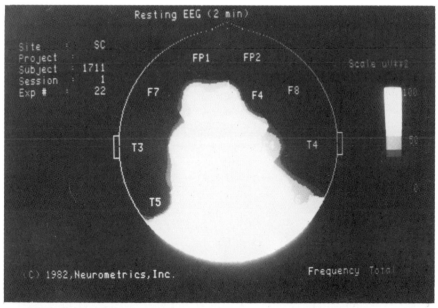

Fig. 68. EEG topography: distribution of 'total energy' recorded during 120 seconds of a resting EEG. This 14-year-old boy has a clinical history of significant learning disorder, normal intelligence as measured by conventional methods, and psychomotor seizures. The data in this photograph, displayed on a video monitor in color, represent information from more than 12 pages of traditional EEGs (artifacts have been removed). Density (black to white) is related to 'microvolts squared' and is a way of showing the amplitude on the conventional EEG. The amount of energy recorded in each area is represented on the tomographic map.

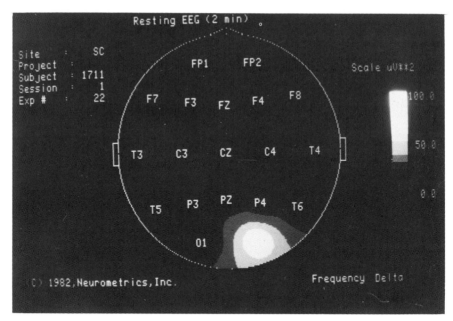

Fig. 69. EEG topography: distribution of 'total delta' energy during the same 120 seconds of artifact-free resting EEG as in Figure 68.

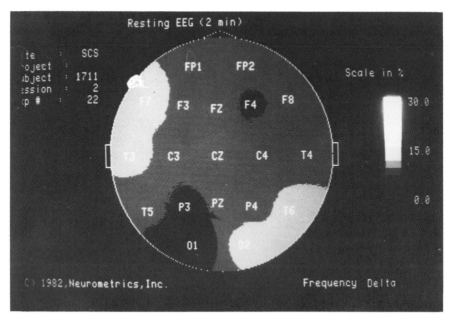

Fig. 70. EEG topography: distribution of 'relative energy', percentage of 'delta energy'/'total energy' during the same 120 seconds as in Figures 68 and 69. These are the same data as in Figure 69, displayed in a different way. Normal subjects tend to have symmetrical patterns of distribution. [Figures 68-70 by courtesy of Dr. Michael Bergelson, Neurometrics, Inc., New York.]

224

Results
A complete neurometric report consists of a numerical analysis and a computer-generated report.

Numerical analysis

    EEG: (1) actual values for relative power and symmetry of amplitude and wave-shape;

           (2) normalized spectral and symmetry values, referenced to an age matched healthy population (z-transformed).

    ER: (1) signal to noise ratio of average evoked responses;

           (2) symmetry values of evoked responses;

           (3) evaluation of morphology of average evoked response wave-shape;

           (4) reactivity differences in ER measures between different stimulus conditions.

    Summary table of severity of deviation from normal values for quantitative EEG and ER features.

Clinic report

    The computer generates a report consisting of:

           (1) head diagram for every EEG and ER feature, which presents density coding of the probability that the value observed might exist in the normal population;

           (2) summary test describing major findings;

           (3) implications for functional impairment, based on neurometric findings, and referrals for further testing when indicated.

Limitations
A neurometric evaluation *does not* replace a neurological examination or a conventional EEG for the diagnosis of neurological diseases such as epilepsy. Although 'maps' of the kind shown in Figures 68-70 may be helpful in quickly orienting interesting professionals, they have not yet proven to be superior to conventional EEGs interpreted by skilled electroencephalographers. Neither does this method of evaluation recommend specific methods of remediation. However, such an evaluation can aid qualified professionals in the development of prescriptive remedial procedures.

At present neurometric evaluation is still primarily a research tool, so facilities for performing it are limited in distribution.

Further reading
Ahn, H., Prichep, L., John, E. R., Baird, H., Trepetin, M., Kaye, H. (1981) 'Developmental equations reflect brain dysfunctions.' *Science.* **210**, 1259-1262.

Baird, H. W., John, E. R., Ahn, H., Maisel, E. (1980) 'Neurometric evaluation of epileptic children who do well and poorly in school.' *Electroencephalography and Clinical Neurophysiology.* **48**, 683-693.

John, E. R., Ahn, H., Prichep, L., Trepetin, M., Brown, D., Kaye, H. (1981) 'Developmental equations for the electroencephalogram.' *Science.* **210**, 1255-1258.

'TENSILON' TEST

This test is used in the diagnosis of myasthenia gravis. A positive diagnosis is made by watching the effect of the intravenous administration of edrophonium chloride ('Tensilon'), an anticholinesterase drug. The drug should be given carefully after reading the directions. The initial dose is 1mg (1ml), followed a minute later by 4mg (4ml) if there is no response and if there are no side-effects. Possible side-effects include lacrimation, sweating, salivation, abdominal cramps, nausea, vomiting and diarrhea. Atropine sulfate should be available in case of excessive parasympathetic stimulation. A positive response, indicated by disappearance of the ptosis and diminution of ocular weakness, occurs within 30 to 60 seconds.

In older children, other conditions besides myasthenia gravis may have myasthenic symptoms which respond to 'Tensilon'. Among these are pontine tumors, leukemia, botulism, neuroblastoma, dermatomyositis, polymyositis, muscular weakness caused by a dystrophic process, and peripheral nerve disease.

APPENDIX A

Neurological evaluation

Name: **Examiner:**   **Date:**

Head circumference: **Chest circumference:**

Length or height: **Weight:**   **BP**   **P**   **R**

Indirect examination: (activity, mobility, co-ordination, physical and apparent mental development in relation to age, communication, response to sound, co-operation, attention span, personality, family resemblance)

General Inspection: (obvious congenital anomalies, body proportions indicative of specific syndrome, body symmetry, skin texture, pigmentation, sexual development, abnormal movements, tremors, tics)

General examination: *Head:* (shape, position, sutures, fontanelle, bruit, transillumination)

Hair: (color, texture, distribution)

Eyes: (lids, sclerae, conjunctivae, pupils, iris, interpupillary distance)

Ears: (shape, position, canals, tympanic membranes, Rinne test, Weber test)

Nose, oral cavity and pharynx swallowing: (tongue, tongue movements, palate, dental development and hygiene)

Neck: (range of motion, thyroid)

Chest (shape)   *Heart:*   *Lungs:*

Abdomen:

Genitalia:

Spine: (structure, flexibility)

Upper extremities: (arms, hand shape, fingers, fingernails, palmar crease)

Lower extremities: (legs, calf development, ankle range of motion, shape of feet)

227

Tests of neurological function:
Cranial nerves:

I smell

II visual acuity
    visual fields
    binocular vision
    pick up thread
    Snellen

III, IV, VI pupils (size and equality)

	R	L
Reaction to light (direct)		
(consensual)		
Reaction to accommodation (direct)		
(consensual)		

Eye movements:

V corneal reflex   jaw jerk

VII facial symmetry: upper   lower   smile

      facial movements   taste

VIII auditory:
  high pitch
  low pitch

Vestibular

IX, X palatal arch   palate elevation   voice quality

      gag reflex

XI sternocleidomastoid strength   shoulder elevation

XII tongue protrusion   atrophy

Funduscopic examination:

	R	L
cornea		
lens		
vessels		
retina		
discs		

Head and back control:

Muscle size, tone, strength, range of motion:

	R	L
upper extremities		
lower extremities		

Deep tendon reflexes

	R	L
Biceps		
Triceps		
Quadriceps		
Achilles tendon		

Clonus: R   L

Plantar response: R   L

Superficial reflexes: R
  abdominal   cremasteric   anocutaneous

Infant automatisms:
  Moro   neck-righting   tonic neck reflex
  grasp   placing   stepping
  parachute   ventral suspension

Fine motor co-ordination:

Gross motor co-ordination:

Tests of minor neurological dysfunction and balance:
  Finger-to-nose   finger-to-finger
  rapid pronation-supination
  heel-to-knee
  Romberg: balance 1 foot eyes open   R   L
                    balance 1 foot eyes closed R   L
  hop   R   L
  walk straight line

Stereognosis:

Graphesthesia:

Laterality   R   L
  sight
  throw
  write
  kick

Gait

Sensory testing:

Communication skills: (speech and language—clarity and content)

Developmental screening

APPENDIX B

Denver Developmental Screening Test

The directions for administration and interpretation of the Denver Developmental Screening Test (DDST) are included in the test kit* and are clear and concise. The test is designed to be used in clinical practice, to ascertain whether an infant's or child's development is within normal limits at the time of examination. It is not an intelligence test. Questionable results demand re-examination, and abnormal findings indicate the need for further investigation.

Infants and children are tested for gross motor, fine motor, adaptive, language and personal-social development by groups of carefully selected items. The standards used for passing and failing a test item are explicit and are set out in detail in the manual.

In interpreting the test results, delay is defined as failure to pass an item which is passed by 90 per cent of children of the same age. Performance is abnormal if (a) two or more sectors have two or more delays, or (b) if one sector has two or more delays and one other sector has one delay and no 'passed' item intersected by the age-line. If one sector shows a delay but the age-line intersects a 'passed' item, the test is considered normal.

Caution

The infants and children included in the original report lived in one area of the United States. Other papers on further standardization of the DDST in many other countries and cultures have been published (e.g. Bryant et al. 1973, Ueda 1978). Many of these attempts to define items of the DDST across cultural and language barriers also have made important contributions to developmental medicine. Some studies have included more children and more statistical information than were in the original report.

A strong feature of the test is that it need not be administered exclusively by physicians or psychologists. The directions are clear, so that usually merely 'yes' or 'no' is required for each item. By definition, the DDST is a screening or identification test, so it will allow a small number of infants or children to pass or fail who would have been identified more clearly by more sophisticated tests (e.g. Gesell or Bayley).

*See p. 4 for supplier's address.

APPENDIX C

Genetic history

General comments

A pedigree is a graphic record in symbolic shorthand of a family's medical history. If the pedigree is drawn up to follow the inheritance of a particular disease (suspected or known) or trait, it can help the physician to confirm the diagnosis, ascertain the pattern of inheritance and provide the basis for genetic counseling of the family.

Many families become tense when being questioned about hereditary diseases and conditions, so the examiner should be tactful and the purpose of the questions should be explained. Questions should be asked about one family member at a time, in order to keep the focus of the pedigree on individuals rather than on the whole family unit. Information should be sought about every member of the family, including first, last and married names, dates of birth and death, cause of death, all pregnancies, stillbirths, miscarriages, elective abortions, premature births and deaths in infancy. Physical signs and symptoms which have a similarity to or bearing on the condition being studied should be enquired about.

Procedure

Figure C1 gives the commonly accepted symbols used in setting down a pedigree.

Begin with the generation of the propositus (proband or index case). The propositus is indicated by an arrow, the siblings are enumerated in birth order and, if known, their actual ages and birth-dates are indicated (Fig. C2). The parents are described next and they are represented above their offspring on the chart (Fig. C3) joined by a single marital bar if they are unrelated and by double lines if there is consanguinity. Then aunts and uncles are considered, taking the father's siblings first (Fig. C4). If they are numerous, it is allowable merely to give the numbers of normal or affected siblings of each sex. The offspring of these are documented, but normal offspring need not be detailed unless a complete genetic analysis is to be undertaken. The next step is to obtain as much information as possible about the grandparents. The complete pedigree can then be depicted graphically, as in Figure C5*.

Modes of inheritance

Sex-linked

The pedigree depicted in Figures C1-5 shows inheritance of an x-linked recessive trait, such as Duchenne muscular dystrophy. Traits due to mutant genes on the x chromosome can be either dominant or recessive. The essential feature of inheritance of these so-called x-linked conditions is that males cannot pass on the condition to their sons because the single x chromosome of the male is inherited only by daughters. Females having two x chromosomes may be heterozygous or homozygous

*This pedigree is simplified for clarity: a complete pedigree would include other information, such as names, dates of birth and death, causes of death, etc.

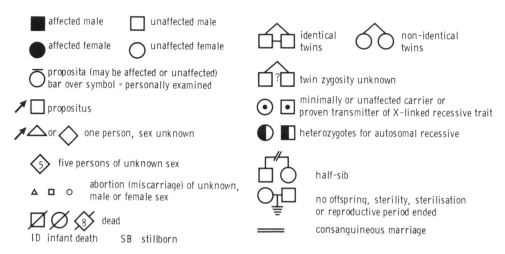

Fig. C1. Symbols used for compiling pedigree.

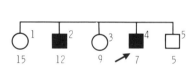

Fig. C2. The propositus is the fourth child of five. An older brother also is affected; two older sisters and a younger brother are not.

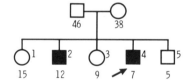

Fig. C3. The parents are alive, are not related and show no sign of the trait being investigated.

for the gene, and clinical effects depend on this and on whether the gene is dominant or recessive. The male, however, can only be hemizygous for X-borne genes and will always have the gene expressed.

The majority of X-borne diseases are inherited as recessives and are transmitted by normal carrier females to affected males. Dominant inheritance of X-borne genes is not so easily demarcated from autosomal dominant transmission, because both males and females are affected and the condition appears in each generation. The crucial distinction between X-borne dominant and autosomal dominant inheritance is that in the former an affected male transmits the gene to all his daughters but to none of his sons, whereas in the latter, affected males and females transmit the gene equally to half their offspring, irrespective of sex.

Autosomal dominant

When the clinical characteristics of a condition are found in individuals possessing the responsible gene on only one of a pair of autosomes, the pattern of inheritance is said to be dominant. The condition will be inherited from generation to generation, as one affected parent will pass on the gene to approximately half the offspring. The defective gene is carried on one chromosome of the pair and there is an

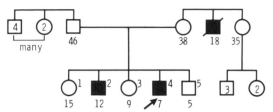

Fig. C4. The pedigree now shows that the father has four normal brothers and two normal sisters, who have had many normal children. On the other hand, the mother had an affected brother who died at 18 years and she has a surviving sister with five normal children (three male, two female).

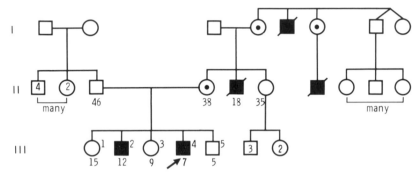

Fig. C5. The mother of child III 4 can now be diagnosed presumptively as the heterozygous carrier of a sex-linked trait and has been given the conventional symbol for heterozygosity (see Fig. C1). Inspection of generation I shows additional evidence of sex-linked transmission, and two females can be assigned as probable heterozygotes. [Figs. C1 to C5 redrawn from Paine and Oppé 1966.]

even chance of the child receiving the chromosome bearing the abnormal gene, so in a sufficiently large pedigree about equal numbers of affected and unaffected siblings should occur.

Except in the case of new mutations, affected individuals will be found to have an affected parent; *i.e.* unaffected parents should not have affected children. However, it is characteristic of many dominantly inherited conditions that the gene effect (hence the severity of the clinical state) varies considerably. If there is only minimal clinical evidence of the condition the gene is said to be weakly expressed. Variations in expression may be the result of interaction of other modifying genes or of environmental influences.

Dominant autosomal inheritance is not affected by sex and a pedigree shows equal numbers of males and females affected. However, in several conditions the gene seems to be modified by sex in the intensity of its expression. Sometimes an individual shows no evidence of the trait who, on genetic grounds, must possess the abnormal gene (*e.g.* an apparently normal parent of affected children). In such a case the gene is said to be non-penetrant. However, while non-penetrance may exist, it is probable that often the true reason is inability to detect minor effects of the gene.

Conditions in which there is dominant inheritance tend to be of minor clinical

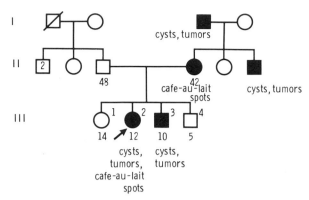

Fig. C6. Simplified pedigree for a child with neurofibromatosis, manifested by *café-au-lait* spots, cysts and tumors.

importance, for they would disappear if they were severe enough to regularly cause death during childhood or to prevent reproduction. However, there are a few exceptions in which disabling conditions can appear in offspring before the parent is affected clinically, and there are also a few diseases which are severe but do not prevent reproduction. Examples from neurology are Huntington's chorea, Charcot-Marie-Tooth disease, myotonic dystrophy and neurofibromatosis (Fig. C6).

Autosomal recessive

A recessively inherited condition only becomes clinically apparent in individuals homozygous for the causative gene: therefore they must inherit the gene from both parents. The parents themselves may be heterozygous (carriers) or homozygous (affected), but it is unusual to find either parent homozygous, so most affected offspring have clinically normal parents. Given two heterozygous parents, the expected distribution of offspring, irrespective of sex, is one half normal but heterozygous (carriers), one quarter normal (homozygous normal) and one quarter affected (homozygous affected) (Fig. C7).

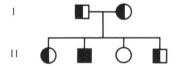

Fig. C7. Expected distribution of children of two heterozygous parents.

The chances of an offspring being affected are one in four for each birth, but is only in large sibships that the expected distribution actually appears. Parents who are clinically normal but carriers of a recessive gene may have several unaffected children, so the presence of the gene is never suspected. Other less fortunate parents may have an affected first child and limit their family because of this. Ascertainment of recessive inheritance by analysis of pedigree therefore is a complicated matter,

234

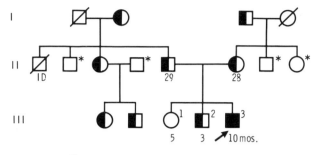

* tested non-carrier

Fig. C8. Simplified pedigree for Tay-Sachs disease.

because only families with affected children will be included, and many of those families will have a disproportionate number of affected children.

There are two ways of detecting autosomal recessive inheritance. If the recessive gene is a rare one, it will be found with much greater frequency among related individuals than in the general population. The likelihood of a child having both parents heterozygous for the gene is much increased if the parents themselves are related, so consanguineous matings are a feature of the rarer recessive genes.

In the case of some of the more common disorders due to recessive genes, such as Tay-Sachs disease, parental consanguinity is less helpful but the heterozygous state can be detected directly by appropriate tests. In Tay-Sachs disease the carrier state can be identified by finding reduced hexosaminidase A activity in blood and tissue samples. These special tests for demonstrating the effects of recessive genes in apparently normal individuals show clearly that dominance and recessiveness are terms of clinical usefulness rather than expressions of biological laws. However, the terms are still valid for genetic prognosis.

REFERENCES

Aase, J. M. (1980) 'Microtia: clinical observations.' *Birth Defects, Original Article Series,* **16,** (4). 283-297; 303-331.

Abe, K., Oda, N. (1980) 'Incidence of tics in the offspring of childhood tiqueurs: a controlled follow-up study.' *Developmental Medicine and Child Neurology,* **22,** 649-653.

Acheson, R. M., Jefferson, E. (1954) 'Some observations on the closure of the anterior fontanelle.' *Archives of Disease in Childhood,* **29,** 196-198.

Altrocchi, P. H., Menkes, J. H. (1960) 'Congenital ocular motor apraxia.' *Brain,* **83,** 576-588.

André-Thomas, Autgaerden, S. (1966) *Locomotion from Pre- to Postnatal Life. Clinics in Developmental Medicine, No. 24.* London: S.I.M.P. with Heinemann Medical.

Baird, H. W., Borofsky, L. G. (1957) 'Infantile myoclonic seizures.' *Journal of Pediatrics,* **50,** 332-339.

Bakwin, H., Bakwin, R. M. (1972) *Behavior Disorders in Children, 4th edn.* Philadelphia: W. B. Saunders.

Baum, J. D., Searls, D. (1971) 'Head shape and size of preterm low birthweight infants.' *Developmental Medicine and Child Neurology,* **13,** 572-575.

Bax, M. C. O. (1972) 'The active or overactive school child.' *Developmental Medicine and Child Neurology,* **14,** 83-86.

—— (1978) 'Who is hyperactive?' *Developmental Medicine and Child Neurology,* **20,** 277-278.

Berenberg, W. (1977) 'Gait analysis in cerebral palsy—an added technique.' *Developmental Medicine and Child Neurology,* **19,** 832.

Bergès, J., Lézine, I. (1965) *The Imitation of Gestures. Clinics in Developmental Medicine, No. 18.* London: S.I.M.P with Heinemann Medical.

Bergsma, D. (Ed.) (1979) *Birth Defects Atlas and Compendium, 2nd edn.* New York: Alan R. Liss for the National Foundation March of Dimes.

Brain, R., Wilkinson, M. (1959) 'Observations on the extensor plantar reflex and its relationship to the functions of the pyramidal tract.' *Brain,* **82,** 297-320.

Brown, J. K. (1977) 'Migraine and migraine equivalents in children.' *Developmental Medicine and Child Neurology,* **19,** 683-692.

Bryant, G.M., Davies, K. J., Richards, F.M., Voorhees, S. (1973) 'A preliminary study of the use of the Denver Developmental Screening Test in a health department.' *Developmental Medicine and Child Neurology,* **15,** 33-40.

Chalfant, J. C., Scheffelin, M. A. (1969) *Central Processing Dysfunctions in Children: A Review of Research.* Bethesda: U.S.D.H.E.W., National Institutes of Health.

Cogan, D. G., Adams, R. D. (1953) 'A type of paralysis of conjugate gaze (ocular motor apraxia).' *Archives of Ophthalmology,* **50,** 434-442.

Cone, T. E., Khoshbin, S. (1978) 'Botticelli demonstrates the Babinski reflex more than 400 years before Babinski.' *American Journal of Diseases of Children,* **132,** 188.

Congdon, P. J., Forsythe, W. I. (1979) 'Migraine in childhood: a study of 300 children.' *Developmental Medicine and Child Neurology,* **21,** 209-216.

Conners, C. K. (1969) 'A teacher rating scale for use in drug studies with children.' *American Journal of Psychiatry,* **126,** 884-888.

Crothers, B., Paine, R. S. (1959) *The Natural History of Cerebral Palsy.* Cambridge, Mass.: Harvard University Press.

DeJong, R. N. (1958) *The Neurologic Examination, 2nd edn.* New York: Hoeber.

Drillien, C. M., Drummond, M. B. (Eds.) (1977) *Neurodevelopmental Problems in Early Childhood.* Oxford: Blackwell.

Dubowitz, V. (1980) *The Floppy Infant, 2nd edn. Clinics in Developmental Medicine, No. 76.* London: S.I.M.P. with Heinemann Medical; Philadelphia; Lippincott.

Dunn, H. G., Daube, J. R., Gomez, M. D. (1978) 'Heredofamilial brachial plexus neuropathy (hereditary neuralgic amyotrophy with brachial predilection) in childhood.' *Developmental Medicine and Child Neurology,* **20,** 28-46.

Dyken, P., Kolár, O. (1968) 'Dancing eyes, dancing feet: infantile polymyoclonia.' *Brain,* **91,** 305-320.

Fenichel, G. M. (1982) 'Neurological complications of immunization.' *Annals of Neurology.* **12,** 119-128.

Fishman, R. A. (1980) *Cerebrospinal Fluid in Diseases of the Central Nervous System.* Philadelphia: W. B. Saunders.

Frankenburg, W. K., Dodds, J. B. (1967) 'The Denver Developmental Screening Test.' *Journal of Pediatrics,* **71,** 181-191.

—— Goldstein, A. D., Camp, B. W. (1971) 'The Revised Denver Developmental Screening Test.' *Journal of Pediatrics,* **79,** 988-995.

Fridman, J., John, E. R., Bergelson, M., Kaiser, J. B., Baird, H. W. (1982) 'Application of digital filtering and automatic peak detection to brain stem auditory evoked potential.' *Electroencephalography and Clinical Neurophysiology,* **53,** 405-416.

Gastaut, H. (1969) 'Classification of the epilepsies. Proposal for an international classification.' *Epilepsia,* **10,** (Suppl.) S14-S21.

Goodenough, P. L. (1926) *Measurement of Intelligence by Drawing.* New York: World Books.

Goodman, R. M., Gorlin, R. J. (1977) *Atlas of the Face in Genetic Disorders.* St. Louis: C. V. Mosby.

Greenberg, R. P., Ducker, T. B. (1982) 'Evoked potentials in the clinical neurosciences.' *Journal of Neurosurgery.* **56,** 1-18.

Hardie, J. de Z., Macfarlane, A. (1980) 'Late-walking children: a review of 160 late walkers in the Oxford area.' *Health Visitor,* **53,** 466-468.

Hart, H., Bax, M., Jenkins, S. (1978) 'The value of a developmental history.' *Developmental Medicine and Child Neurology,* **20,** 442-452.

Hoffmann, J. (1893) 'Über chronische spinale Muskelatrophie in Kindesalter auf familiarer Basis.' *Deutsche Zeitschrift für Nervenheilkunde,* **3,** 427-470.

Ingraham, F. D., Matson, D. D. (1954) *Neurosurgery of Infants and Children.* Springfield, Ill.: Charles C. Thomas.

Illingworth, R. S. (1958) 'The early diagnosis of cerebral palsy.' *Cerebral Palsy Bulletin,* **2,** 6-8.

—— (1966) *The Development of the Infant and Young Child: Normal and Abnormal, 3rd edn.* Edinburgh: E. & S. Livingstone.

—— (1977) *Basic Developmental Screening, 2nd edn.* Oxford: Blackwell.

John, E. R. (1974) 'Assessment of acuity, color vision and shape perception by statistical evaluation of evoked potentials.' *Annals of Ophthalmology,* **6,** 55-66.

—— (1977) *Functional Neuroscience. Vol. 2: Neurometrics: Clinical Applications of Electrophysiology.* Hillsdale, N.J.: Lawrence Erlbaum.

Kahn, E., Cohen, L. (1934) 'Organic drivenness: a brain-stem syndrome and an experience.' *New England Journal of Medicine,* **210,** 748-756.

Kas, C. (1966) *Paper presented to Conference on Learning Disabilities, Lawrence, Kansas, November 1966.* (Quoted in Chalfont and Scheffelin 1969.)

Knobloch, H., Pasamanick, B. (Eds.) (1974) *Gesell and Amatruda's Developmental Diagnosis, 3rd edn.* Hagerstown, Md.: Harper & Row.

Koppitz, E. M. (1964) *The Bender Gestalt Test for Young Children.* New York: Grune & Stratton.

Korobkin, R., Berg, B. O., Wilson, C. B. (1975) 'Facial myokymia in association with medulloblastoma.' *Developmental Medicine and Child Neurology,* **17,** 340-357.

Kugelberg, E., Welander, L. (1956) 'Heredofamilial juvenile muscular atrophy simulating muscular dystrophy.' *Archives of Neurology and Psychiatry,* **75,** 500-509.

Kulenkampff, M., Schwartzman, J. S., Wilson, J. (1974) 'Neurological complications of pertussis immunization.' *Archives of Disease in Childhood,* **49,** 46-49.

Lawrence, K. M. (1964) 'Megalencephaly.' *Developmental Medicine and Child Neurology,* **6,** 638-640.

Leibowitz, D., Dubowitz, V. (1981) 'Intellect and behaviour in Duchenne muscular dystrophy.' *Developmental Medicine and Child Neurology,* **23,** 577-590.

Little, W. J. (1861) 'On the influence of abnormal parturition, difficult labours, premature birth, and asphyxia neonatorum on the mental and physical condition of the child, especially in relation to deformities,' *Transactions of the Obstetrical Society of London,* **3,** 293. (*Reprinted: Cerebral Palsy Bulletin,* (1958) **1,** 5-36.)

Lorber, J., Priestley, B. L. (1981) 'Children with large heads: a practical approach to the diagnosis of 557 children with special reference to 109 children with megalencephaly.' *Developmental Medicine and Child Neurology,* **23,** 494-504.

Mayo, O., Nelson, M., Townsend, H. R. (1973) 'Three more "happy puppets".' *Developmental Medicine and Child Neurology,* **15,** 63-69.

McArtor, R., Saunders, B. (1979) 'Iatrogenic second-degree burns caused by a transilluminator.' *Pediatrics,* **63,** 422-424.

Mac Keith, R. C. (1959) 'A note on the clasp-knife phenomenon.' *Cerebral Palsy Bulletin,* **6,** 32-33.

Meadows, A., Gordon, J., Massari, D. J., Littman, P., Fergusson, J., Moss, K. (1981) 'Declines in IQ scores and cognitive dysfunctions in children with acute lymphocytic leukaemia treated with cranial irradiation.' *Lancet,* **2,** 1015-1018.

Medical Research Council (1963) *Aids to the Investigation of Peripheral Nerve Injuries. War Memorandum No. 7, 2nd Edn.* London: H.M.S.O.

Melnick, M., Myrianthopoulos, N. C. (1979) *External Ear Malformations: Epidemiology, Genetics and Natural History.* New York: Alan R. Liss.

Menkes, J. H. (1980) *Textbook of Child Neurology. 2nd edn.* Philadelphia: Lea and Febiger.
Moosa, A. (1974) 'Muscular dystrophy in childhood.' *Developmental Medicine and Child Neurology.* **16**, 97-111.
Moore, R. Y., Baumann, R. J. (1969) 'Intracranial bruits in children.' *Developmental Medicine and Child Neurology.* **11**, 650-652.
Nelson, K. B., Ellenberg, J. H. (1976) 'Predictors of epilepsy in children who have experienced febrile seizures.' *New England Journal of Medicine.* **295**, 1029-1033.
—— —— (1978) 'Epidemiology in cerebral palsy.' *Advances in Neurology.* **19**, 421-435.
Osler, W. (1889) *The Cerebral Palsies of Children—a Clinical Study from the Infirmary for Nervous Diseases. Philadelphia.* Philadelphia: P. Blakiston, Son & Co.
Otis, J. C., Root, L., Pamilla, J. R., Kroll, M. A. (1983) 'Biomechanical measurement of spastic plantarflexors.' *Developmental Medicine and Child Neurology.* **25**, 60-66.
Paine, R. S. (1957) 'Facial paralysis in children, review of the differential diagnosis and report of ten cases treated with cortisone.' *Pediatrics.* **19**, 303-316.
—— (1960) 'Neurologic examination of infants and children.' *Pediatric Clinics of North America.* **7**, 471-510.
—— Oppé, T. E. (1966) *Neurological Examination of Children. Clinics in Developmental Medicine. Nos. 20/21.* London: S.I.M.P. with Heinemann Medical.
—— Brazelton, T. B., Donovan, D. E., Drorbaugh, J. E., Hubbell, J. P., Sears, E. M. (1964) 'Evolution of postural reflexes in normal infants, and in the presence of chronic brain syndromes.' *Neurology.* **14**, 1036-1048.
Pashayan, H., Pruzansky, S., Putterman, A. (1973) 'A family with blepharo-naso-facial malformations.' *American Journal of Diseases of Children.* **125**, 389-393.
Pollack, M. A., Shprintzen, R. J., Zimmerman-Manchester, K. L. (1979) 'Velopharyngeal insufficiency: the neurological perspective. A report of 32 cases.' *Developmental Medicine and Child Neurology.* **21**, 194-201.
President's Committee on Mental Retardation (1976) *Mental Retardation: The Known and the Unknown. DHEW Publication, 76.* 21008. Washington: DHEW.
Rapin, I. (1982) *Children with Brain Dysfunction—Neurology. Cognition. Language and Behavior.* New York: Raven Press.
Richman, N., Graham, P. J. (1971) 'A behavioral screening questionnaire for use with three-year-old children.' *Journal of Child Psychology and Psychiatry.* **12**, 5-33.
Rosenbloom, L., Horton, M. E. (1971) 'The maturation of fine prehension in young children.' *Developmental Medicine and Child Neurology.* **13**, 3-8.
Rushton, A. R., Shaywitz, B. A., Duncan, C. A., Geehr, R. B., Manuelidis, E. E. (1981) 'Computed tomography in the diagnosis of Canavan's disease.' *Annals of Neurology.* **10**, 57-60.
Rutter, M., Tizard, J., Whitmore, K. (1970) *Education, Health and Behaviour.* London: Longmans.
Salmon, M. A. (1978) *Developmental Defects and Syndromes.* Aylesbury: H. M. Publishers.
Sandberg, S. T., Rutter, M. Taylor, E. (1978) 'Hyperkinetic disorder in psychiatric clinic attenders.' *Developmental Medicine and Child Neurology.* **20**, 279-299.
Shapiro, A. K., Shapiro, E. S., Braun, R. D., Sweet, R. D. (1978) *Gilles de la Tourette Syndrome.* New York: Raven Press.
Sheridan, M. D. (1976a) *Manual for the STYCAR Vision Tests, 3rd edn.* Windsor: N.F.E.R.
—— (1976b) *Manual for STYCAR Hearing Tests, 3rd edn.* Windsor: N.F.E.R.
—— (1976c) *Manual for STYCAR Language Tests.* Windsor: N.F.E.R.
Slosson, R. L. (1967) *Slosson Drawing Co-ordination Test (SDCT) for Children and Adults.* East Aurora, N.Y.: Slosson Educational Publications.
Smithells, R. (1979) 'Fetal alcohol syndrome.' *Developmental Medicine and Child Neurology.* **21**, 244-248.
Stephenson, J. B. P. (1980) 'Reflex anoxic seizures and ocular compression.' *Developmental Medicine and Child Neurology.* **22**, 380-386.
Sutherland, D. H., Olshen, R., Cooper, L., Wyatt, M., Leach, J., Mubarak, S., Schultz, P. (1981) 'The pathomechanics of gait in Duchenne muscular dystrophy.' *Developmental Medicine and Child Neurology.* **23**, 3-22.
Swaiman, K. F., Wright, F. S. (1982) *The Practice of Pediatric Neurology. 2nd edn.* St. Louis: C. V. Mosby.
Taylor, C. J., Green, S. H. (1981) 'Menkes' syndrome (trichopoliodystrophy): use of scanning electronmicroscope in diagnosis and carrier identification.' *Developmental Medicine and Child Neurology.* **23**, 361-368.
Till, K. (1968) 'Spinal dysraphism: a study of congenital malformation of the back.' *Developmental Medicine and Child Neurology.* **10**, 471-477.

238

Touwen, B. (1976) *Neurological Development in Infancy. Clinics in Developmental Medicine, No. 58.* London: S.I.M.P. with Heinemann Medical; Philadelphia: Lippincott.

—— (1979) *Examination of the Child with Minor Neurological Dysfunction, 2nd edn. Clinics in Developmental Medicine, No. 71.* London: S.I.M.P. with Heinemann Medical; Philadelphia: Lippincott.

Tyrer, J. H., Sutherland, J. M. (1961) 'The primary spinocerebellar atrophies and their associated defects, with a study of the foot deformity.' *Brain,* **84,** 289-300.

Ueda, R. (1978) 'Study of the Denver Developmental Screening Test on Tokyo children.' *Developmental Medicine and Child Neurology,* **20,** 647-656.

Weingarten, K. (1968) 'Observations on the tic problem.' *Wiener Klinische Wochenschrift,* **80,** 83-87.

Werdnig, G. (1891) 'Zwei frühinfantile hereditäre Fälle von progressiver Muskelatrophie unter dem Bilde der Dystrophie, aber auf neurotischer Grundlage.' *Archiv für Psychiatrie und Nervenkrankheiten,* **22,** 437-481.

Worster-Drought, C. (1974) Suprabulbar paresis.' *Developmental Medicine and Child Neurology,* **16,** Suppl. 30.

Yannet, H., Horton, F. (1952) 'Hypotonic cerebral palsy in mental defectives.' *Pediatrics,* **9,** 204-211.

243

245

Opsoclonus 47
Optic atrophy 51
Optic disc 49-51
  congenitally raised 50
Optic nerve, hyaline bodies *(drüsen)* 50
Optic neuritis 50-1
Organic drivenness 181
Osteogenesis imperfecta, blue sclerae 36
Oxycephaly 24

P

Palate, lesions 64
Palmomental reflex 63
Parachute reaction 145-7, 155
Paraplegia 108
Paresis, definition 108
Parietal lobe lesions 91
Parinaud syndrome 42
Parkinsonism 83, 104
  arm swinging 102
Peabody Picture Vocabulary Test 162, 176, 188
Peripheral neuropathy 100
Peroneal muscular atrophy (Charcot-Marie-
    Tooth disease) 68, 105
Pertussis vaccination, infantile myoclonic seizures
    associated 8-9
Pes cavus 67-8, 69 *(fig.)*
Phenothiazines: catatonia due to 83
  dyskinetic movements due to 71
Phenylketonuria: hair 26
  odor 17
Phenytoin (diphenylhydantoin), side effects 65,
    101, 103
Phytanic acid storage disease (Refsum syndrome)
    49 *(table)*, 100
Pierre-Robin syndrome 32, 63
Pithed fog posture, 117, 118 *(fig.)*
Placing reactions 143-5, 153, 154 *(fig.)*
Plagiocephaly (positional cranial asymmetry) 24,
    123
Platybasia 26, 66
  downbeat nystagmus 46
Plegia, definition 108
Pons, glioma 44
Porencephaly 28
Positional cranial asymetry (plagiocephaly) 24
Positron-emission tomography (PET) 200, 201
    (fig.)
Postencephalitic states 83
Posterior fossa cyst/tumour 25, 100
Posture 98
  examination 96-7
Prader-Willi syndrome 19 *(fig.)*, 124
Preschool children, developmental level checklist
    165 *(table)*
Progressive external ophthalmoplegia 48, 49
    (table)
Progressive spinal muscular atrophy *See* Werdnig-
    Hoffmann disease

Pseudoataxia 100
Pseudobulbar palsy 64
Pseudohypertelorism 31-2
Pseudoseizures 134
Pseudostrabismus 39
Pseudotumor cerebri 25, 100
Psychological tests 168
Ptosis 34-5
  complete 35
  congenital 34-5, 149
    partial 43
  hysterical 35
  in infancy 148-9
  upside-down 35
Puncta, placement 32
Pupil 36-8
  Argyll-Robertson 37-8
  distance to midline 30 *(fig.)*
  interpupillary distances 29 *(table)*
  response 150
  white 35
Pure tone audiometry 177-8

Q
Quadriplegia 108-9

R
Radioisotope imaging 196-202
  brain scan 197-8
  cisternography 199
  CSF leak test 202
  CSF shunt elevation 201 *(fig.)*, 202
  nuclear tomography 199-202
Rag doll position 153
Raymond-Cestan syndrome 44
Recording information 3
Referral 1
Reflexes, infantile 139-43
  percentage of normal, with increasing age 140
    (table)
Reflex rigidity 83
Refsum syndrome (phytanic acid storage disease)
    49 *(table)*, 100
Responsibility, diffusion and overlap 193
Retina 48-9
  angiomatosis 48
  cherry-red spot 49
  hemorrhages 49, 147
  hyperpigmentation 48
  melanosis 48
  pepper and salt 48
  primary dystrophy 49 *(table)*
Retinal artery narrowing 48
Retinitis pigmentosa 48-9, 100
  associated disorders 49 *(table)*
  secondary 49 *(table)*
Retrobulbar masses 35
Rigidity, types 82-3
Riley-Day syndrome (familial dysautonomia) 36,
    48, 63